The
Administrative
Dental Assistant

The
Administrative
Dental Assistant

Linda J. Gaylor, RDA, BPA, MEd

Coordinator, Curriculum and Instruction
San Bernardino County Superintendent of Schools
Regional Occupational Program, Career Training, and Support Services
San Bernardino, California

4th Edition

ELSEVIER

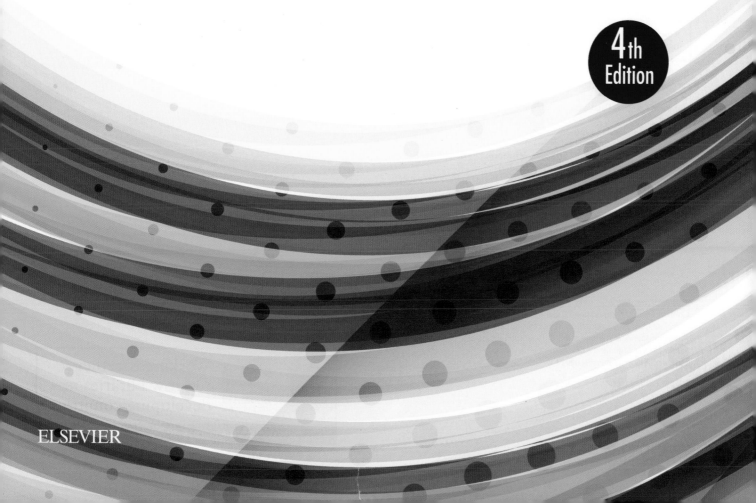

ELSEVIER

3251 Riverport Lane
St. Louis, Missouri 63043

THE ADMINISTRATIVE DENTAL ASSISTANT, FOURTH EDITION ISBN: 978-0-323-29444-7

Previous editions copyrighted 2012, 2007, 2000.

Library of Congress Cataloging-in-Publication Data

Names: Gaylor, Linda J., author.
Title: The administrative dental assistant / Linda J. Gaylor.
Description: Fourth edition. | St. Louis, Missouri : Elsevier, [2017] | Includes bibliographical references and index.
Identifiers: LCCN 2015040164 | ISBN 9780323294447 (pbk. : alk. paper)
Subjects: | MESH: Dental Assistants. | Dental Offices--organization & administration.
Classification: LCC RK60.5 | NLM WU 90 | DDC 617.6/0233--dc23
LC record available at http://lccn.loc.gov/2015040164

Content Strategist: Kristin Wilhelm
Content Development Manager: Luke Held/Ellen-Wurm Cutter
Associate Content Development Specialist: Katie Gutierrez
Publishing Services Manager: Jeff Patterson
Senior Project Manager: Anne Konopka
Designer: Xiaopei Chen/Renée Duenow

Printed in China

Last digit is the print number: 9 8 7 6 5 4 3 2 1

To Diane Gaylor, daughter-in-law, friend, and colleague, whom we lost far too soon. Diane holds a special place in the hearts of family, friends, and educational professionals from coast to coast. Diane's ability to connect with all of us, just when we needed it the most, enriched our lives each and every day.

LJG

REVIEWERS

Susan Bowen, CDA, BS
Instructor
Dental Assisting Program
Wayne Community College
Goldsboro, North Carolina

Jamie Collins, CDA, RDH
Instructor
Dental Assisting Program
College of Western Idaho
Eagle, Idaho

Nadine Danyluk, CDA
Instructor
Dental Assisting Program
Okanagan College
Kelowna, British Columbia

Joseph W. Robertson, DDS
Dentist in Private Practice
Troy, Michigan;
Co-Director and Instructor
Dental Hygiene Program
Oakland Community College
Waterford, Michigan

Tara Swift, CDA, MS
Adjunct Faculty
Dental Assisting Program
Community College of Rhode Island
Lincoln, Rhode Island

ABOUT THE AUTHOR

Linda Gaylor holds a Bachelor of Science degree in Public Administration, with a minor in Organizational Management, and a Master of Education degree in Educational Management from the University of La Verne in La Verne, California. Ms. Gaylor has served on numerous national, state, and local boards and committees in the advancement of dental assisting and health science education. She currently holds RDA licensure from California and membership in the American Dental Assistants Association. Ms. Gaylor has worked extensively in private practice as an administrative assistant, office manager, and registered dental assistant for more than 20 years and brings a comprehensive perspective to the writing of *The Administrative Dental Assistant*. Ms. Gaylor's career also includes 15 years of classroom and clinical instruction preparing students for careers in all areas of dental assisting.

Currently Ms. Gaylor works in an administrative role as a curriculum and instructional coordinator. One of her many duties is the coordination of curriculum and instruction for countywide dental assisting programs and health science courses. She works with teachers and business members to develop and revise course content, providing students with the latest skills and techniques needed for a career in the twenty-first century. In addition to her curriculum work, she also designs and facilitates professional development workshops for teachers.

PREFACE

In today's dental practices, organizing and operating an efficient dental business presents many challenges. A well-qualified administrative dental assistant will understand basic business concepts, understand all facets of the dental practice, and be a loyal and active member of the dental healthcare team. The purpose of this book is to provide a comprehensive textbook that illustrates the functions of the dental business office and to provide information on how to organize tasks, complete procedures, develop effective communication skills, and acquire a professional outlook toward dentistry. In addition, this edition introduces students to Career-Ready Practices that build a foundation for essential skills needed for success in today's world, such as critical thinking, problem solving, communication, and collaboration. These practices will provide the skills and knowledge required to be a flexible employee who is able to work in diverse groups and adapt to the rapidly changing dental profession.

The fourth edition of *The Administrative Dental Assistant* continues to provide the basic skills and knowledge necessary to work in a progressive dental office. The continued focus of this edition is the transition from a paper-based dental practice to a dental practice that incorporates technology to perform basic and advanced functions of the dental business office. As we move further and further away from the traditional paper-based dental practice toward a computer-based environment, it will become increasingly more important for the administrative dental assistant to understand how to work in a digitally integrated dental practice. As a member of the dental healthcare team, the administrative dental assistant will need to become proficient in essential skills, such as problem solving, critical thinking, teamwork, and leadership, to adapt to the new and emerging technology. Although the technology is changing, the basic procedures and routines remain the same. For an administrative dental assistant to move beyond the role of a data-entry technician, he or she must become skilled in communication, basic bookkeeping, appointment control, and records management, as well as fundamental dental procedures and terminology. With a solid foundation, the administrative dental assistant will be able to adapt quickly to the rapidly changing role of technology in the field of dental practice management.

Specifically, in this fourth edition the reader will find the following:
- Integration and use of technology in the dental business office
- Communication skills that take into consideration the entire dental healthcare team, patient relations, record management, and risk management
- Basic dental anatomy, charting, terminology, and common dental procedures
- Application of Health Insurance Portability and Accountability Act of 1996 (HIPAA) and Health Information Technology for Economic and Clinical Health (HITECH) Act regulations in securing patient information and the implementation of the electronic health record

- Controlled record management, with examples of paper-based charts and electronic files
- Effective scheduling, insurance processing, recall systems, and inventory control, with suggested steps for developing a routine in both paper-based and computer-based formats
- Examples to illustrate the transition from a paper-based procedure to a computer-based procedure
- A basic foundation in bookkeeping accounts receivable and accounts payable in which theories can be applied to a manual system and transferred to a computerized system, with examples provided in both formats
- An overview of an integrated computerized dental practice management system that is linked to perform many functions
- An Introduction to Dentrix, a leading dental practice management software system
- Employment skills necessary to obtain a position as an administrative dental assistant and assistance in cultivating the skills necessary to remain employed

The Administrative Dental Assistant package includes a textbook, a workbook (practical application of a variety of tasks, both manual and computerized), and an informational and interactive companion Evolve website. The textbook and accompanying ancillaries include many features that encourage learning and cultivate comprehension. Career-Ready Practices challenge the student to reach beyond basic learning, to research subjects, and to express an opinion based on knowledge obtained in the textbook, additional resources, and interactive discussions. In addition, the Evolve website includes an interactive tool that simulates a week in the life of a typical administrative dental assistant to provide a wealth of realistic practice.

✳ CAREER-READY PRACTICES

CCTC—Common Career Technical Core

1. *Act as a responsible and contributing citizen and employee.*
   Career-ready individuals understand the obligations and responsibilities of being a member of a community, and they demonstrate this understanding every day through their interactions with others. They are conscientious of the impacts of their decisions on others and the environment around them. They think about the near-term and long-term consequences of their actions and seek to act in ways that contribute to the betterment of their teams, families, community, and workplace. They are reliable and consistent in going beyond the minimum expectation and in participating in activities that serve the greater good.

2. *Apply appropriate academic and technical skills.*
   Career-ready individuals readily access and use the knowledge and skills acquired through experience and education to be more productive. They make connections between abstract concepts and real-world applications, and they

make correct insights about when it is appropriate to apply the use of an academic skill in a workplace situation.

3. *Attend to personal health and financial well-being.*
   Career-ready individuals understand the relationship between personal health, workplace performance, and personal well-being; they act on that understanding to regularly practice healthy diet, exercise, and mental health activities. Career-ready individuals also take regular action to contribute to their personal financial well-being, understanding that personal financial security provides the peace of mind required to contribute more fully to their own career success.

4. *Communicate clearly, effectively, and with reason.*
   Career-ready individuals communicate thoughts, ideas, and action plans with clarity, whether using written, verbal, and/or visual methods. They communicate in the workplace with clarity and purpose to make maximum use of their own and others' time. They are excellent writers; they master conventions, word choice and organization, and use effective tone and presentation skills to articulate ideas. They are skilled at interacting with others; they are active listeners and speak clearly and with purpose. Career-ready individuals think about the audience for their communication and prepare accordingly to ensure the desired outcome.

5. *Consider the environmental, social, and economic impacts of decisions.*
   Career-ready individuals understand the interrelated nature of their actions and regularly make decisions that positively impact and/or mitigate negative impact on other people, organizations, and the environment. They are aware of and utilize new technologies, understandings, procedures, materials, and regulations affecting the nature of their work as it relates to the impact on the social condition, the environment, and the profitability of the organization.

6. *Demonstrate creativity and innovation.*
   Career-ready individuals regularly think of ideas that solve problems in new and different ways, and they contribute those ideas in a useful and productive manner to improve their organization. They can consider unconventional ideas and suggestions as solutions to issues, tasks or problems, and they discern which ideas and suggestions will add greatest value. They seek new methods, practices, and ideas from a variety of sources and seek to apply those ideas to their own workplace. They take action on their ideas and understand how to bring innovation to an organization.

7. *Employ valid and reliable research strategies.*
   Career-ready individuals are discerning in accepting and using new information to make decisions, change practices, or inform strategies. They use a reliable research process to search for new information. They evaluate the validity of sources when considering the use and adoption of external information or practices. They use an informed process to test new ideas, information, and practices in their workplace situation.

8. *Utilize critical thinking to make sense of problems and persevere in solving them.*
   Career-ready individuals readily recognize problems in the workplace, understand the nature of the problem, and devise effective plans to solve the problem. They are aware of problems when they occur and take action quickly to address the problem. They thoughtfully investigate the root cause of the problem prior to introducing solutions. They carefully consider the options to solve the problem. Once a solution is agreed upon, they follow through to ensure the problem is solved, whether through their own actions or the actions of others.

9. *Model integrity, ethical leadership, and effective management.*
   Career-ready individuals consistently act in ways that align to personal and community-held ideals and principles while employing strategies to positively influence others in the workplace. They have a clear understanding of integrity and act on this understanding in every decision. They use a variety of means to positively impact the direction and actions of a team or organization, and they apply insights into human behavior to change others' actions, attitudes and/or beliefs. They recognize the near-term and long-term effects that management's actions and attitudes can have on productivity, morale, and organizational culture.

10. *Plan education and career path aligned to personal goals.*
    Career-ready individuals take personal ownership of their own educational and career goals, and they regularly act on a plan to attain these goals. They understand their own career interests, preferences, goals, and requirements. They have perspective regarding the pathways available to them and the time, effort, experience, and other requirements to pursue each, including a path of entrepreneurship. They recognize the value of each step in the educational and experiential process, and they recognize that nearly all career paths require ongoing education and experience. They seek counselors, mentors, and other experts to assist in the planning and execution of career and personal goals.

11. *Use technology to enhance productivity.*
    Career-ready individuals find and maximize the productive value of existing and new technology to accomplish workplace tasks and solve workplace problems. They are flexible and adaptive in acquiring and using new technology. They are proficient with ubiquitous technology applications. They understand the inherent risks—personal and organizational—of technology applications, and they take actions to prevent or mitigate these risks.

12. *Work productively in teams while using cultural/global competence.*
    Career-ready individuals positively contribute to every team, whether formal or informal. They apply an awareness of cultural differences to avoid barriers to productive and positive interaction. They find ways to increase the engagement and contribution of all team members. They plan and facilitate effective team meetings.

THE TEXTBOOK

The following features are included in the textbook to help the student learn facts, apply procedures, synthesize concepts, and evaluate outcomes.

- Objectives clearly state what you need to know and be able to do.
- HIPAA boxes identify where regulations need to be applied.
- *Remember* icons alert you to important information.
- *Food for Thought* boxes emphasize relevant principles.
- *What Would You Do?* boxes use common situations to encourage you to apply what you have learned and to develop your problem-solving skills.
- Boxed information is used to highlight key points, organize information, and give examples for easy reference.
- Examples show what or what not to say or do as an administrative dental assistant.
- *Anatomy of . . .* illustrations are used to describe the function and information needed to complete forms, identify specific equipment, or explain the varied elements of computerized forms.

- Illustrations and figures offer visual support in the explanation of information and procedures.
- Step-by-step procedures show you how to perform business office tasks correctly and completely.
- A patient file folder provides samples of 15 forms that would be found in a typical patient file folder—both traditional paper forms and the electronic versions with an explanation of how the forms are used and the required information needed to complete the forms.
- *Key Points* at the end of each chapter summarize the chapter and can be used as a study tool.
- *Career-Ready Practices* exercises help you to build and practice the skills you will need in a more complex life and work environment. There is a focus on creativity, critical thinking, communication, and collaboration.
- Screen shots of Dentrix and other computer-based functions show you what you will see when you use these applications.
- The Glossary at the end of the textbook defines terms and concepts as they apply to the text.

Anatomy of... images with annotated text are used to explain the varied elements of common office functions, computerized forms, and dental office equipment.

Procedure boxes provide step-by-step instructions on a wide variety of dental office duties.

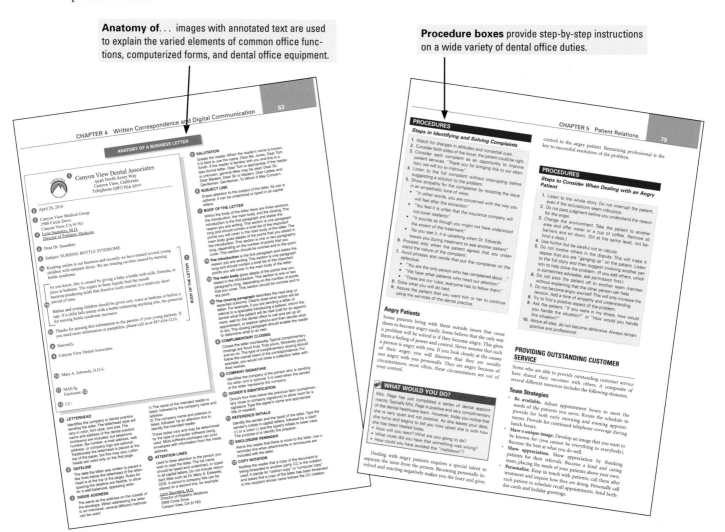

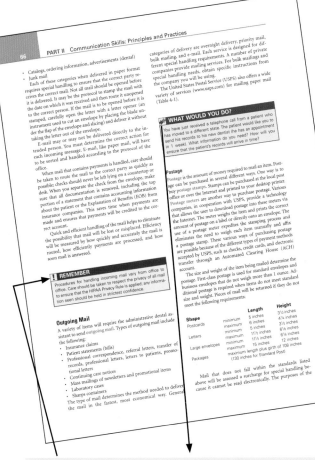

HIPAA boxes highlight specific standards and give examples where regulations need to be applied.

Remember icons are used to alert the reader to important information.
Food for Thought boxes emphasizes relevant principles.
What Would You Do? boxes use common situations to encourage the reader to apply what they have learned and to develop critical thinking and problem solving skills.

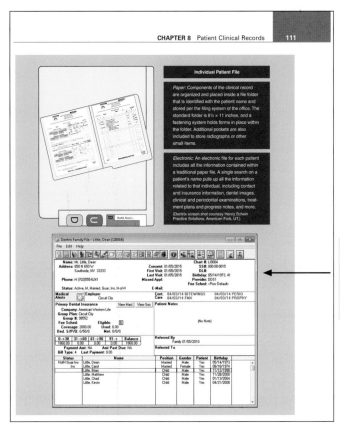

Patient Records provide examples of forms in electronic and traditional paper format with an explanation of how the forms are used and the required information needed to complete the forms.

Key Points help students ensure that they have grasped the key content and prompt them to go back into the chapter for any topic they need to review before "graduating" to the next chapter.

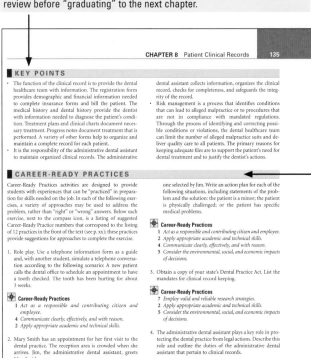

Career Ready Practices are exercises that focus on 21st century job skills including creativity, critical thinking, communication, and collaboration. They are included at the end of each chapter, asking readers to complete assignments that will help them practice specific skills that are needed in a more complex life and work environment.

THE WORKBOOK

Included with the Workbook is a fully functional copy of the Dentrix Learning Edition DVD, a student-focused, modified version of a leading dental practice management software program. The student will be able to manage a dental practice, create patient files, and perform common tasks required in a computerized dental practice with the ability to access existing patients from a prepopulated database or create new patient files and work with them.

The design of the Workbook helps students to apply information they have learned in a fun and stimulating way. The activities are project-based and simulate a real-world application. Each activity is integrated and provides the student with guided and independent practice. At the conclusion of the project, the student will have completed a variety of routine daily functions of a dental business office.

- Objectives are stated at the beginning of the chapter and identify what the student will accomplish.
- Exercises include listing and defining terms, multiple-choice questions, short answers, and, when applicable, completing relevant forms and computer application.
- *What Would You Do?* exercises are included to help apply what students have learned to solve problems that may have multiple solutions.
- Activities are designed to be completed sequentially, simulating real-world conditions and applications.
- New to this edition is the creation of a Dental Practice Manual. In small groups (or individually), students will develop a practice philosophy, create a dress code and code of conduct for employees, and write a variety of job descriptions.
- Dentrix practice management software activities include guided practice through structured tutorials and independent practice with real-world routines and applications.

THE COMPANION EVOLVE SITE

The companion Evolve website for *The Administrative Dental Assistant* was created specifically to enhance the experiences of both students and instructors using the textbook and workbook. Accessible via http://evolve.elsevier.com/Gaylor/ada, the following resources are provided.

For the Instructor

- **TEACH Instructor Resource Manual:** Detailed and customizable chapter support materials based on textbook learning objectives
  - Lesson Plans
  - Lecture Outlines
  - PowerPoint Presentations
  - Test Bank (500 questions with answers, rationales, and page references for remediation)
  - Image Collection
  - Rubrics for Career-Ready Practices

For the Student

- Practice Quizzes
- Dental Office Online Simulation Tool

Plus . . .

"Day in the Life" Simulation Tool

The features of this interactive software are designed to guide the student through simulated tasks typical in a dental business office. Each day of the week in the program increases the difficulty of the tasks and introduces new concepts. Concepts are directly related to material in the textbook. Later days in the week will require students to independently apply information and concepts that they have learned in the textbook. Students may find that the exercises have more significance after completing Chapters 3 through 17.

The interactive program simulates a "Day in the Life of an Administrative Dental Assistant" and challenges students to complete tasks as they would occur in the workplace. Students organize functions, prioritize tasks, solve problems, and complete daily tasks typical of an administrative dental assistant. Exam and study modes incorporated into the program provide flexibility in teaching and learning. The exam mode requires students to log in and complete the tasks in order from Monday through Friday, tracking their progress and outputting a results sheet, whereas the study mode allows students to enter any day and time throughout the weeklong exercise to practice or review specific procedures.

- Students select a variety of tasks that are typical in practice management software: enter and update patient data, post payment and treatment procedures, submit insurance e-claims for payment, evaluate reports, and schedule appointments.
- Patients arrive for appointments and the student must complete related tasks, such as updating patient information and completing the checkout process. The mail arrives on a daily basis and must be processed. The telephone rings and the student must take care of the caller.
- Pop-ups ask the student questions about a particular subject relevant to the task at hand. Prompts inform students if they have answered the question correctly or incorrectly and provide a rationale. (Students are able to go back and view the correct response if they have answered incorrectly.)

TEXTBOOK ADAPTATION

The textbook and ancillaries have been carefully designed to provide the skills and knowledge necessary for the efficient operation of a dental business office and can be adapted and adopted for the following:

- A one-semester course for the administrative dental assistant
- To fulfill the business component of a dental assisting course
- As a resource for dental assistants who want to upgrade their skills

- As a resource for review before an examination
- As a resource for an administrative dental assistant trained on the job
- As a basic course with real-world application for dental hygiene and dental students

The fourth edition of this textbook has been edited and written at a time when it is common to see a paper-based dental practice and a paperless dental practice side by side.

Because this workplace environment is common, I felt it was necessary to include basic elements of both systems to better prepare you for the transition to a totally paperless system. Whether you are new to the dental profession or have many years of experience, *The Administrative Dental Assistant* will provide you with resources that you can use in today's dental practice.

Linda J. Gaylor

ACKNOWLEDGMENTS

A project such as this one does not happen in a vacuum. It is the result of countless hours of hard work by all those involved. First and foremost I need to acknowledge the support of my family and friends. Their understanding and encouragement provided the motivation that kept me going.

I acknowledge the contributions of the entire publishing team at Elsevier: Kristin Wilhelm, Katie Gutierrez, Joe Gramlich, Jeff Patterson, Anne Konopka, and Renee Duenow.

Thank you to the entire group of professionals, family, and friends who have made the dream of *The Administrative Dental Assistant* a reality.

CONTENTS

Preface, viii

PART I Introduction to the Dental Profession

1 Orientation to the Dental Profession, 2
Introduction, 2
Your Role as the Administrative Dental Assistant, 2
Types of Administrative Assistants, 4
  Office Manager, 4
  Business Manager, 4
  Receptionist, 4
  Insurance Biller, 4
  Records Manager, 4
  Data Processor, 4
  Bookkeeper, 5
  Appointment Scheduler, 5
Personal Traits of an Administrative Dental
  Assistant, 5
Education, 5
Members of the Dental Healthcare Team, 6
  Dentist, 6
  Dental Hygienist, 6
  Dental Assistant, 7
Health Insurance Portability and Accountability
  Act of 1996, 7
  Background, 7
  Administrative Simplification, 7
  Transactions and Code Sets, 8
  Electronic Data Interchange (EDI), 8
  Standards for Privacy of Individually Identifiable
    Health Information (The Privacy Rule), 8
  Standards for Security of Individually Identifiable
    Health Information (The Security Rule), 9
  National Provider Identifier Standard, 10
The HITECH Act, 10
The 2013 HIPAA Omnibus Final Rule, 10
Occupational Safety and Health Administration
  (OSHA), 10
  Professional Ethics, 10
Legal Standards, 10
  Licensure, 10
  Registration, 11
  Certification, 11
Patient's Rights, 11
Professional Organizations, 12
  American Dental Assistants Association, 12
  HOSA–Future Health Professionals, 13

2 Dental Basics, 15
Introduction, 15
Basic Dental Office Design, 15
  Nonclinical Areas, 15
  Clinical Areas, 17

Basic Dental Anatomy, 20
  Basic Structures of the Face and Oral Cavity, 20
  Basic Anatomical Structures and Tissues of the
    Teeth, 24
  Dental Arches, 25
  Occlusion, 26
  Types of Teeth, 26
  Surfaces of the Teeth, 26
Numbering Systems, 27
  Universal/National Numbering System, 27
  International Standards Organization Designation
    System, 27
  Symbolic Numbering System (Palmer System), 28
Charting Methods, 29
  Color Coding, 29
  Charting Symbols, 29
  Types of Dental Charts, 29
Dental Procedures, 33
  Basic and Preventive Dental Procedures, 33
  Restorative Procedures, 33
  Prosthetic Procedures, 34
  Surgical Procedures, 35
  Endodontic Procedures, 36
  Other Common Procedures, 36
Basic Chairside Dental-Assisting Duties, 37
  Seating and Dismissing a Patient, 37
  Digital Images and Radiographs, 38
  Occupational Safety and Health Administration
    (OSHA), 38
  Infection Control, 39

PART II Communication Skills: Principles and Practices

3 Communication Skills and Telephone Techniques, 42
Introduction, 42
Elements of the Communication Process, 42
Mediums of Communication, 42
  Verbal Communication, 42
  Nonverbal Communication, 43
  Nonverbal Cues from the Dental Healthcare Team, 43
Interpersonal Communication, 44
Barriers to Effective Communication, 44
  Semantics, 44
  Jargon, 45
  Credibility, 45
  Preconceived Ideas, 45
  Other Barriers, 45
Improving Communication, 46
  Responsibilities of the Sender, 46
  Responsibilities of the Receiver, 46

Telephone Techniques, 47
   Developing a Positive Telephone Image, 47
   Active Scripts, 49
   Answering the Telephone, 50
   Placing Outgoing Telephone Calls, 50

4 Written Correspondence and Digital Communication, 53
Introduction, 53
Letter Writing Style, 53
   Tone, 53
   Outlook, 54
   Personalizing Letters, 54
   Organization, 55
Letter Style (Appearance), 55
   Appearance, 55
   Stationery, 55
   Lettering, 57
   Paragraphing, 57
   White Space, 57
   Line Spacing, 57
Letter Style (Format), 57
Punctuation Styles, 59
Types of Correspondence Used in Dentistry, 62
   Letters to Patients, 62
   Letters between Professionals, 64
   Correspondence between Staff Members, 64
Writing Resources, 64
Letter Templates, 64
Digital Communications, 64
   Electronic Mail (E-Mail), 65
Mail, 65
   Incoming Mail, 65
   Outgoing Mail, 66
   Postal Cards (Postcards), 69
Dictation, 69

5 Patient Relations, 71
Introduction, 71
Psychology: Humanistic Theory, 71
   Maslow: Hierarchy of Needs, 71
   Rogers: Fully Functioning Human Beings, 71
   Humanistic Theory in the Dental Office, 72
Practice Branding: Creating a Positive Image, 72
   Investigation Stage: Where Should I Go? 72
   Initial Contact Stage: What Are They Like? 73
   Confirmation of Initial Impression Stage: What Are They Really Like? 75
   Final Decision Stage, 76
   Managing Patient Expectations, 77
Problem Solving, 78
   Noncompliance, 78
   Complaints, 78
   Angry Patients, 79
Providing Outstanding Customer Service, 79
   Team Strategies, 79
   Personal Strategies for Providing Exceptional Patient Care, 80

6 Dental Healthcare Team Communications, 82
Introduction, 82
Dental Practice Procedural Manual, 82
Communications, 83
   Personal Communications, 83
   Organizational Communications, 83
   Channels, 83
   Organizational Barriers to Communication, 86
Organizational Conflicts, 86
   Constructive, 86
   Destructive, 86
   Classifying Conflict, 86
   Conflict-Handling Styles, 87
Staff Meetings, 87
   Before the Meeting, 88
   During the Meeting, 88
   After the Meeting, 88

PART III Managing Dental Office Systems

7 Computerized Dental Practice, 92
Introduction, 92
Basic Systems, 92
   Patient Dental Records Management, 92
   Basic Business Functions, 93
   Additional Software Suites, 93
Selecting a Practice Management System, 95
Functions to Consider when Selecting a Software Package, 95
   General Requirements, 95
   Patient Information, 95
   Patient Billing, 96
   Treatment Planning, 96
   Insurance Processing, 96
   Recall and Reactivation, 96
   Management Reports, 97
   Electronic Scheduler, 97
   Database Management and Word Processing, 97
   Clinical Integration, 97
Basic Operation of a Software Package, 98
Roles of the Administrative Dental Assistant, 98
   Recording Patient Demographics, 98
   Creating an Account, 98
   Maintaining Patient Records, 99
   Posting Transactions, 99
   Using a General Database, 99
   Processing Insurance Claims, 99
   Scheduling Electronically, 101
   Producing Reports, 101
Daily Procedures with a Computerized System, 101
   Backup System, 101

8 Patient Clinical Records, 107
Introduction, 107
Electronic Clinical Records, 107
   Clinical Records, 108
   Electronic Health Records, 108

Components of the Clinical Record, 108
Collecting Information, 127
   Privacy Practices Notice, 127
   Registration Forms, 127
   Other Diagnostic Records, 127
   Diagnostic Models, 127
Clinical Records Risk Management, 127
   Maintaining Clinical Records (Manual and
      Electronic), 127
   Procedures for Specific Tasks, 132

9 Information Management, 136
Introduction, 136
Filing Methods, 136
   Alphabetic, 137
   Numeric, 139
   Geographic, 139
   Subject, 139
   Chronological, 139
   Electronic, 139
Types of Information, 141
   Business Records, 141
   Patient and Insurance Information, 142
Filing Equipment for a Paper System, 142
   Vertical Files, 142
   Lateral Files, 142
   Card Files, 142
Filing Supplies, 142
   File Folders, 142
   Vertical File Folders, 142
   Lateral File Folders, 143
   Guides, 143
   Out-Guides, 143
   File Labels, 143
   Color Coding, 143
   Aging Labels, 143
Preparing the Paper Clinical Record, 144
   General Guidelines, 144
   Preparing the Label, 144
   Coding the File Folder, 144
   Cross-Referencing (Numeric Indexing), 144
Preparing Business Documents for Filing, 144
Preparing Paper Documents for Filing, 145
   Inspecting, 145
   Indexing, 145
   Coding, 145
   Filing Procedures, 145
   Sorting, 145
   Putting Records and Documents in Their Final
      Place, 145
   How to Safeguard Records, 145
   Retention and Transfer of Records, 146

10 Dental Patient Scheduling, 149
Introduction, 149
Mechanics of Scheduling, 149
   Selecting the Appointment Book (Manual
      and Electronic), 149
   Common Features of an Appointment Book, 150

The Art of Scheduling, 151
   Productivity, 154
   Scenarios for Scheduling, 155
   Results of Poor Scheduling, 157
Making Appointments, 157
Time-Saving Functions, 159
   Develop Call Lists, 159
   Maintain Daily Schedule Sheets, 160
   Establish a Daily Routine, 160

11 Recall Systems, 163
Introduction, 163
Classification of Recalls, 164
Methods for Recalling Patients, 164
   General Information Needed for a Recall
      System, 164
   Prescheduled Recall System, 164
   Telephone Recall System, 167
   Mail Recall System, 168
   Automated Recall Systems, 169

12 Inventory Management, 173
Introduction, 173
Establishing an Inventory Management
   System, 173
   Data Communication Technology, 174
   Manual Inventory Management Systems, 175
   Inventory Management System Protocol, 177
Types of Supplies, Products, and
   Equipment, 178
   Consumable Supplies and Products, 178
   Nonconsumable Products, 178
   Major Equipment, 178
Selecting and Ordering Supplies, Products, and
   Equipment, 179
   Selecting Supplies and Products, 179
   Purchasing Major Equipment, 180
   Selecting the Vendor, 180
   Information to Consider Before Placing
      an Order, 181
   Receiving Supplies and Products, 182
   Storage Areas, 183
Occupational Safety and Health Administration
   (OSHA), 183

13 Office Equipment, 188
Introduction, 188
Electronic Business Equipment, 188
   Hardware, 188
   Software, 189
   Data, 191
   Personnel, 191
   Procedures, 191
Telecommunication, 191
   Telephone Systems, 191
   Mobile Communication Devices, 194
Intraoffice Communications, 194
   Electronic Systems, 194
   Manual Systems, 195
Office Machines, 195

Business Office Environment, 196
  *Questions to Consider When Organizing
    a Business Office, 196*
  Safety, 198

PART IV Managing Dental Office Finances

14 Financial Arrangement and Collection Procedures, 201
Introduction, 201
Designing a Financial Policy, 201
  Elements of a Financial Policy, 201
  Community Standards, 201
  Practice Philosophy, 201
  Business Principles, 201
Financial Policies, 201
  Payment in Full, 202
  Insurance Billing, 202
  Extended Payment Plans, 202
  Third-Party Finance Plans, 202
  Credit Cards, 203
  Financial Policy Communications, 203
Managing Accounts Receivable, 205
  Gather Financial Data, 206
  Prepare a Treatment Plan, 207
  Monitor the Accounts Receivable Report, 208
  Collection Process, 208

15 Dental Insurance Processing, 213
Introduction, 213
Types of Dental Insurance, 213
  Fee for Service, 213
  Capitation Programs, 217
  Closed Panel Programs, 217
  Franchise Dentistry, 217
  Direct Reimbursement, 217
  Preferred Provider Organization, 217
  Health Maintenance Organization, 217
  Managed Care, 218
  Individual Practice Association, 218
  Union Trust Funds, 218
Other Types of Insurance Coverage, 218
  Secondary Coverage, 218
  Government Assistance, 218
  Workers' Compensation, 218
  Auto Accidents, 218
  Other Accidents, 218
Insurance Claims Processing, 218
  *Collecting Information and Determining
    Benefits, 219*
  Maximum Coverage, 219
  Deductible, 219
  Percentage of Payment, 219
  Copayment, 219
  Limitation to Coverage, 219

Eligibility, 219
Preauthorization or Pretreatment, 219
Electronically Submitted Forms, 220
Practice Management Systems, 220
Application Service Providers, 220
E-Claims Service Providers, 220
Insurance Provider Claims Processing, 221
Paper Dental Claim Forms, 221
Superbills and Encounter Forms, 221
Insurance Payments, 221
Insurance Tracking Systems, 222
Completing a Dental Claim Form, 223
Insurance Coding, 223
  *Documentation Needed for Insurance
    Processing, 224*
Fraudulent Insurance Billing, 233
  Advisory Opinions, 233

16 Bookkeeping Procedures: Accounts Payable, 235
Introduction, 235
Organizing an Accounts Payable System, 235
Verification of Expenditures, 235
Check Writing, 236
  Payment Authorization and Transfer, 236
  Electronic Check Writing, 236
  Making a Deposit, 236
Reconciling a Bank Statement, 241
  Information Listed on a Bank Statement, 241
  Items Needed for Reconciling the Account, 242
  Steps in Reconciling the Account, 242
Payroll, 245
  Creating the Payroll Record, 245
  Payroll Records, 245
  Computerized Payroll, 248
  Payroll Services, 250
  Calculating Payroll, 250
  Calculating Net Salary, 252
  Payroll Taxes: Reports and Deposits, 254
  Employer Identification Number, 256

17 Bookkeeping Procedures: Accounts Receivable, 258
Introduction, 258
Components of Financial Records Organization, 258
  Patient Information, 258
  Methods of Recording Transactions, 258
Billing, 260
  Electronic Financial Record, 262
  Pegboard System, 262
Daily Routine for Managing Patient Transactions, 263
  Identify Patients, 263
  Produce Routing Slips, 263
  Post Transactions, 263
  Routine for Managing Financial Transactions, 270
Reports, 270
  Types of Reports, 270
  Additional Reports, 271

PART V Managing Your Career

18 Employment Strategies, 273
   Introduction, 273
   Career Opportunities for Administrative Dental
      Assistants, 273
      Private Practice, 273
      Insurance Companies, 274
      Management and Consulting Firms, 274
      Teaching, 274
      Future Career Opportunities, 274
   Steps for Developing Employment Strategies, 274
      Assessing Yourself and Your Career Options, 274

      Gathering Information, 274
      Composing a Resume, 275
      Writing Cover Letters, 280
      Looking for a Job, 280
      Going on an Interview, 283
      Accepting a Job Offer, 284
   Leaving a Job, 284

Glossary, 286
Index, 297

PART I

Introduction to the Dental Profession

1 Orientation to the Dental Profession, 2

2 Dental Basics, 15

Orientation to the Dental Profession

LEARNING OBJECTIVES

1. Define dental healthcare team and identify the business duties expected of the administrative dental assistant.
2. Describe the eight roles of an administrative dental assistant.
3. List the personal traits and educational background of an administrative dental assistant.
4. Name the various members of the dental healthcare team and discuss the roles they play in the delivery of dental care.
5. Explain the rules and function of the Health Insurance Portability and Accountability Act of 1996 (HIPAA), including Administrative Simplification, as it applies to the dental healthcare system.

6. Describe the role of the Occupational Safety and Health Administration (OSHA) in dentistry.
7. Identify the five sections of the American Dental Association's *Principles of Ethics and Code of Professional Conduct* and demonstrate an understanding of its content by explaining, discussing, and applying the principles.
8. Explain the legal standards of dentistry, including licensure, registration, and certification.
9. Explain the rights of dental patients.
10. Describe the roles of the American Dental Assistants Association (ADAA) and the HOSA—Future Health Professionals.

INTRODUCTION

The dental profession in the twenty-first century is a complex healthcare delivery system. It uses the latest technology and demands caring, well-trained, multiskilled dental auxiliaries. The dental assistant is required to know all phases of the dental practice and the daily business operations. Those who excel and become vital members of the dental healthcare team will have mastered multiple skills, will be flexible, and will work well in a team environment.

The primary objective of dentistry is to provide quality care for all patients. This care is given without regard to social standing, insurance coverage, ethnic background, or ability to pay. A dentist can provide quality care for all patients only if the total picture of dentistry is taken into consideration.

Dentistry is a service of providing dental care to improve and maintain dental health. Dental professionals of the twenty-first century will need to consider the business side of dentistry in the total treatment of their patients. Without a well-developed business plan, the dental healthcare team will not be able to satisfy the needs of their patients. Patients want and will demand that they be treated by qualified professionals who provide quality care while treating them as individuals. Patients will expect to be treated with respect for themselves and their time, they will expect that the dental healthcare team members will be skillful in the performance of their duties, and they will expect the dental healthcare team to work in harmony. A service-based business is considered successful when it meets the needs of the people it serves.

An effective dental healthcare team can be described as a group of dental professionals, including dentists and dental auxiliaries, who work together to provide a service (Figure 1-1). This service blends technical skills with "people skills." The dental healthcare team is technically competent, compassionate, caring, fair, and well rooted in strong ethical principles. The dental healthcare team works in harmony and always places the needs of the patients first. The dental healthcare team considers patients as whole persons and attends to their needs accordingly.

YOUR ROLE AS THE ADMINISTRATIVE DENTAL ASSISTANT

Fifty years ago, the role of the dental receptionist was simplistic. The duties included greeting patients, answering the telephone, scheduling appointments, performing basic bookkeeping tasks, and occasionally filing a dental insurance claim form. As the twentieth century progressed, the receptionist's role evolved. As the duties have changed, so has the title. Today, the role of the administrative dental assistant is complex. The assistant may be required to manage office staff, organize a marketing campaign, be familiar with several types of healthcare delivery systems, and perform computerized tasks daily.

Because of the wide range of duties and responsibilities of the administrative dental assistant, dental professionals are not in agreement on the type of training that is required. Some believe that the duties of the administrative dental

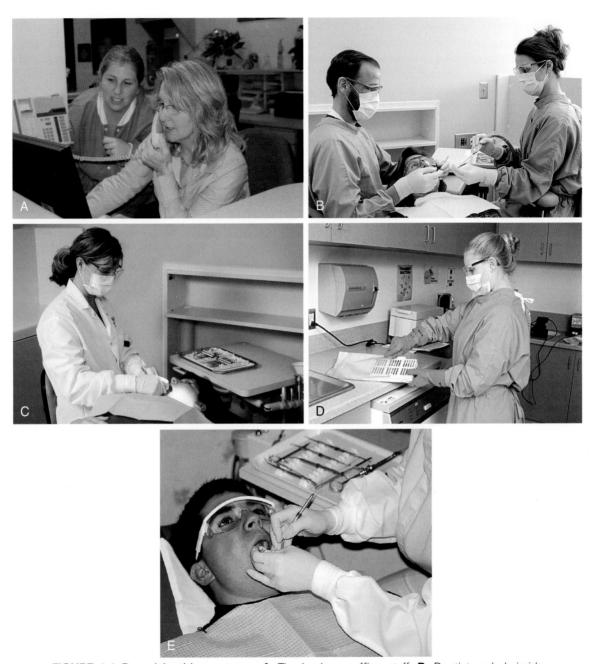

FIGURE 1-1 Dental healthcare team. **A,** The business office staff. **B,** Dentist and chairside assistant. **C,** Dental hygienist. **D,** Circulating (roving) assistant. **E,** Expanded (extended) function assistant. (**A,** Courtesy William C. Domb, Upland, Calif. **B, C, D,** and **E,** From Bird DL, Robinson DS: *Modern dental assisting*, ed 11, St. Louis, 2015, Saunders.)

assistant are business in nature and therefore do not require an understanding of technical dentistry. Business duties that can be expected of the administrative dental assistant may include

- Knowledge of computers and several different software packages, computerized patient databases, insurance claims, word processing, accounting, electronic transfers via online services, web page development, and the Internet
- Operation of electronic business machines, such as fax machines, calculators, photocopiers, electronic credit card transmission devices, voice mail, and multiline telephones

- Knowledge of bookkeeping practices, such as accounts receivable, accounts payable, banking, payroll, and accounting reports and records
- Ability to communicate, both in writing and verbally, with patients, dental healthcare team members, and other dental professionals
- Use of business management skills for staff development and supervision, marketing strategies, contract negotiations, and legal and ethical issues

Other dental professionals believe that the duties of the administrative dental assistant can be carried out efficiently by a chairside dental assistant. The knowledge and skills of the chairside assistant are needed to schedule appointments efficiently, to communicate using dental terminology, to process dental insurance claims, to correctly code procedures for posting, to make entries in patients' clinical records, and to perform chairside assistant duties when additional help is needed in the clinical area. However, all dental professionals agree that the administrative dental assistant must be talented in patient and staff relations and must be an outstanding communicator and an active participant on the dental healthcare team.

TYPES OF ADMINISTRATIVE ASSISTANTS

The role of an **administrative dental assistant** is important, multifaceted, and complex. Depending on the size of the dental practice, the range of duties varies. In small dental practices, all of the business office duties may be assigned to one or two administrative assistants. These duties overlap and are woven into the daily activities of the business office. It is difficult sometimes to discern where one job description begins and the other leaves off. In larger dental practices, duties are divided and given specific job titles. These titles and their corresponding duties are described below.

Office Manager

The **office manager** typically organizes and oversees the daily operations of the office staff. In a small office or a solo practice, this may be required in addition to other administrative assistant duties. In the larger, multipractitioner practice, this could be the sole responsibility of one person. The office manager's duties include:

- Formulating and carrying out office policy
- Managing business and clinical staff
- Scheduling staff
- Resolving conflicts
- Hiring and terminating business office and clinical staff
- Organizing and conducting staff development
- Being a liaison between the owner or dentist and the staff

Business Manager

In large practices, the owner of the business may be a dentist, a group of dentists, or a corporation with several locations. The business operation of the dental practice may be assigned to a **business manager.** The business manager's duties include:

- Managing the fiscal operation
- Creating and interpreting reports
- Developing marketing campaigns
- Negotiating contracts with managed care providers
- Overseeing compliance with insurance, managed care, and government programs

Receptionist

In the past, the duties of the business office were assigned to the **receptionist.** With the growth of dental practices and increased business responsibilities, the role of the receptionist has changed and is vital to the success of the dental practice.

During a patient's initial telephone call, the voice and attitude of the receptionist help to determine whether the patient will have a positive or negative opinion of the dental practice. When a patient arrives for his or her first appointment, the receptionist is the first to greet him or her. If the receptionist conveys a negative impression, in either appearance or attitude, a patient may develop a negative opinion about the remainder of the staff and the quality of the dental care he or she is about to receive. The single most important role of the receptionist is to help the patient formulate a positive impression of the dental practice by projecting a positive and helpful attitude. Without a positive reception, patients may seek dental treatment elsewhere.

The responsibilities of the receptionist include:

- Projecting a positive attitude
- Greeting patients
- Answering the telephone
- Managing incoming and outgoing mail
- Collecting patient data
- Answering patient questions
- Being a liaison between the patient and the dentist
- Making financial arrangements

Insurance Biller

The **insurance biller or coder** has one of the most important functions in the dental practice. It is the responsibility of the insurance biller to oversee the filing of insurance claims. Before claims can be processed, the insurance biller must gather all necessary information and documentation. In addition to filing insurance claims, the insurance biller tracks and monitors claims to ensure that they are paid in a timely manner.

An insurance biller's duties include:

- Collecting insurance data
- Verifying eligibility
- Determining benefits
- Communicating benefits to the patient
- Filing preauthorization forms
- Coding procedures
- Filing completed claims for payment
- Tracking the progress of insurance claims
- Collecting copayments from patients

Records Manager

The **records manager** organizes and maintains all aspects of patients' clinical charts according to preset standards. He or she establishes and maintains an efficient filing system, ensuring that all clinical records have been placed in their correct locations. This task may be the primary responsibility of one administrative assistant or be part of the daily routine for several assistants.

The records manager's duties include:

- Collecting patient histories
- Ensuring compliance with industry standards
- Ensuring confidentiality and accuracy
- Keeping records safe from destruction and loss

Data Processor

When a computerized system is used in a dental practice, it is necessary for the information to be keyed into the computer.

In the majority of dental practices this procedure is the responsibility of several assistants; administrative and clinical. The data processor or dental assistant is responsible for entering data into the computer system. This information is collected from various sources, such as patient registration forms, direct entry from the patient, and clinical treatment notes. This information is integrated together to form a comprehensive patient record.

The data processor uses various computer skills to perform different tasks, such as:
- Generating accounting reports
- Generating dental insurance claims
- Transmitting dental insurance claims electronically
- Recording chairside dental treatment
- Managing patient clinical records
- Generating letters of referral to specialists
- Producing newsletters
- Maintaining a recall system
- Sending electronic mail

Bookkeeper

All bookkeeping entries must be made according to an approved method of record keeping. The purpose of bookkeeping is to track all fees, all money collected, and all money paid out. A bookkeeping system shows the amount charged for a service (fee), the amount collected for a service (income), and the amount still owed for a service (accounts receivable). It would be very difficult to understand a dental practice's financial status if it had no bookkeeping system. The Internal Revenue Service (IRS) uses bookkeeping information to calculate the amount of money owed for taxes. As discussed in greater detail later, bookkeeping records are considered legal documents. They should never be altered or changed.

In addition to tracking the monies collected and the monies owed, the bookkeeper records and maintains the accounts payable. Accounts payable is a record of the money that the dental practice owes to others. These accounts include payroll, taxes, and unpaid bills. The bookkeeper maintains records of the money deposited in checking and savings accounts and uses a checking system (manual check writing or electronic debit accounts) to pay vendors.

Not all dental practices hire a full-time bookkeeper. In some practices, an administrative assistant or assistants maintain the basic records and an accountant is hired to audit the records, prepare reports, and file tax returns.

The bookkeeper's duties include:
- Maintaining accounts receivable records
- Maintaining accounts payable records
- Writing checks (written or electronic transfer)
- Depositing money collected in checking and savings accounts
- Maintaining accurate and truthful records
- Paying employees
- Filing tax and payroll reports with the IRS
- Depositing tax money according to IRS and state regulations (payroll and income taxes)

Appointment Scheduler

It is vital to the efficiency and success of a dental practice that appointments be scheduled so that the productivity of the dental team is maximized. Efficient scheduling minimizes the patient's stress, resulting in a positive dental experience.

The appointment scheduler's duties include:
- Organizing and maintaining the daily patient schedule
- Assigning patients to appointment times that meet the needs of both patients and the dental practice
- Scheduling patients in a timely manner
- Maximizing the daily schedule so that personnel can work smarter, not harder
- Balancing the schedule to reduce stress among the dental healthcare team and patients
- Tracking dental treatments (determining which treatments have not been completed)
- Maintaining a recall system

PERSONAL TRAITS OF AN ADMINISTRATIVE DENTAL ASSISTANT

The administrative dental assistant's duties may be assigned to several people or to a few, depending on the size and complexity of the practice. It is clear that a successful dental practice in the twenty-first century depends on careful selection of those who play key roles in the daily operation of the practice.

The personal traits of the administrative dental assistant are varied. The assistant should:
- Be flexible and able to do more than one job at a time
- Be multiskilled to handle both dental assisting and business needs
- Be able to work in a diverse culture and maintain patient relations
- Have a strong work ethic
- Understand and apply dental professional ethics
- Maintain good communication, both written and verbal, between patients and all members of the dental healthcare team
- Be tactful with patients, *placing patients first*
- Be productive by performing jobs quickly and efficiently
- Work effectively in a team environment
- Apply initiative
- Prioritize duties
- Make decisions and know what needs to be done without direction (but also know when to ask for direction)

EDUCATION

To meet the qualifications for an administrative dental assistant in the twenty-first century, applicants should acquire dental assisting and business skills through a training program. Such programs enable the student to understand the complexity of a dental practice and to develop the skills necessary to become a successful member of a dental healthcare team.

No licensure is available for the duties of an administrative dental assistant. Those assistants who are required to take dental radiographs, perform direct patient care, or engage in infection control procedures (cleaning treatment rooms or preparing instruments for sterilization), however, must consult their state's Dental Practice Act. The Dental Practice Act outlines the duties that can be performed by dental auxiliaries, the type of education needed, and what licensure (if any) is required.

MEMBERS OF THE DENTAL HEALTHCARE TEAM

Dentist

General Dentistry

Heading the dental healthcare team is the dentist. He or she has completed 7 or 8 years of college, including 4 years of undergraduate studies with a strong emphasis in the biological sciences and 3 to 4 years of postgraduate studies in the field of dentistry. Those who attend an American Dental Association (ADA)–accredited dental school earn a Doctor of Dental Surgery (DDS) or a Doctor of Dental Medicine (DMD) degree.

All dentists, regardless of training, are required to pass both a written and a practical examination, which are regulated by each state, before practicing dentistry. Dentists who receive their degree in a foreign country may require additional training before practicing in the United States. In addition to following the regulations outlined in each state's Dental Practice Act, members of organizations such as the ADA and the Academy of General Dentistry must adhere to the organizations' codes of conduct and ethical standards.

Specialization

All dentists may perform the duties described in the Dental Practice Act. When the treatment becomes too complex for the general dentist, however, he or she is required to refer the patient to a specialist. The ADA recognizes nine specialties.

Dental public health. Dentists who specialize in dental public health help to organize and run dental programs for the general public. These programs may require knowledge of how to establish and maintain educational programs within a school system or a dental clinic in an area where people have limited access to dental care. Such a clinic can be located in an inner city, on a Native American reservation, or in a rural community.

Endodontics. Endodontics involves the tissues of the tooth (pulp). *Endodontists* perform root canal procedures and other surgical procedures that are needed to prevent the loss of a tooth.

Oral and maxillofacial pathology. Oral pathologists are specialists in oral and maxillofacial pathology. They diagnose and treat diseases of the mouth and oral structures.

Oral and maxillofacial radiology. *Radiologists* who specialize in oral and maxillofacial radiology produce and interpret images and data generated by all modalities of radiant energy (x-rays and other types of imaging) that are used for the diagnosis and management of diseases, disorders, and conditions of the oral and maxillofacial region.

Oral and maxillofacial surgery. *Oral surgeons* are specialists in oral and maxillofacial surgery. They perform both simple tasks, such as extractions of teeth, and complex surgical procedures, such as facial reconstruction. These specialists perform surgical procedures of the head and neck.

Orthodontics and dentofacial orthopedics. An *orthodontist* treats conditions of malocclusion (teeth that meet in a disordered way) and is a member of a complex team of medical and dental doctors who have specialized in orthodontics and dentofacial orthopedics and who restore facial features and oral functions.

Pediatric dentistry. *Pedodontists* are specialists in pediatric dentistry. In all phases of dentistry, they treat patients from newborns through adolescence. Some provide treatment in a hospital setting to patients who are under general anesthesia or who have special needs. Others provide preventive and restorative dental treatment to children.

Periodontics. *Periodontists* (specialists in periodontics) treat patients who have diseases of the soft tissue surrounding the teeth (periodontal disease). Periodontal disease occurs in various stages, which vary in severity. The periodontist focuses treatment on correcting and preventing progression of the disease.

Prosthodontics. *Prosthodontists* receive advanced training in prosthodontics and perform procedures that replace lost and damaged tooth structure. Replacement of tooth structure is accomplished by placing crowns over the remaining structures. In addition to replacement of tooth structure, prosthodontists replace teeth. Tooth replacement includes the placement of partial dentures (fixed and removable), full dentures, or crowns over implants.

An additional 2 to 4 years of education is required for a dentist to become a board-certified specialist. Those who choose a specialty may do so for a variety of reasons. Some enjoy the challenge of the complexity of a given specialty, whereas others, such as those who practice pediatric dentistry, enjoy working with a select group of patients. The work of the specialist and of the general dentist in the delivery of dental healthcare involves a team effort. The general dentist refers a patient to a specialist for complex treatment and the specialist in turn returns the patient to the general dentist for all other phases of dentistry. Such teamwork ensures that the patient receives total quality care.

Advanced training is not limited to the nine recognized specialties; dentists can receive advanced training in all areas of dentistry. Most members of the dental healthcare team are required by the Dental Practice Act to continue their education through approved coursework.

Dental Hygienist

The dental hygienist provides oral hygiene instruction and oral prophylaxis to dental patients. One of the key roles of the hygienist is to instruct and motivate patients in the area of preventive dentistry. Hygienists may also perform other duties as assigned to the dental assistant by the state's Dental

Practice Act. The expanded duties of the hygienist may include:

- Administering local anesthesia
- Applying pit and fissure sealant
- Root planing, scaling, and polishing
- Processing and evaluating radiographs
- Performing all duties assigned to the dental assistant

The educational requirements for a dental hygienist vary from a 2-year to a 4-year post–high school program. Each program must be accredited by the Commission on Dental Accreditation as specified by the Council on Dental Education of the ADA. Each hygienist must pass a written and a practical examination before he or she is issued a license.

Dental Assistant

The duties of the dental assistant are essential to the efficient operation of successful dental practices. Dental assistants provide a link between the patient and the dentist. There are several types of dental assistants or dental auxiliaries (persons who provide a service in a dental practice other than the dentist).

Chairside Dental Assistant

The chairside dental assistant helps the dentist during patient treatment in such areas as maintaining a clean and clear operating field, passing instruments, and manipulating dental materials. In addition, a chairside dental assistant who is registered or certified can perform intraoral duties under the direct or indirect supervision of the dentist (according to standards outlined in the state's Dental Practice Act). In addition to direct patient care, the assistant performs many necessary adjunct duties.

Expanded (Extended) Function Assistant

The expanded (extended) function assistant has received additional training and education in functions that provide more independent patient care under direct or indirect supervision of the dentist. Procedures that can be performed by an expanded function assistant are outlined in the Dental Practice Act, are usually reversible, and can be redone if necessary. Some states may require an expanded function assistant to receive licensure or certification.

Circulating (Roving) Assistant

The circulating (roving) assistant performs a variety of duties, such as helping dentists, hygienists, or assistants as needed; taking dental radiographs; and maintaining responsibility for sterilization and infection control procedures.

HEALTH INSURANCE PORTABILITY AND ACCOUNTABILITY ACT OF 1996

The responsibility of enforcing the regulations and compliance issues mandated by the Health Insurance Portability and Accountability Act of 1996 (HIPAA) in a dental office ultimately belongs to the dentist, but this is not a one-person job; each member of the dental healthcare team has a role. Most compliance issues fall under the domain of the business office; therefore most of the responsibility falls to the administrative dental assistant. Compliance issues are numerous and include the way in which insurance claims are coded, how patient information is shared with others, who has access to protected health information, how records are stored, and how patients are contacted outside the dental office.

Background

In 1991, the Workgroup for Electronic Data Interchange (WEDI) was created by the U.S. Department of Health and Human Services (HHS) to study the impact of replacing paper-generated healthcare transactions with electronically generated transactions. The purpose of the study was to find ways in which the rising costs of healthcare could be contained. The prepared report, published in 1993, stated that savings in healthcare costs would be substantial if paper-generated transactions were replaced by electronically generated transactions. This report became the foundation for the Administrative Simplification provisions incorporated in the HIPAA document that President Clinton signed in August 1996.

As specified in its title, HIPAA consists of sections on two major topics: portability and accountability. The portability section of the Act simply guarantees that a person covered by health insurance provided by an employer can obtain health insurance through a second employer should he or she change jobs. The accountability section of the Act answers the question of who and what should be accountable for specific healthcare activities. The Administrative Simplification portion of the accountability section addresses issues regarding administrative systems and the business issues of healthcare.

Administrative Simplification

Administrative Simplification was designed to make the business of healthcare easier through the development of standards for transaction code sets, privacy of patient information, security of patient information, and national provider identifiers. These standard sets were implemented from October 2002 to May 2007. Officially, HIPAA applies to a healthcare provider who transmits any health information in electronic form in connection with a transaction identified by HIPAA. Electronic forms may include diskette, CD, and FTP (file transfer protocol). Some common transactions are electronic claims, eligibility requests, and claims status inquiries made to administrators of dental plans.

✚ HIPAA

Four Sets of HIPAA Standards

- Electronic Transactions and Code Sets
- Privacy Rule
- Security Rule
- National Provider Identifier Standard

Transactions and Code Sets

Almost all dental practices fall under the rules and regulations of HIPAA in one form or another. HIPAA states that any practice that sends or receives certain transactions electronically must send or receive them in a standard format. This means that all transactions and codes must be transmitted in the same format. Transactions and code sets are primarily a set of alpha and numeric codes used to report specific treatment, procedures, and diagnoses to insurance carriers. Before HIPAA, more than 400 different transactions and code sets could be used when medical and dental claims forms were submitted. Most insurance companies and government agencies had their own sets of codes. This high number of code sets resulted in increased costs of medical and dental services because it was very time consuming and labor intensive to manage them. One recommendation provided by the WEDI report was that code sets should be standardized to reduce the amount of time and labor needed to process the claim. This change reduced not only the number of hours required to process claims on the medical and dental side but also the workload of the insurance company or government agency that processes these claims. Today, only seven transaction code sets are used across all sectors of the healthcare industry. Another recommendation for saving costs was to make the transition from paper claims to electronic claims.

! REMEMBER

HIPAA requires that all providers who do business electronically must use the same healthcare transactions, code sets, and identifiers.

Electronic Data Interchange (EDI)

The move away from paper-generated claims toward electronically generated claims required the standardization of electronic data sets used to transfer and process insurance claims. Computer programs are built with these transaction data sets, which contain the information needed to code electronic transmissions. It is through these sets of codes that a computer is able to translate and process information received and transmitted. These data sets are transparent in the work that administrative dental assistants do; it is the responsibility of the computer programmer to program them into applicable systems. The final product that results from these standardized data sets is a common language that can be interpreted by all computer systems and software programs, both large and small.

HIPAA also states that all codes used to report treatment must be standardized (these are the codes used by insurance billers and coders to identify procedures that have been completed by the dentist). The national standard for codes used to report dental treatment is the Code on Dental Procedures and Nomenclature (the Code). The Code is defined in the latest edition of Current Dental Terminology (CDT), which is published by the ADA (discussed in detail in Chapter 15). In addition to the Code for dental treatment, codes are provided for all segments of the healthcare system.

✚ HIPAA

HIPAA Transactions and Code Set Standards

- Dental Codes: CDT
- Diagnosis Codes: ICD-10-CM
- Procedures Codes: CPT-4
- Physician Service Codes: CPT-4
- Inpatient Service Codes: ICD-CM
- Other Service Codes: HCPCS
- Drug Codes: NDC

✚ HIPAA

Types of Electronic Transactions

- Submission of Dental Insurance Claims or Equivalent Encounters
- Receipt of Remittance and Payment Reports
- Query Regarding and Receipt of Claims Status from Insurance Company
- Status Reports on Enrollment and Disenrollment in a Dental Health Plan
- Query Regarding and Receipt of Patient Eligibility
- Referral Certification and Authorization
- Receipt of Coordination of Benefits Reports

Standards for Privacy of Individually Identifiable Health Information (The Privacy Rule)

Once it was determined that the efficiency and effectiveness of healthcare could be improved through electronic transmissions, Congress expressed concern for the privacy of patient health information. The final result was that Congress incorporated into HIPAA provisions that mandated the adoption of federal privacy protections for individually identifiable health information. After several revisions and public hearings, the HHS adopted the final Privacy Rule and ensured that it would work as intended. The intent of the rule is to protect patient health information; it applies to three types of covered entities: health plans, healthcare clearinghouses, and healthcare providers who use an electronic method of transferring information. It should be noted that the federal Privacy Rule (with a compliancy date of April 13, 2003) is a minimum standard (that is, it is the least that should be done) and does not supersede federal, state, or other laws that grant individuals even greater privacy protections. Covered entities are free to retain or adopt more protective policies or practices.

To comply with the Privacy Rule, it is necessary for individual dental offices (as well as other identified entities) to establish day-to-day administrative policies and procedures by which protected health information (PHI) can be safeguarded. PHI must be protected in all formats and in all locations; this includes the transfer of information provided in oral, written, and electronic formats and when stored (paper and electronic copies). Another component of the rule requires a written policy and procedure manual for handling PHI and the appointment of one person (Privacy Officer) who will be responsible for overseeing the process.

Some safeguards designed to control unauthorized disclosure of PHI include locking of file drawers or doors at night, assignment of computer passwords, security of passwords, and protection of patient files at all times. To keep passwords secure, a system must be established for changing passwords on a regular schedule and keeping them private. It is advised that staff members do not post or share passwords with one another. Protecting PHI in patient files may require (1) ensuring that PHI does not appear on the outside of the patient record file, (2) taking care not to leave files where they can be viewed by patients, or (3) refraining from discussion of PHI when it may be overheard by other patients.

The Privacy Rule provides patients with the following rights.

Access to Medical Records

Patients should be able to see and obtain copies of their medical records and to request corrections if they detect errors and mistakes. Providers should grant access to these patient records within 30 days of a request and may charge patients for the cost of copying and sending records.

Notice of Privacy Practices

Covered healthcare plans must provide notice to patients regarding how they may use personal medical information and their rights under the new privacy regulations. Patients also may ask covered entities to restrict the use or disclosure of their information beyond the practices included in the notice, but the covered entities would not have to agree to this request.

Limits on Use of Personal Medical Information

The Privacy Rule sets limits on how healthcare plans and covered providers may use individually identifiable health information. In addition, patients must sign a specific authorization form before a covered entity is permitted to release their medical information to a life insurer, a bank, a marketing firm, or another outside business for purposes not related to healthcare.

Prohibition on Marketing

The final Privacy Rule sets new restrictions and limits on the use of patient information for marketing purposes. Pharmacies, healthcare plans, and other covered entities must first obtain an individual's specific authorization before patient information can be disclosed for marketing purposes.

Confidential Communications

Under the Privacy Rule, patients may request that their doctors, healthcare plans, and other covered entities take reasonable steps to ensure that their communications with the patient are kept confidential.

Complaints

Consumers may file a formal complaint regarding the privacy practices of a covered healthcare plan or provider.

In addition to the privacy rules stated earlier that apply to the patient, all healthcare plans, pharmacies, doctors, and other covered entities must establish polices and procedures for protecting the confidentiality of PHI related to their patients.

Steps to Protect Patient Privacy

Written privacy procedures.
- Identify staff members who have access to PHI
- Explain how PHI will be used and when it may be disclosed
- Ensure that any business associates who have access to PHI agree to the same limitations on the use and disclosure of PHI

Employee training and privacy officer.
- Train employees in the established privacy procedures
- Designate an individual to be responsible for ensuring that procedures are followed (Privacy Officer)
- If an employee fails to follow established procedures, administer appropriate disciplinary action

Public responsibilities. Limited circumstances may require the disclosure of health information for specific public responsibilities.
- Emergency circumstances
- Identification of the body of a deceased person or determination of the cause of death
- Public health needs
- Research that involves limited data or that has been independently approved by an institutional review board
- Judicial and administrative proceedings
- Limited law enforcement activities
- Activities related to national defense and security

Standards for Security of Individually Identifiable Health Information (The Security Rule)

The Security Rule requires that covered providers protect the integrity, confidentiality, and availability of electronic health information. The Security Rule is divided into three standards: administrative, physical, and technical. For covered providers to meet these standards, they must perform a risk analysis and decide how to manage risks by establishing a risk management protocol, develop a sanction policy, and provide ongoing review of the established protocol to ensure compliance. The Security Rule addresses only **electronically protected health information (ePHI)** that is shared electronically, in contrast to the Privacy Rule, which covers PHI provided in oral, written, and electronic forms.

> **! REMEMBER**
>
> The Privacy Rule refers to what patient health information must be kept confidential. The Security Rule addresses how to keep patient health information confidential.

> **➕ HIPAA**
>
> *Security Rule: Protecting Electronic Personal Health Information (ePHI)*
>
> **Confidentiality:** Only authorized individuals may access electronic health information.
> **Integrity:** The information does not change except when changed by an authorized person.
> **Availability:** Authorized persons can always retrieve ePHI, regardless of circumstances.

National Provider Identifier Standard

The National Provider Identifier (NPI) standard is the final standard established under HIPAA. The NPI is given to all individual healthcare providers and provider organizations such as group practices, clinics, hospitals, and schools. The NPI, a distinctive standard identification number, is issued by the U.S. government and was mandated to appear on all electronic transactions no later than May 23, 2007. The NPI replaces the Social Security Number, the Individual Tax ID, and other identifiers used with standard electronic healthcare transactions such as dental insurance claim forms.

THE HITECH ACT

The Health Information Technology for Economic and Clinical Health Act (HITECH Act) is part of the American Recovery and Reinvestment Act of 2009 (ARRA). ARRA contains incentives related to health care information technology in general as well as specific incentives designed to accelerate the adoption of electronic health record (EHR) systems among providers.

Because this legislation anticipates a massive expansion in the exchange of electronic protected health information (ePHI), the HITECH Act also widens the scope of privacy and security protections available under HIPAA, increases the potential legal liability for noncompliance, and provides for more enforcement.

Highlights of the HITECH Act pertaining to dentistry:
- Individuals have the right to obtain PHI in an electronic format
- Patients can assign a third party as the recipient of the ePHI
- Business associates (vendors who provide electronic health records systems and others) are directly responsible for privacy and security of PHI
- New requirements for marketing communications
- New reports for security breaches
- Possibility of civil and criminal penalties

THE 2013 HIPAA OMNIBUS FINAL RULE

The HIPAA Omnibus Final Rule was enacted to strengthen the Privacy and Security Rules for health information that were established under HIPAA. The Omnibus Final Rule greatly enhances a patient's privacy protections, provides individuals with new rights to their health information, and strengthens the government's ability to enforce the law.

Highlights of HIPAA Omnibus Final Rule include:
- Expands patient rights by allowing patients to ask for a copy of their electronic medical and dental records in electronic form
- When patients pay out of pocket in full, allows patients to instruct their provider to refrain from sharing information about their treatment with their health plan
- Sets limits on how information can be used and disclosed for marketing and fundraising purposes and prohibits the sale of individuals' health information without their permission
- Requires that Notice of Privacy Practices forms inform patients that they will be notified if their PHI is subject to breach

OCCUPATIONAL SAFETY AND HEALTH ADMINISTRATION (OSHA)

The Occupational Safety and Health Administration (OSHA) is a government agency within the U.S. Department of Labor that fulfills the mission of assuring the safety and health of America's workers by setting and enforcing standards. Before employees in a dental practice can perform any duty that has been identified by OSHA as hazardous, they must first take a safety course and pass a test administered by the employer. This information is outlined in the dental practice's Hazard Communication Program and is available to all employees.

Professional Ethics

Both laws and ethics must be observed in the daily operation of a dental practice. This responsibility is assigned to each member of the dental healthcare team. Ethics deals with moral judgments as determined by a professional organization. When an organization establishes a high standard of ethical and moral judgment, which is reflected in the way it treats and serves members of society, society in turn will grant the organization the opportunity to practice self-government. According to the ADA, self-government is a privilege and an obligation.

An excerpt from the preamble of the ADA's *Principles of Ethics and Code of Professional Conduct* is given on page 13, followed by the five Principles of Ethics.

LEGAL STANDARDS

In addition to the ethical standards established by a professional organization to outline the ideal standards for care, practitioners must adhere to the legal standards established by society to regulate all of its members. Legal standards are expressed as laws and regulations. These standards are enacted by legislators and regulated by boards and commissions. The profession of dentistry is regulated and controlled by individual state Dental Practice Acts. Each state enacts a Dental Practice Act, which outlines the duties of members of the dental profession, including dentists, dental hygienists, dental assistants, and dental laboratory technicians. Included in the Dental Practice Act are educational requirements, specific duties, and licensure requirements. Each state has its own Dental Practice Act and all members of the dental profession who practice must uphold the state's specified standards. When a practitioner moves from one state to another, it is his or her responsibility to obtain any needed licenses and to follow the standards of the new state.

Licensure

Licensure is a method used to identify members of a profession who meet minimum standards and are qualified to perform the duties outlined in regulations and standards (Dental Practice Act). The Board of Dental Examiners is the agency that has been assigned the authority to issue state licenses. Once a license has been issued, it must be renewed at established intervals. Continued education is one

AMERICAN DENTAL ASSOCIATION PRINCIPLES OF ETHICS AND CODE OF PROFESSIONAL CONDUCT

Principles of Ethics

The Association believes that dentists should possess not only knowledge, skill, and technical competence but also those traits of character that foster adherence to ethical principles. Qualities of honesty, compassion, kindness, integrity, fairness, and charity are part of the ethical education of a dentist and practice of dentistry and help define the true professional. As such, each dentist should share in providing advocacy to and care of the underserved. It is urged that the dentist meet this goal, subject to individual circumstances.

The ethical dentist strives to do that which is right and good. The *ADA Code* is an instrument to help the dentist in this quest.

Section 1—Principle: Patient Autonomy ("Self-Governance")

The dentist has a duty to respect the patient's rights to self-determination and confidentiality.

This principle expresses the concept that professionals have a duty to treat the patient according to the patient's desires, within the bounds of accepted treatment, and to protect the patient's confidentiality. Under this principle, the dentist's primary obligations include involving patients in treatment decisions in a meaningful way, with due consideration being given to the patient's needs, desires, and abilities and safeguarding the patient's privacy.

Section 2—Principle: Non-Maleficence ("Do No Harm")

The dentist has a duty to refrain from harming the patient.

This principle expresses the concept that professionals have a duty to protect the patient from harm. Under this principle, the dentist's primary obligations include keeping knowledge and skills current, knowing one's own limitations and when to refer a patient to a specialist or other professional, and knowing when and under what circumstances delegation of patient care to auxiliaries is appropriate.

Section 3—Principle: Beneficence ("Do Good")

The dentist has a duty to promote the patient's welfare.

This principle expresses the concept that professionals have a duty to act for the benefit of others. Under this principle, the dentist's primary obligation is service to the patient and the public-at-large. The most important aspect of this obligation is the competent and timely delivery of dental care within the bounds of clinical circumstances presented by the patient, with due consideration given to the needs, desires, and values of the patient. The same ethical considerations apply whether the dentist engages in a fee-for-service, managed care, or some other practice arrangement. Dentists may choose to enter into contracts governing the provision of care to a group of patients; however, contract obligations do not excuse dentists from their ethical duty to put the patient's welfare first.

Section 4—Principle: Justice ("Fairness")

The dentist has a duty to treat people fairly.

This principle expresses the concept that professionals have a duty to be fair in their dealings with patients, colleagues, and society. Under this principle, the dentist's primary obligations include dealing with people justly and delivering dental care without prejudice. In its broadest sense, this principle expresses the concept that the dental profession should actively seek allies throughout society on specific activities that will help improve access to care for all.

Section 5—Principle: Veracity ("Truthfulness")

The dentist has a duty to communicate truthfully.

This principle expresses the concept that professionals have a duty to be honest and trustworthy in their dealings with people. Under this principle, the dentist's primary obligations include respecting the position of trust inherent in the dentist–patient relationship, communicating truthfully and without deception, and maintaining intellectual integrity.

Excerpted from ADA principles of ethics and code of professional conduct, with official advisory opinions, © 2012 American Dental Association. All rights reserved. Reprinted with permission.

requirement for license renewal. Another condition of renewal is that all requirements must have been met and documented. Renewal periods are specified in the Dental Practice Act.

> **! REMEMBER**
>
> When dental auxiliaries perform duties that are not assigned to them in the Dental Practice Act, they are committing a criminal act.

Registration

Registration is a form of licensure that has been established by some states as a method of protecting the public. Requirements for registration are outlined in the Dental Practice Act. Some states mandate registration for such duties as exposing radiographs, performing intraoral tasks, and handling the expanded duties of the dental auxiliary. Registrations must be renewed periodically through additional required training.

Certification

In some states, it is a condition of licensure that the dental assistant must be a Certified Dental Assistant (CDA). Certification is granted by the Dental Assisting National Board (DANB). To qualify for certification, the dental assistant must graduate from a Commission on Dental Accreditation (CODA)–accredited program or must meet the work experience requirements and pass a written examination. DANB has created different "pathways" by which qualifications and requirements can be met. It offers a CDA certificate as well as certification in various specialty areas.

PATIENT'S RIGHTS

During the past 20 years there have been numerous healthcare initiatives, and professional organizations that have identified key patient rights that should be extended to medical and dental patients. It is important to know the context of these rights as it applies to the treatment of patients in the dental practice. As discussed earlier, patients want and demand to be treated in a professional manner. The following is a composite of key rights and how they may apply to dental patients.

PATIENT'S BILL OF RIGHTS

Patients have the Right to be Seen for Treatment in a Reasonable Length of Time.

It is not acceptable for a patient to have to wait several days to a few weeks before seeing the dentist in an emergency. Scheduling is very important and time should be allowed daily for emergency patients to be seen. Patients need to know that the dentist will see them in an emergency. The purposes of an emergency appointment are to relieve pain, eliminate the possibility of further health damage, and temporize an affected tooth structure. If further treatment is necessary, the patient will be scheduled (within a few days, not weeks) for further treatment and will receive a comprehensive dental examination. Patients who are made to wait several weeks to months to be seen for routine preventive care (prophylaxis) will seek treatment elsewhere. Creative scheduling and working within the matrixed appointment book will help the administrative dental assistant to achieve this goal (see Chapter 10).

Patients have the Right to See the Dentist when they Receive Dental Treatment.

When patients are scheduled for procedures with the dental hygienist, it is necessary that the dentist also be available at that time to see the patient. If the patient is returning for scheduled treatment and has been examined by the dentist recently, it is good patient management to have the dentist step into the treatment room and ask whether the patient has any questions. Depending on the state's Dental Practice Act, the dentist may not need to be present when the patient is receiving treatment for a problem that was first diagnosed by the dentist.

> ### ❗ REMEMBER
>
> Dental auxiliaries cannot diagnose and treat patients. If a patient will be seen by an auxiliary without a dentist present, the procedure must be performed according to the Dental Practice Act and one must ask whether the patient has any questions. Depending on the state's Dental Practice Act, the dentist may not have to be present when the patient is receiving treatment for a problem that was first diagnosed by the dentist.

Patients have the right to know what treatment is recommended, the cost, and what alternative options are available.

The patient must be informed of and must agree to all treatment in advance of receiving the treatment. This is accomplished when open communications exist between the dentist, the dental auxiliary, and the patient. The dentist and members of the dental healthcare team must take the time to discuss and answer all questions regarding treatment. Written treatment plans that list each procedure and its fee must be given to the patient. Consent forms outline the nature of the procedure, expectations, and possible complications.

Patients have the Right to Expect that they will be Safe.

Providing complete infection control is a duty of the entire dental healthcare team. The administrative dental assistant must ensure an adequate amount of time between patient visits to allow quality infection control procedures. The dental assistant and the dentist must follow strict infection control protocol for the protection of patients. Patients also expect that the dentist will keep them safe by using materials and procedures that have been approved and meet industry standards.

Patients have the Right to Expect that the Dental Healthcare Team will Communicate in a way that they can Understand.

Communications between the dentist, the dental auxiliary, and the patient must be spoken in a language that is understood by the patient. The dental staff must be prepared to explain all procedures using common terminology. This may be accomplished by development of scripts, use of visual aids, and provision of educational information that has been prepared for patients.

Patients have the Right to Know the Dentist and Dental Auxiliary Team are Licensed.

All dentists and dental auxiliaries should post their diplomas, certificates, and licenses in easy view of patients. Members of the dental healthcare team should be prepared to answer questions about the dentist's and the dental auxiliary's training and licensure background. A script that contains all of these details would be helpful. This information can also be transmitted to patients via newsletters, brochures, and letters of introduction about new dental healthcare team members.

Patients have the Right to Choose their Dentist.

Members of the dental profession believe that every patient has the right to choose his or her own dentist. A third-party may direct patients to a network of providers, where the patient can choose a dentist within the network.

Patients have the Right to Expect that their Medical and Dental Information is Kept Private.

The dental healthcare team will follow all laws and regulations to ensure that all patients' personal information is secure. The dental practice will have a written policy, identify key personnel, and provide training in privacy procedures.

Patients have the Right to View their Medical and Dental Information.

The dental healthcare team will grant access to patient records and follow applicable laws and regulations.

PROFESSIONAL ORGANIZATIONS

American Dental Assistants Association

The American Dental Assistants Association (ADAA) is a professional organization for dental assistants. It has a variety of functions, including promoting professional growth and facilitating community involvement. The ADAA provides continuing education to dental assistants through home study courses; professional journals; and local, state, and national meetings. Membership in the ADAA provides many benefits, such as:

- Professional liability insurance
- Accidental death insurance
- Discounts on home study continuation courses
- Subscription to *Dental Assistant Journal*
- Discounted membership dues for students
- Scholarship opportunities

AMERICAN DENTAL ASSISTANTS ASSOCIATION PRINCIPLES OF PROFESSIONAL ETHICS AND CODE OF MEMBER CONDUCT

American Dental Assistants Association Principles of Professional Ethics (2011)

- Cause no harm;
- Uphold all federal, state, and local laws and regulations;
- Be truthful and honest in verbal, financial, and treatment endeavors;
- Recognize and report signs of abuse to proper authorities;
- Assist in informed decision-making of treatment options; while respecting the rights of patients to determine the final course of treatment to be rendered;
- Do not discriminate against others;
- Support, promote and participate in access to care efforts through education, professional activities and programs;
- Deliver optimum care utilizing professional knowledge, judgment and skill within the law;
- Be compassionate, respectful, kind and fair to employers, co-workers, and patients;
- Refrain from denigrating by word, print, or in electronic communication his/her employer, workplace, or colleagues at all times;
- Create and maintain a safe work environment;
- Assist in conflict management when necessary to maintain harmony within the workplace;
- Strive for self-improvement through continuing education;
- Strive for a healthy lifestyle which may prevent physical or mental impairment caused by any type of illness;
- Refrain from any substance abuse;
- Never misrepresent professional credentials or education.

American Dental Assistants Association (ADAA) Code of Member Conduct

As a member of the American Dental Assistants Association, I pledge to:

- Abide by the Bylaws of the Association;
- Maintain loyalty to the Association;
- Pursue the objectives of the Association;
- Hold in confidence the information entrusted to me by the Association;
- Serve all members of the Association in an impartial manner;
- Maintain respect for the members and the employees of the Association;
- Exercise and insist on sound business principles in the conduct of the affairs of the Association;
- Use legal and ethical means to influence legislation or regulation affecting members of the Association;
- Issue no false or misleading statements to fellow members or to the public;
- Refrain from disseminating malicious information concerning the Association or any member or employee of the American Dental Assistants Association;
- Maintain high standards of personal conduct and integrity;
- Cooperate in a reasonable and proper manner with staff and members;
- Accept no personal compensation from fellow members, except as approved by the Association;
- Assure public confidence in the integrity and service of the Association;
- Promote and maintain the highest standards of performance in service to the Association.

The ADAA has adopted its own *Principles of Ethics and Professional Conduct* as a guide for its members.

HOSA–Future Health Professionals

HOSA is a student organization that is sponsored by the U.S. Department of Education and 48 state departments of education. HOSA's mission is to promote career opportunities in healthcare and to enhance the delivery of quality healthcare to all people. HOSA provides a unique program of leadership development, motivation, and recognition designed exclusively for secondary, postsecondary, adult, and collegiate students enrolled in Health Science Technology programs.

Programs are started at the local school level, where members have the opportunity to participate in a wide range of leadership and skill development activities. Most states offer local, regional, and state conferences at which members can network with healthcare professionals, participate in leadership workshops, and compete in a number of individual and team leadership and skill events. Those who rank in the top three at the state level can go on to represent their state at the National Leadership Conference (NLC). During the NLC, members represent their home state and the top 10 at each event earn national recognition. In addition to its competitive events program, HOSA annually awards thousands of dollars in scholarships to members.

▌ KEY POINTS

- Role of an administrative dental assistant: The role of the administrative dental assistant is multifaceted and requires a broad range of skills. These assistants work in a collaborative environment with other members of the dental healthcare team. They are directly involved in patient communication and in communications with other members of the dental community. Administrative dental assistants often perform duties that are otherwise assigned to the:
  - Office Manager
  - Business Manager
  - Receptionist

  - Insurance Biller
  - Records Manager
  - Data Processor
  - Bookkeeper
  - Appointment Scheduler
- Members of the dental healthcare team: Members of the dental healthcare team work together to provide quality dental care for all patients. Members include the:
  - Dentist
  - Hygienist
  - Dental Assistant

- Subspecialties: Nine dental specialties address the various needs of patients.
- HIPAA: Each member of the dental healthcare team must follow the rules and regulations of HIPAA. The four HIPAA standards are:
  - Transactions and Code Sets Standard
  - Standards for Privacy of Individually Identifiable Health Information (Privacy Rule)
  - Standards for Security of Individually Identifiable Health Information (Security Rule)
  - National Provider Identifier Standard
- Highlights of the HITECH Act pertaining to dentistry:
  - Individuals have the right to obtain PHI in an electronic format
  - Patients can assign a third party as the recipient of the ePHI
  - Business associates (vendors who provide EHR systems and others) are directly responsible for privacy and security of PHI
  - New requirements for marketing communications
  - New reports for security breaches
  - Possibility of civil and criminal penalties

- Highlights of HIPAA Omnibus Final Rule:
  - Expands patient rights by allowing patients to ask for a copy of their electronic medical and dental record in electronic form
  - When patients pay out of pocket in full, allows patients to instruct their provider to refrain from sharing information about their treatment with their health plan
  - Sets limits on how information can be used and disclosed for marketing and fundraising purposes and prohibits the sale of individuals' health information without their permission
  - Requires that Notice of Privacy Practices forms inform patients that they will be notified if their PHI is subject to breach
- Professional ethical and legal responsibilities: In the daily operation of the dental practice, the dental healthcare team is faced with both legal and ethical issues. Ethical issues are those that involve principles of moral judgment. Legal issues are outlined in each state's Dental Practice Act. These include:
  - ADA *Principles of Ethics and Code of Professional Conduct*
  - ADAA *Principles of Ethics and Professional Conduct*
  - Patient's Bill of Rights

CAREER-READY PRACTICES

Career-Ready Practices activities are designed to provide students with experiences that can be "practiced" in preparation for skills needed on the job. In each of the following exercises, a variety of approaches may be used to address the problem, rather than "right" or "wrong" answers. Below each exercise, next to the compass icon, is a listing of suggested Career-Ready Practice numbers that correspond to the listing of 12 practices in the front of the text (see p. viii-ix); these practices provide suggestions for approaches to complete the exercise.

1. Research the job description for an administrative dental assistant, including but not limited to the knowledge, skills, abilities, work activities, work styles, and work values required for a career as an administrative dental assistant. Search hint: Do a web search at onetonline.org for medical secretaries.
   a. Using the information from your search and the information in the text, what do you think a typical day of an administrative dental assistant would look like?
   b. What skills and technology will be needed?
   c. How will you interact with patients and dental healthcare team members?

Career-Ready Practices
   7 *Employ valid and reliable research strategies.*
   8 *Utilize critical thinking to make sense of problems and persevere in solving them.*
   10 *Plan education and career path aligned to personal goals.*

2. Research job opportunities in your region for administrative dental assistants and identify what skills, tasks, and experience are desired.

Career-Ready Practices
   7 *Employ valid and reliable research strategies.*
   10 *Plan education and career path aligned to personal goals.*
   12 *Work productively in teams while using cultural/global competence.*

3. In a group, compare the information you researched in 1 and 2 above and prepare a job description for an administrative dental assistant, identifying what you feel are the most important skills, knowledge, and work styles necessary.

Career-Ready Practices
   4 *Communicate clearly, effectively, and with reason.*
   6 *Demonstrate creativity and innovation.*
   12 *Work productively in teams while using cultural/global competence.*

4. Reflect on the ADAA and ADA's Principles of Ethics and Professional Conduct and write a minimum of three paragraphs on why you feel it is important to follow these codes (for both patients and members of the dental healthcare team).

Career-Ready Practices
   1 *Act as a responsible and contributing citizen and employee.*
   4 *Communicate clearly, effectively, and with reason.*
   9 *Model integrity, ethical leadership, and effective management.*

Dental Basics

LEARNING OBJECTIVES

1. List and describe the different areas of a dental office.
2. Identify the basic structures of the face and oral cavity, including the basic anatomical structures and tissues of the teeth.
3. Distinguish between different tooth-numbering systems.
4. Interpret dental-charting symbols.
5. Categorize basic dental procedures.
6. List basic chairside dental assisting duties and identify Occupational Safety and Health Administration (OSHA) and state regulations.

INTRODUCTION

The administrative dental assistant has a unique opportunity to communicate in several "languages." You will be a translator between the dental community and the patient. As part of your job, you will represent the dentist when you communicate with dental professionals, dental insurance companies, patients, vendors, and fellow team members. Patients are often unwilling or unable to ask the dentist questions directly, so they will turn to the assistants for clarification. To be an effective communicator, you must first understand the language of dentistry.

During a typical day, you may have to explain a procedure to a patient, give postoperative instructions, review tooth-brushing instructions, answer many patient questions, communicate instructions to a dental laboratory technician, speak to a pharmacist, refer a patient to a specialist, or speak to other dental professionals. In addition, you may need to clarify a treatment for a dental insurance company or other team members. Effective communication is promoted by an understanding of the language that is spoken by all diverse professionals and patients with whom you interact on a daily basis.

If you are unable to understand the dental language, it will be very difficult for you to carry out the fundamental duties of your job, such as appointment scheduling, insurance coding, clinical chart management, and billing. Therefore it is necessary that you have a basic understanding of the dental language—the terms used to identify procedures, dental materials, and equipment. The development of a professional dental vocabulary is essential to successful communication.

! REMEMBER

Tools are found in the garage.
Utensils are found in the kitchen.
Instruments are found in the dental office.

BASIC DENTAL OFFICE DESIGN

Dental offices, similar to people, come in all shapes and sizes. Although many variables may influence the architectural design of a dental office, all consist of the same basic work areas, which can be divided between the business of dentistry and the practice of dentistry, or the nonclinical and clinical areas (Figure 2-1).

Nonclinical Areas

Reception Area

The first area that a patient sees is the reception area (Figure 2-2). When patients enter the reception area for the first time, they begin to formulate thoughts and opinions about the dental practice. They are concerned about the cleanliness of this area because it may reflect the condition of the treatment area. Patients often perceive their dental experience in terms of the impression they develop during the first few seconds after entering the reception area. (This is discussed further in Chapter 5.)

Business Office and Administrative Area

The reception area usually opens into the business office (Figure 2-3). Most duties of the administrative dental assistant are carried out in this area. The configuration shown in Figure 2-3 is preferred by most dental practitioners but it is not free of disadvantages. When the business area is open, all conversations can be overheard by waiting patients. For this reason, some designs include a sliding glass window in a wall between the two areas; this allows the administrative dental assistant to view and monitor the reception area while reducing the possibility that the patient will overhear conversations.

Consultation Area

When privacy is needed, such as when one is interviewing patients, establishing financial agreements, or speaking with

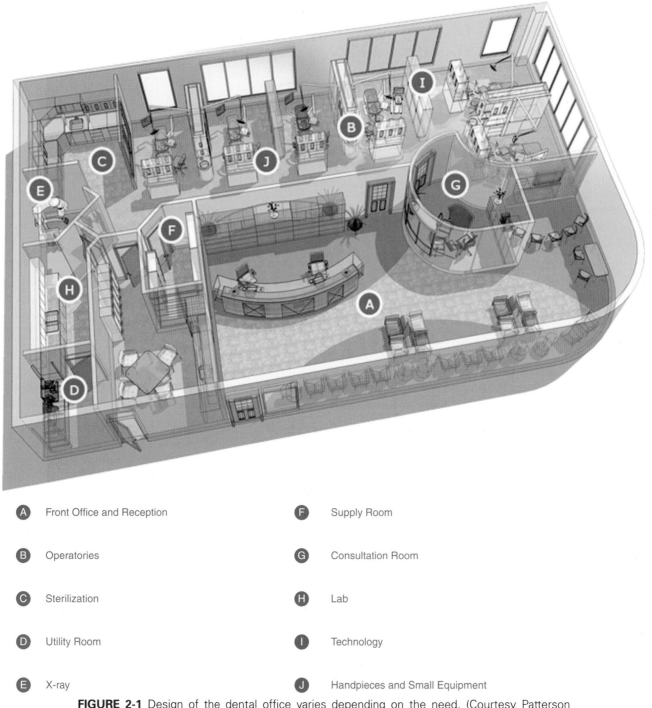

Ⓐ	Front Office and Reception		Ⓕ	Supply Room
Ⓑ	Operatories		Ⓖ	Consultation Room
Ⓒ	Sterilization		Ⓗ	Lab
Ⓓ	Utility Room		Ⓘ	Technology
Ⓔ	X-ray		Ⓙ	Handpieces and Small Equipment

FIGURE 2-1 Design of the dental office varies depending on the need. (Courtesy Patterson Dental, St. Paul, Minn.)

patients about private matters, an area away from other patients is recommended (Figure 2-4). Because the consultation area is used for patient contact, it should be designed with the comfort of the patient in mind. A table should be provided for the dental staff and the patient to sit down together. When all participating parties sit at a table, the environment created is nonthreatening to the patient.

This room can double as a very comfortable work area. When equipped with a telephone, computer, and workspace,

it can be used as an additional office, where phone calls and other work can be conducted without interruption.

Doctor's Private Office

A private office provides space and an area where the dentist can work quietly. This area is the private domain of the occupant and you should not enter it unless you are specifically invited. It is advisable to ask the doctor about the status of this area and how it should be treated. Some doctors

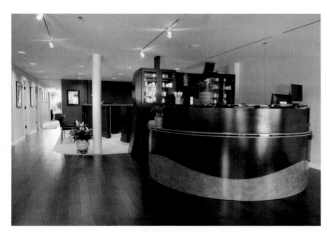

FIGURE 2-2 Typical reception area. (Copyright © 2011 leezsnow, iStock.com. All rights reserved.)

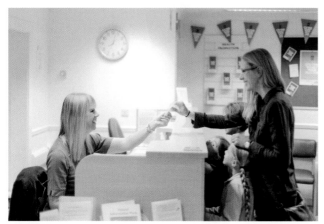

FIGURE 2-3 Administrative dental assistant performing daily tasks such as scheduling appointments, making financial arrangements, and following bookkeeping procedures. (Copyright © 2013 urbancow, iStock.com. All rights reserved.)

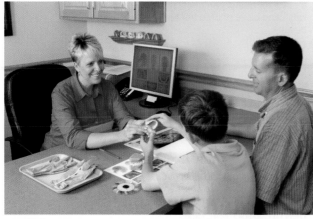

FIGURE 2-4 Dentist discussing treatment options in the consultation area. (Copyright © 2009 jacomstephens, iStock.com. All rights reserved.)

maintain an "open door" policy and welcome your entrance. Others consider this area very private and do not allow intrusion or entrance when they are not present.

Private offices may be staffed by office managers, business managers, and other specified personnel. Always respect the privacy of these areas. Papers, documents, and computer information may not be for all eyes; therefore obtain clear direction on how these areas are to be respected.

Staff Room

The staff room is an area set aside for the exclusive use of the staff. This room can be used as a lunchroom or a meeting area. Depending on the size of the staff and the office, this room may be as simple as a very small eating area or as large as a small apartment. Responsibility for maintaining the area is usually assigned to the dental auxiliary.

Additional Nonclinical Areas

Larger practices may provide areas for record and supply storage. These areas often include storage shelves and large file cabinets. Locker rooms provide a place for changing from street clothes into uniforms. The Occupational Safety and Health Administration (OSHA) has mandated that clothing worn during dental treatment cannot be worn outside the dental office. The dentist should provide a laundry service so that the dental assistant does not have to take contaminated uniforms home.

Clinical Areas

Dental and support activities take place in clinical areas. The dentist, dental assistant, hygienist, and laboratory technician perform their duties in these areas.

Treatment Rooms

Treatment rooms may also be referred to as "operatories." (Although the latter term is fading from use because patients associate the term with "surgical operating room," it may still be used by some dental personnel.) The treatment room is the area in which patients are treated by the dentist, dental hygienist, and dental assistant.

Depending on the size and type of a dental practice, the basic practice will consist of two or more treatment rooms. While the dentist is attending to a patient in one room, the other room can be prepared for the next patient. In larger practices with several treatment rooms, more than one patient can be seated at the same time. Simultaneously, the hygienist may treat one patient, an expanded function assistant can finish a procedure with a second patient, and one or more dentists may be attending to their patients. Anatomy of a Treatment Room shows the basic equipment found in the treatment room. Treatment rooms may be configured slightly differently but the goals remain the same: provide adequate equipment for use in treating the patient, allow for proper infection control, and ensure the comfort and safety of employees and patients.

In addition to basic equipment, the room may include a media system that is used to entertain and educate patients. An intraoral camera, which involves a digitized system that allows the dentist to take intraoral images (Figure 2-5), also may be present. Intraoral images are used to illustrate some problems for which dental treatment is needed that cannot be detected radiographically.

These images can be stored digitally and are a valuable diagnostic tool.

Offices also use a variety of decorating media to enhance the beauty of the office and to create a comfortable environment for patient treatment.

ANATOMY OF A TREATMENT ROOM

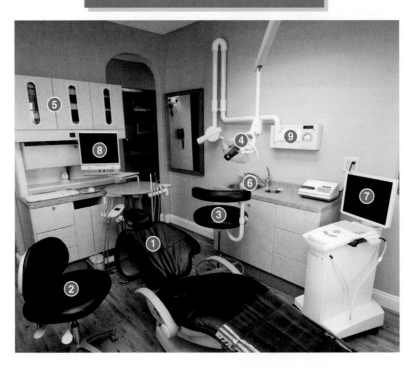

❶ PATIENT CHAIR

Typically this is a lounge type chair so that the patient can be placed in a supine position. Control panels are used to place the chair in various positions. Arms are attached to the chair or to a portable unit to provide the dentist and the assistant easy access to the necessary tubing for handpieces, oral evacuation, and air-water syringe. Additional arms provide an overhead light and a tray for instrument placement.

❷ OPERATOR'S STOOL

This stool is adjustable, including the backrest, and moves on rollers. It is used by the dentist, dental hygienist, or expanded function assistant while they are attending to the patient.

❸ ASSISTANT'S STOOL

This stool is used by the assistant and is slightly different from the operator's stool. It typically includes a footrest because it is raised higher than the operator's stool. The abdominal arm of the stool is used for balance and to provide a rest for forearms.

❹ OPERATING LIGHT

This light is either attached to the chair or suspended from the ceiling. It is high intensity and illuminates the oral cavity.

❺ CABINETS

Cabinets designed for storage of equipment and supplies may be either built-in or mobile. The assistant and the dentist need areas to place the instruments they are using and to manipulate dental materials.

❻ HANDWASHING SINK

A sink is placed in the room or just outside the entrance. The sink provides a place for dental personnel to properly wash and glove prior to treating the patient.

❼ CAD/CAM

Computer Aided Design/Computer Aided Manufacturing: This technology is used to design and create restorations such as veneers, onlays, crowns, and bridges. This technology is a time and cost savings to the dental practice, allowing the dentist or lab tech to complete these restorations in one visit.

❽ COMPUTER MONITOR

The monitor is used to view digital radiographs, complete chart entries, and schedule appointments.

❾ DENTAL X-RAY MACHINE

This machine is used for taking intra-oral radiographs.

(Image courtesy Patterson Dental, St. Paul, Minn.)

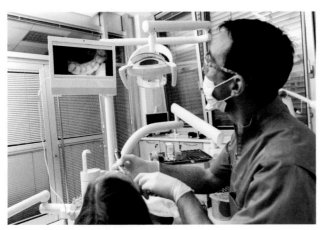

FIGURE 2-5 A dentist using an intraoral camera. (Copyright © 2013 choja, iStock.com. All rights reserved.)

Sterilization Area

In the sterilization area, contaminated instruments are cleaned, packaged, sterilized (all microorganisms completely killed), and prepared for reuse. The room is separated into two areas (Figure 2-6). The contaminated area is where cleaning, packaging, and sterilization take place. Once packages have been removed from the sterilizer, they are placed in the clean area, which is used for the assembly and storage of

treatment trays. During processing and storage, sterile instruments remain packaged. So that sterility is ensured, they are opened only in the treatment room in the presence of the patient.

Dental Laboratory Area

In the dental laboratory, the dentist and the assistant can perform duties that do not require patient contact. In small practices, this area may be used for basic laboratory functions, such as preparing diagnostic casts, pouring models, and fabricating trays used for bleaching and other procedures. In larger practices that employ a dental laboratory technician, the dental laboratory would be much larger and crowns, bridges, partials, and dentures would be made there.

Additional Clinical Areas

Radiology and imaging area. The x-ray room or imaging area is the place where the dental assistant will take digital images or radiographs. The difference between a digital image and a radiography (x-ray film) is the technology used to create and process the image. Digital imaging uses the same x-ray machine but the image is captured using electronic signals and sensors and can be displayed on a computer monitor almost immediately. A conventional radiograph or film is created by exposing film to x-rays and processing them using chemicals, typically taking 10 to 20 minutes. Equipment includes a standard dental x-ray machine used to take intraoral (inside the mouth) films (conventionally and digitally) and a computer if using a digital imaging system. The area may also include a film-based or digital panographic unit used to take extraoral (outside the mouth) films (Figure 2-7). Imaging or radiographic equipment is often located in each treatment room. A darkroom or daylight loader will be needed to process conventional x-ray film.

Patient education room. The patient education room is a separate area that is designated for use in patient education

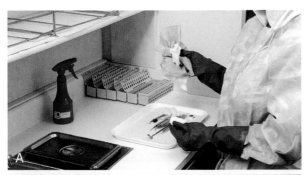

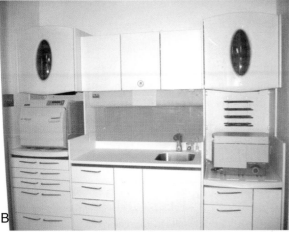

FIGURE 2-6 Sterilization area, contaminated **(A)** and clean **(B)**. (From Bird DL, Robinson DS: *Modern dental assisting*, ed 11, St. Louis, 2015, Saunders.)

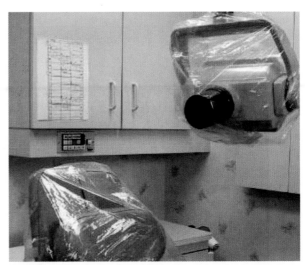

FIGURE 2-7 Radiographic area. (From Bird DL, Robinson DS: *Modern dental assisting*, ed 11, St. Louis, 2015, Saunders.)

and motivation. The room includes equipment that demonstrates correct brushing and flossing techniques. With the use of technology, additional information can be streamed to a television screen, allowing the dental office to take advantage of an endless library of educational and motivational material. Brochures and pamphlets may be given to patients for home study.

BASIC DENTAL ANATOMY

Knowledge of basic dental anatomy helps the administrative dental assistant to communicate with other dental professionals, patients, and insurance companies.

Basic Structures of the Face and Oral Cavity
Skull

The skull is made up of two sections. The cranium consists of 8 bones that form a protective structure for the brain and the face consists of 14 bones (Table 2-1, Figure 2-8).

Oral Cavity

The oral cavity, or the mouth, is the anatomical area where dentistry is performed (Figure 2-9). This cavity is regarded as the beginning of the digestive system; it contains sensory receptors, is used to create speech patterns, and serves as a vehicle for human pleasure and as a weapon that can be used for defense (both verbal and physical).

Lips and Cheeks

The lips surround the opening to the oral cavity. The corners of the mouth, where the upper and lower lips meet, are the commissures. The vermilion border represents the junction of the tissue of the face with the mucous membrane of the lips (Figure 2-10). The cheeks form the side of the face. The insides of the cheeks are covered with moist mucous membrane. The junction of the mucous membrane of the cheek and the gingiva is the buccal vestibule. The junction of the lips and the gingiva is the labial vestibule (Figure 2-11).

Frenum

The frenum (plural, frena) is a strip of tissue that connects two structures. Five frena are located in the oral cavity. Two—maxillary and mandibular—are labial frena. These connect the tissue of the lips (labia) to the gingival tissue. Two buccal frena (right and left) connect the cheek to the gingiva in the area of the maxillary first molar. One lingual frenum connects the tongue to the floor of the mouth (Figure 2-12). (Run your tongue around the vestibule of your mouth and you will feel the labial and buccal frena.)

TABLE 2-1	Bones of the Skull	
Bone	**Number**	**Location**
Eight Bones of the Cranium		
Frontal	1	Forms the forehead, most of the orbital roof, and the anterior cranial floor
Parietal	2	Form most of the roof and upper sides of the cranium
Occipital	1	Forms the back and base of the cranium
Temporal	2	Form the sides and base of the cranium
Sphenoid	1	Forms part of the anterior base of the skull and part of the walls of the orbit
Ethmoid	1	Forms part of the orbit and the floor of the cranium
Fourteen Bones of the Face		
Zygomatic	2	Form the prominence of the cheeks and part of the orbit
Maxillary	2	Form the upper jaw
Palatine	2	Form the posterior part of the hard palate and the floor of the nose
Nasal	2	Form the bridge of the nose
Lacrimal	2	Form part of the orbit at the inner angle of the eye
Vomer	1	Forms the base for the nasal septum
Inferior conchae	2	Form part of the interior of the nose
Mandible	1	Forms the lower jaw
Six Auditory Ossicles		
Malleus, incus, stapes	6	Bones of the middle ear

From Bird DL, Robinson DS: *Modern dental assisting*, ed 11, St. Louis, 2015, Saunders.

Tongue

The tongue, which is covered with taste buds, is a strong muscle that aids in the digestive process and contributes to speech formation. The posterior (back) of the tongue is connected to the hyoid bone. The anterior portion is attached only to the lingual frenum.

DID YOU KNOW?
When the maxillary labial frenum is too thick or wide, it keeps the two front teeth from coming into contact. This creates a diastema.

DID YOU KNOW?
A short lingual frenum keeps the tongue from extending as far as is needed for speech formation. This condition is referred to as "tongue tied." A simple procedure of clipping the frenum corrects the problem.

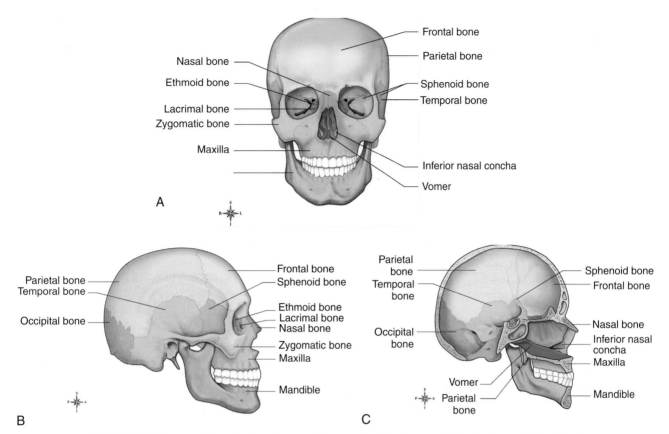

FIGURE 2-8 Views of the skull and cranial bones. **A,** Anterior view. **B,** Lateral view. **C,** Left half of skull views from within. (From Patton KT, Thibodeau GA: *Anthony's textbook of anatomy & physiology*, ed 20, St. Louis, 2013, Mosby.)

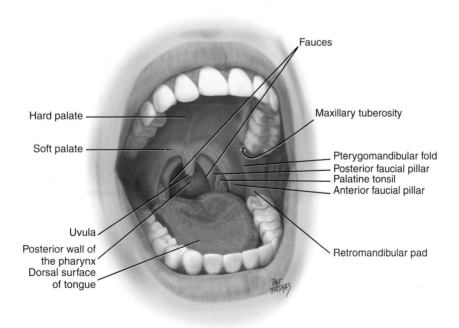

FIGURE 2-9 Features of the oral cavity. (From Fehrenbach MJ, Herring SW: *Illustrated anatomy of the head and neck*, ed 4, St. Louis, 2012, Saunders.)

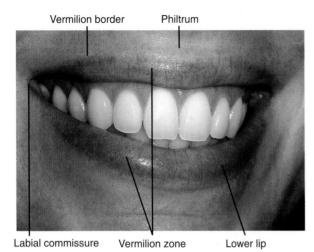

FIGURE 2-10 Landmarks of the mouth. (From Bird DL, Robinson DS: *Modern dental assisting*, ed 11, St. Louis, 2015, Saunders.)

Salivary Glands

The salivary glands produce saliva, which provides moisture for the mucous membrane, lubricates food, cleans the teeth, supplies an enzyme (amylase) that begins the digestive process, and is the source of minerals (fluorides, calcium, and phosphate) needed for the remineralization of tooth structure. The three pairs of salivary glands are parotid glands, submandibular glands, and sublingual glands (Figure 2-13).

Hard and Soft Palates

The hard palate, or roof of the mouth, is covered with masticatory mucosa. Located within the hard palate are the rugae, or folds of tissue, behind the maxillary anterior teeth. Located straight behind (posterior) the central incisors is the incisive papilla (Figure 2-14). (With your tongue, press on the hard palate. Behind the anterior teeth, you should be able to feel the rugae, incisive papilla, and hard bony structure that forms the hard palate.)

The soft palate is the posterior continuation of the hard palate. The soft and flexible region located on the back (posterior) of the soft palate is the uvula (see Figure 2-9), which is a projection of tissue that hangs in the center of the throat. Both the soft palate and the uvula move upward during swallowing to direct food downward into the oropharynx and not upward into the nasal cavity.

During dental procedures, one must be careful not to stimulate the gag reflex. Tissue located in the posterior portion of the mouth, including the soft palate and the uvula, forms the gag reflex area. When this area is touched by a foreign object or is stimulated by the taste of some foods or materials, gagging can occur.

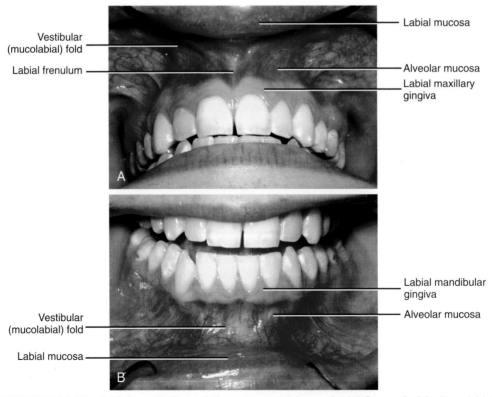

FIGURE 2-11 The labial vestibule and the upper and lower labial frena. **A,** Maxillary labial mucosa and attachments of the frenum. **B,** Mandibular labial mucosa and attachments of the frenum. (From Liebgott B: *The anatomical basis of dentistry*, ed 3, St. Louis, 2010, Mosby.)

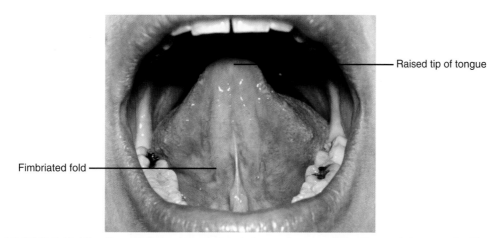

FIGURE 2-12 The lingual frenum and the delicate tissues of the floor of the mouth. (From Liebgott B: *The anatomical basis of dentistry,* ed 3, St. Louis, 2010, Mosby.)

- Raised tip of tongue
- Fimbriated fold

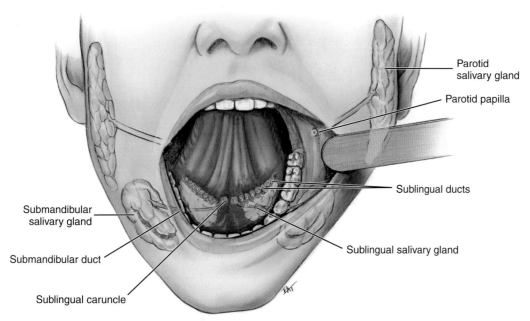

- Parotid salivary gland
- Parotid papilla
- Sublingual ducts
- Submandibular salivary gland
- Submandibular duct
- Sublingual caruncle
- Sublingual salivary gland

FIGURE 2-13 Salivary glands. (From Fehrenbach MJ, Herring SW: *Illustrated anatomy of the head and neck,* ed 4, St. Louis, 2012, Saunders.)

Oral Mucosa

The tissue that lines the oral cavity is the oral mucosa. Two types of oral mucosa are present. Lining mucosa covers the cheeks, lips, vestibule, ventral surface (underside) of the tongue, and soft palate. This tissue is very thin and can be injured easily.

Masticatory mucosa is much thicker and denser and is attached tightly to bone (with the exception of the tongue). It is designed to resist the pressure of chewing food and is not easily injured. This tissue type forms the gingivae (gums), hard palate, and dorsum (top) of the tongue.

Gingiva

Gingiva (*plural,* gingivae) is the term that refers to the masticatory mucosa and the tissue that surrounds the teeth. Normal healthy gingival tissue is firm and attached tightly around the teeth; in white people, it is coral or salmon pink in color. In nonwhites, the color is commonly darker.

DID YOU KNOW?
Gingivitis is an inflammation of the gingival tissue that results in red, swollen, and bleeding gums. This condition is the result of poor brushing and flossing habits but is reversible with a regular regimen of correct brushing and flossing techniques. If gingivitis goes untreated, it will progress into periodontal disease, which is the destruction of bone and tissue. Periodontal disease, when untreated, results in tooth loss.

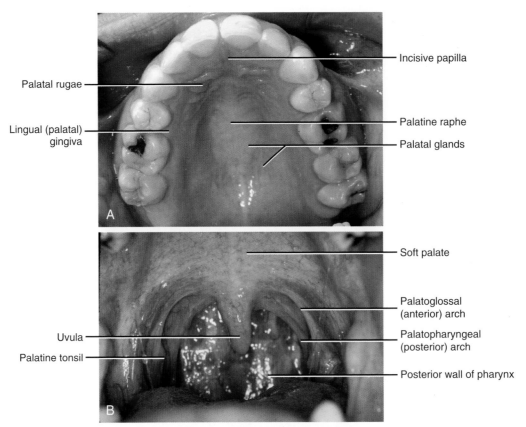

FIGURE 2-14 A, Surface features of the hard palate. **B,** Surface features of the soft palate. (From Liebgott B: *The anatomical basis of dentistry,* ed 3, St. Louis, 2010, Mosby.)

Basic Anatomical Structures and Tissues of the Teeth

Anatomical Structures

The shape, size, and functions of teeth vary but teeth are made of the same component structures. In fact, each tooth

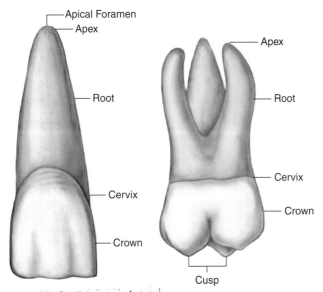

FIGURE 2-15 Anatomical structures of an incisor *(left)* and a molar *(right).* (From Fehrenbach MJ, Popowics T: *Illustrated dental embryology, histology, and anatomy,* ed 4, St Louis, 2016, Elsevier.)

consists of three anatomical structures: crown, cervix, and root (Figure 2-15). The **crown** of the tooth is covered with enamel. Crowns vary in size according to the type and function of the tooth. The **cervix,** or the neck of the tooth, is the narrow portion of the tooth at which the root and the crown meet. Each **root** is covered by a thin, hard shell called the **cementum.** Each tooth consists of one to four roots.

Tissues of a Tooth

The crown is covered with a hard, mineralized substance called **enamel** (Figure 2-16). Enamel is 99% inorganic matter and it cannot regenerate. This means that once enamel has been damaged by extensive caries or trauma, it cannot repair itself; the function of the tooth can be restored only by means of a dental restoration procedure.

The bulk of a tooth is made of **dentin**—a living cellular substance similar in structure to bone. It is softer than the hard outer shell of the crown (enamel) and the covering of the root surface (cementum).

The **periodontal ligament** (connective fibers that help to hold the tooth in the alveolar socket while providing protection and nourishment for it) may attach to the tooth at the cementum— the thin, hard covering of the root surface of a tooth.

In the center of the crown is the **pulp chamber.** Within the pulp chamber is the **pulpal tissue,** which is composed of connective tissue, blood vessels, and nerves. Blood vessels and nerves enter the tooth through the **apical foramen** (a small opening) at the **apex** (tip) of the root and they fill the **root canal** (pulp cavity).

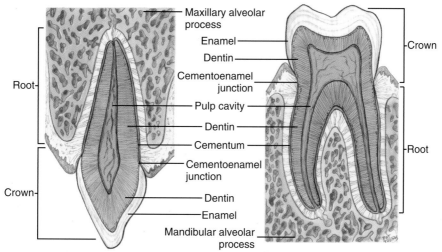

FIGURE 2-16 Longitudinal section of a tooth. (From Fehrenbach MJ, Popowics T: *Illustrated dental embryology, histology, and anatomy*, ed 4, St Louis, 2016, Elsevier.)

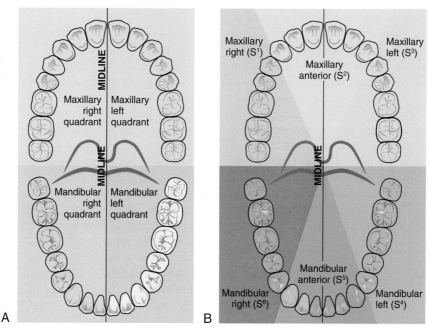

FIGURE 2-17 A, Oral cavity quadrants. **B,** Oral cavity sextants. View shown leads into the oral cavity.

Dental Arches

The anatomical structure of the mouth is divided into sections. The upper section is referred to as the maxillary arch and the lower section is the mandibular arch. Each dental arch contains the same number of teeth.

Quadrants

The dental arches are divided into four sections, or quadrants. Each quadrant consists of the same number and type of teeth as the opposite quadrant. These quadrants are maxillary right, maxillary left, mandibular left, and mandibular right (Figure 2-17, *A*).

DENTAL CARIES

Dental caries (tooth decay) is a progressive disease that demineralizes enamel, enters the dentin, and quickly reaches the pulp of the tooth. Bacteria within the mouth metabolize sugars and give off toxins (acid) that dissolve (demineralize) the calcium salts in the tooth. The process can be stopped by removing the carious lesion and replacing the lost tooth structure with a variety of dental materials (fillings). If caries are not stopped before they reach the pulp, the condition is irreversible and the tooth will die. Options available at this time include extracting (removing) the diseased tooth or performing a root canal procedure (replacing all pulpal tissue with appropriate dental material) to save the function of the tooth.

Sextants

Dental arches are sometimes divided into sextants (six sections). This method of division is most commonly used in periodontal evaluations. Sextants are maxillary right posterior, maxillary anterior, maxillary left posterior, mandibular left posterior, mandibular anterior, and mandibular right posterior (Figure 2-17, B).

Occlusion

Occlusion is the relationship between the maxillary arch and the mandibular arch in terms of the way they meet or touch. In perfect occlusion, teeth meet at specific contact points, allowing space and room for the teeth to properly chew and grind food (mastication). In malocclusion, the teeth are out of alignment or occlusion.

Types of Teeth

Functions, sizes, and locations of the teeth are important factors in the digestive process. Each human has two sets of teeth. The first set, or primary dentition (Figure 2-18, A), consists of 20 teeth. When these teeth are lost or shed, they are replaced with permanent dentition, which consists of 32 teeth (Figure 2-18, B). Not all of the primary teeth are lost and replaced at the same time. The presence of both primary and permanent dentition is referred to as mixed dentition (Table 2-2).

Anterior Teeth

The size and function of teeth vary according to where they are located in the dental arch (see Figure 2-18). Anterior teeth (toward the front) consist of central incisors, lateral incisors, and cuspids (canines). Incisors are characterized by thin, sharp, incisal edges that aid in food cutting. Cuspids, which are very strong and have a sharp point (cusp), are designed for grasping and tearing food.

Posterior Teeth

Posterior teeth (toward the back) consist of the first premolar, second premolar (bicuspid), first molar, second molar, and third molar (wisdom tooth). These teeth have flat surfaces with rounded projections and are used for grinding and crushing.

Surfaces of the Teeth

Each tooth is divided into sections, which are referred to as the surfaces of the tooth (Figure 2-19). Each surface has a name that is used by a dental professional to describe the exact location of tooth decay, restorations, and other conditions.

- Proximal refers to the surfaces (distal and mesial) that are adjacent or next to another surface of a tooth.
- Interproximal is the space created by two proximal surfaces.
- Mesial refers to the proximal surface (of a tooth) that is facing toward the midline (a vertical line that divides the face into two sections, running between the eyes, down the center of the nose, and between the right and left centrals).
- Distal refers to the proximal surface that faces away from the midline.
- Buccal refers to the surfaces of posterior teeth that face or touch the cheeks.
- Lingual refers to the surfaces of teeth that face the tongue, or the inside of the mouth.
- Occlusal refers to the broad, flat chewing surface of posterior teeth (premolars and molars).
- Incisal refers to the sharp cutting edges of the anterior teeth (incisors and cuspids).
- Labial refers to the surfaces of anterior teeth that face or touch the lips.
- Facial is an interchangeable term used to describe the buccal and labial surfaces.

Without knowledge of these surfaces, the dental assistant is unable to interpret directives given by the dentist during clinical examinations and dental procedures. It is the responsibility of the administrative dental assistant to transfer information about these conditions from the clinical record to other forms and to correctly bill the patient and the insurance carrier.

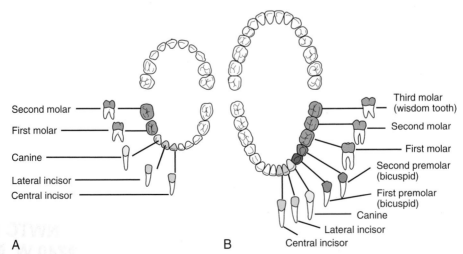

Second molar

First molar

Canine

Lateral incisor

Central incisor

A

Third molar (wisdom tooth)

Second molar

First molar

Second premolar (bicuspid)

First premolar (bicuspid)

Canine

Lateral incisor

Central incisor

B

FIGURE 2-18 A, Deciduous teeth. **B,** Permanent teeth. (Modified from Applegate E: *The anatomy and physiology learning system,* ed 4, St. Louis, 2011, Saunders.)

TABLE 2-2 Ages at Which Teeth Erupt and Are Shed

Tooth Type	Age at Eruption	Age at Shedding
Deciduous Teeth		
Central incisors	6-8 months	5-7 years
Lateral incisors	8-10 months	6-8 years
First molars	12-16 months	9-11 years
Canines	16-20 months	8-11 years
Second molars	20-30 months	9-11 years
Permanent Teeth		
First molars	6-7 years	
Central incisors	6-8 years	
Lateral incisors	7-9 years	
Canines	9-10 years	
First premolars	9-11 years	
Second premolars	10-12 years	
Second molars	11-13 years	
Third molars	15-25 years	

In addition to singular surfaces, names for combinations of surfaces further identify and locate dental conditions and restorations. When two surface names are combined, the *-al* of the first surface name is replaced with an *-o-*, which is followed by the second surface name in full (e.g., distolingual).

When more than two surface names are combined, the *-al* is replaced with *-o-* for all names, except the last (e.g., mesio-occlusodistal). Note that when the surface name *occlusal* follows another *-o-*, a hyphen must be inserted between the two *o*'s. Table 2-3 provides a complete list of surface name combinations and their corresponding abbreviations.

NUMBERING SYSTEMS

Universal/National Numbering System

The Universal/National Numbering System was developed in the United States to ensure consistency in identification of individual teeth (Figure 2-20). Instead of calling out the name of a tooth, such as maxillary right second molar or mandibular right second premolar, the dentist can simply call out tooth numbers 2 and 29. This system begins with the maxillary right third molar and assigns number 1 to this tooth and continues across the maxillary arch, ending with tooth number 16 (maxillary left third molar). Numbering of the mandibular arch is continued by assignment of number 17 to the mandibular left third molar tooth and of number 32 to the mandibular right third molar.

International Standards Organization Designation System

The International Standards Organization (ISO) numbering system is also called the Fédération Dentaire Internationale

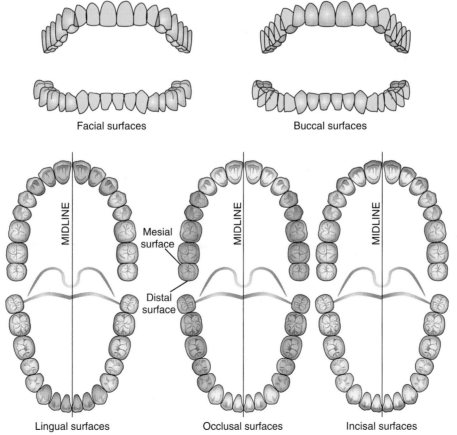

Facial surfaces   Buccal surfaces

Lingual surfaces   Occlusal surfaces   Incisal surfaces

FIGURE 2-19 Surfaces of t he teeth. *Top,* Facial and buccal surfaces. *Bottom,* Lingual, occlusal, mesial, distal, and incisal surfaces.

TABLE 2-3	**Tooth Surface Abbreviations**
B	Buccal
D	Distal
F	Facial
I	Incisal
L	Lingual
M	Mesial
O	Occlusal
BO	Bucco-occlusal
DI	Distoincisal
DL	Distolingual
DO	Disto-occlusal
LO	Linguo-occlusal
MI	Mesioincisal
MO	Mesio-occlusal
MOD	Mesio-occlusodistal
MODBL	Mesio-occlusodistobuccolingual

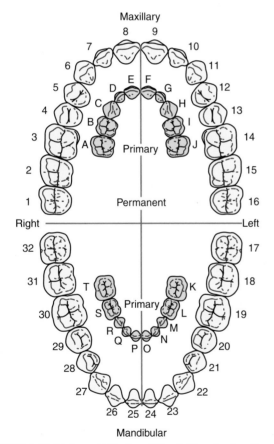

FIGURE 2-20 Universal/National Tooth Numbering System.

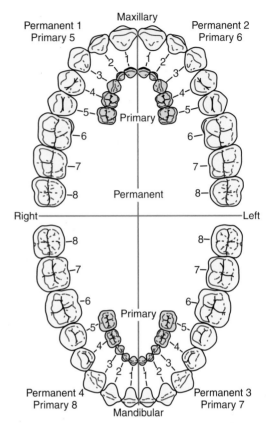

FIGURE 2-21 International Tooth Numbering System.

(Table 2-4). Each number is pronounced individually; for example, 10 is pronounced "one zero," and so forth.

In addition to their use in identifying quadrants and sextants, numbers are used to identify individual teeth. Numbering is the same for each quadrant; therefore identical teeth have the same name and the same number. For example, central incisors are assigned number 1, laterals number 2, and so forth; third molars are assigned number 8. The combination of the quadrant number and the tooth number gives each tooth an individual number configuration.

Symbolic Numbering System (Palmer System)

In the Symbolic Numbering System, each tooth in a quadrant is assigned a number and quadrants are differentiated by a symbol (Figure 2-22). The numbering system begins with the central incisor as number 1 and ends with the third molar as number 8 (permanent dentition). Each quadrant is represented with a symbol and the number or letter is placed within the bracket.

Maxillary right	**Maxillary left**
8 7 6 5 4 3 2 1	1 2 3 4 5 6 7 8
8 7 6 5 4 3 2 1	1 2 3 4 5 6 7 8
Mandibular right	**Mandibular left**

Primary teeth are assigned letters, beginning with the central incisor as A and ending with the second primary molar as E.

(FDI) Numbering System (Figure 2-21). This system is widely used in countries other than the United States. In this system, the quadrants and sextants are assigned numbers. Each configuration is a two-digit number that consists of a 0 and the numbers 1 through 8. Instead of calling out the name of the quadrant or sextant, the dentist refers to the numbers

TABLE 2-4	International Standards Organization Designation System
00	Oral cavity
01	Maxillary arch
02	Mandibular arch
10	Maxillary right quadrant
20	Maxillary left quadrant
30	Mandibular left quadrant
40	Mandibular right quadrant
03	Maxillary right posterior sextant
04	Maxillary anterior sextant
05	Maxillary left posterior sextant
06	Mandibular left posterior sextant
07	Mandibular anterior sextant
08	Mandibular right posterior sextant

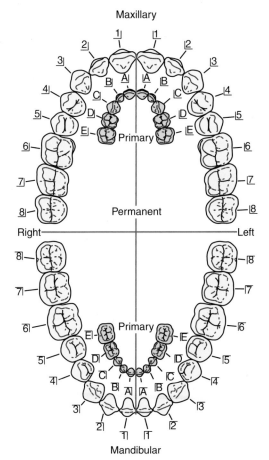

FIGURE 2-22 Symbolic (Palmer) Tooth Numbering System.

Maxillary right	Maxillary left
E D C B A	A B C D E
E D C B A	A B C D E
Mandibular right	**Mandibular left**

This symbolic system is used primarily in orthodontic and pediatric dentistry.

CHARTING METHODS

The primary objective of charting is to express, through symbolism, various conditions that involve individual teeth, or groups of teeth, in their respective arches. Such symbolic writing is referred to as "dental shorthand." The charting process allows existing restorative conditions to be easily recognized; work that needs to be completed is also easily identified. Charting involves several components, such as color coding, symbolization, and type of chart used to record the information.

Color Coding

Red indicates dental conditions that require treatment:
- Dental caries
- Extractions, tooth impactions
- Existing restorations that must be replaced
- Periodontal abscesses
- Fractures
- Endodontic treatment (uncompleted)

Blue or black indicates existing dental restorations or conditions that do not require treatment at this time:
- Amalgam and composite restorations
- Crowns and bridges
- Completed endodontic treatment
- Impacted teeth
- Extracted teeth

Charting Symbols

Information is recorded on a dental chart with a combination of symbols and color. Unlike the numbering systems, which have been standardized, charting conventions still vary widely among practices. It is necessary for all members of the dental healthcare team to follow a standardized method of charting within their own practice to ensure consistency. An example of common charting illustrations is provided.

Types of Dental Charts

Two different types of dental charts are used to record dental conditions. One is the anatomical chart, which uses an anatomical representation of the teeth within the dental arches. The other type is the geometric chart, on which circles are used to represent teeth and which are divided into sections that represent the surfaces of the teeth.

In each of the charting methods, the teeth are arranged in the same configuration as they are in the mouth. In most systems, when you look at the chart it is as though you are looking at the patient. The patient's right is located on your left and the patient's left is located on your right. Occasionally doctors choose to reverse the chart, in which case the patient's right is located on your right and the patient's left is on your left (the numbering system *will not change;* the maxillary right third molar will always be tooth number 1 [Universal/National Numbering System]).

COMMON CHARTING SYMBOLS

The following matrix and the three different chart examples (anatomical, geometric, and computer generated [see charts following this box]) of the same patient's clinical chart symbolize dental procedures and conditions.

The matrix is divided into five columns. The first column categorizes **Dental Procedures** according to the categories listed in *Current Dental Terminology* (CDT). (See Chapter 15 for detailed information on CDT.) The second column, **Description,** represents the subcategories of CDT. The third column, **Charting Instructions,** explains how to illustrate the identified

dental procedure or condition on the patient's clinical chart. With proper illustration of procedures and conditions and use of correct color coding and symbolization, the dental healthcare team will be able to interpret the patient's clinical chart correctly. The fourth column, **Charting Example,** identifies the tooth number on the charting examples (anatomical, geometric, and computer generated). Although they differ in design, all charts present the same information. The fifth column, **Black's Classification,** identifies the corresponding classification and tooth surface.

Dental Procedures and Condition	Description	Charting Instructions	Charting Example	Black's Classification
Restorative Procedures	Amalgam	Dental caries are outlined and filled in with red. Completed amalgam restorations are colored solid blue or black.	Tooth #2 Tooth #18	Class II MO Class I O
	Resin-Based Composite	Dental caries are outlined in red. Completed restorations are filled with blue or black dots.	Tooth #7 Tooth #29 Tooth #4	Class III M Class II MOD Class V B
	Inlay/Onlay Cast metal	Work to be completed is outlined in red and diagonal lines are drawn. Completed restorations are drawn over in blue or black.	Tooth #31	MOD Inlay
	Inlay/Onlay Resin-based	Work to be completed is outlined in red. Completed restoration is filled in with blue or black dots.	Tooth #14	DOL Onlay
	Crown Cast metal	Work to be completed is outlined in red and diagonal lines are drawn. Completed crown is drawn over with blue or black.	Tooth #30	
	Crown Porcelain fused to gold	Work to be completed is outlined in red on the buccal surface or facial surface and diagonal lines are drawn on the occlusal and lingual surface (posterior teeth) and the lingual surface (anterior teeth). Computer-generated chart draws diagonal lines on all surfaces. Completed crown is drawn over in blue or black.	Tooth #19 Tooth #21 Tooth #15	
	Crown Porcelain or resin-based	Work to be completed is outlined in red. Completed crown is filled with blue or black dots (computer-generated chart outlined in blue).	Tooth #13	
	Stainless Steel Crown	Work to be completed is identified by writing **SS** in red on the crown of the tooth (computer-generated chart outlined in red). Completed crown is identified by writing over the SS in blue or black (computer-generated chart outlined in blue).	Tooth #3	
	Veneer Bonding	Work to be completed is outlined in red on the facial surface only (computer-generated chart filled facial surface in red). Completed veneer is filled in with blue or black dots (computer-generated chart filled facial surface in blue).	Tooth #8 Tooth #9	

COMMON CHARTING SYMBOLS—cont'd

Dental Procedures and Condition	Description	Charting Instructions	Charting Example	Black's Classification
	Post and Core Build-up	A red vertical line is drawn through the root (approximating the root canal) and a small inverted triangle is drawn in the gingival third of the crown (approximating the pulp chamber of the tooth). Completed post and core is filled in with blue or black.	Tooth #30	
Endodontic Procedures	Endodontic Therapy (root canal)	When therapy is indicated, a red vertical line is drawn through each root (approximating the root canal). Completed treatment is drawn over in blue or black.	Tooth #28	
	Periapical Abscess	A small, red circle is drawn at the apex of the root of the infected tooth.	Tooth #27	
Implant Services	Implant	When an implant is indicated, horizontal red lines are drawn across the root of the replaced tooth. When an implant is present, blue or black lines are drawn (computer-generated chart outlined root).	Tooth #13	
Prosthodontics Fixed	Fixed Bridge	The charting instructions for the type of crown to be used in the construction of the bridge are followed. In addition, connect the teeth involved with two horizontal lines, and draw an **X** through the roots of the missing teeth. When the bridge has been inserted, it is colored over in blue or black.	Tooth #19 Tooth #20 Tooth #21	(Retainer) (Pontic) (Retainer)
Oral Surgery	Extraction	A single, angled red line is drawn through the tooth (/) (computer-generated chart drew two lines ‖).	Tooth #1 Tooth #32	
	Extracted or Missing Tooth	A blue or black **X** is drawn through the tooth.	Tooth #16	
	Impacted or Unerupted Tooth	A red circle is drawn around the tooth (crown and root).	Tooth #17	
Other Conditions	Rotated Tooth	A red semicircular line is placed at the root of the tooth with an arrow pointing in the direction of the rotation.	Tooth #17	
	Drifting Tooth	A red line is placed above the crown of the tooth with an arrow indicating the direction of the drift.	Tooth #31	
	Fractured Tooth	A red zigzag is placed on the tooth surface where the fracture occurred. If the root is fractured, the zigzag is placed on the root.	Tooth #24	Class IV
	Diastema	When there is more space than normal between two teeth, two vertical red lines are placed between the teeth.	Teeth #8, 9	

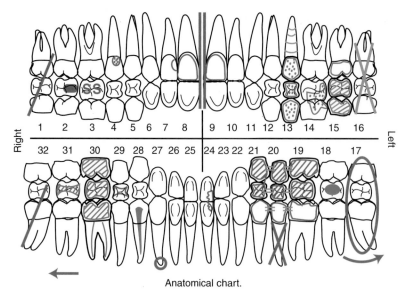

Anatomical chart.

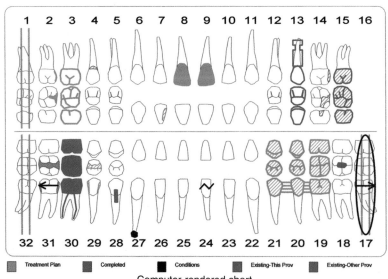

Geometric chart.

Computer-rendered chart.

DENTAL PROCEDURES

It is necessary for the administrative dental assistant to have an understanding of dental procedures if he or she is to be an effective and efficient member of the dental healthcare team. Administrative dental assistants perform several tasks daily that require the identification and understanding of dental procedures. These tasks include:

- Scheduling appointments
- Billing insurance companies and patients
- Corresponding with dental specialists
- Communicating with patients and other dental healthcare team members
- Planning treatments

Basic and Preventive Dental Procedures

The following procedures are just a few of the many that may be performed in a dental practice.

Initial Examination

Initial oral examination is performed during the patient's first visit to the dental practice. Diagnostic aids are used during the examination to help the dentist identify existing conditions and restorations as well as the dental needs of the patient. These aids may consist of digital images or radiographs—both intraoral and extraoral—diagnostic models, and an intraoral camera to digitally document conditions within the oral cavity. In addition to performing the oral examination, the dentist evaluates other tissues and structures of the head and neck to help determine whether any other medical conditions may exist. Included in this procedure is the recording of vital signs and may be referred to a medical laboratory for additional tests.

Prophylaxis

During **dental prophylaxis,** the dentist or dental hygienist removes stains and deposits and polishes teeth. Dental assistants following the rules and regulations set by each state may perfrom coronal polishing. In addition to this cleaning, the patient may receive brushing and flossing instructions, nutritional counseling, and home care instruction. **Fluoride treatments** (to strengthen enamel and protect teeth from developing carious lesions) are normally performed after children's teeth are cleaned.

Restorative Procedures
Restorative Dentistry

During **restorative dentistry,** the dentist removes caries from the tooth. After the caries have been removed, the tooth is prepared to receive a material that will replace the lost tooth structure. The type of restorative material used depends on the location and the size of the restoration.

Amalgam Restorations

Restorative materials fall into two basic categories: amalgam and resin-based composite. **Amalgam** is an alloy of different metals that is silver in color and is used to restore the

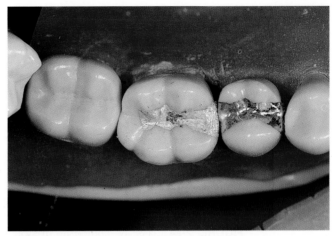

FIGURE 2-23 Example of class II amalgam restoration. (From Hatrick CD, Eakle WS: *Dental materials: clinical applications for dental assistants and dental hygienists,* ed 3, St Louis, 2016, Elsevier.)

function of posterior teeth (Figure 2-23). Because of the color of the restoration, amalgam is used only in posterior teeth or on the lingual surfaces of some anterior teeth. This metal is strong and lasts for 5 to 20 years. Amalgam is inexpensive and its use is covered by most insurance companies.

Resin-Based Composite Restorations

Resin-based composite restorations are tooth colored and are used primarily on anterior teeth (Figure 2-24, *A, B*). New hybrid resin–based composites that are now becoming popular are much stronger than the original composites and are also being used in posterior teeth.

Cast Crown Restorations

Cast crowns are needed when a large amount of tooth structure is removed. Because the design and functions of teeth may vary, if a large amount of tooth structure is removed, amalgam or resin-based composite may not be strong enough to restore the tooth to full function. In these cases, it is necessary to use material that can withstand the stress and force of normal tooth function. Gold is the closest replacement for tooth enamel. Because of the color of gold, it is used only on posterior teeth, especially in the maxillary arch, which is not normally visible. (In some cultures, visible gold teeth are a status symbol.)

A cast restoration is a two-step procedure. On the first visit, the tooth is prepared for the crown, impressions are taken, and a temporary crown is fabricated. Impressions are sent to the dental laboratory, where a technician prepares the casting according to the directions of the dentist (instructions are given on a prescription called a lab slip). There are different types of cast restorations:

Full gold and metal crowns are cast from gold alloy and other metals and are categorized according to the amount of gold

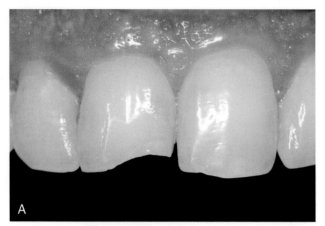
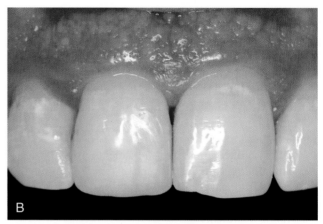

FIGURE 2-24 Class IV composite restoration showing before **(A)** and after **(B)**. (From Heyman HO, Swift EJ, Ritter, AV: *Sturdevant's art and science of operative dentistry*, ed 6, St. Louis, 2013, Mosby.)

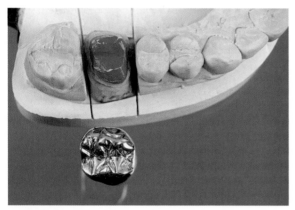

FIGURE 2-25 Posterior gold crown. (From Bird DL, Robinson DS: *Modern dental assisting*, ed 11, St. Louis, 2015, Saunders.)

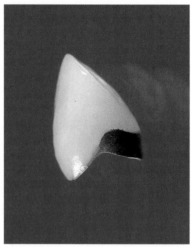

FIGURE 2-26 Anterior porcelain-fused-to-metal (PFM) crown. (From Bird DL, Robinson DS: *Modern dental assisting*, ed 11, St. Louis, 2015, Saunders.)

used: high noble, noble, low noble, and nongold (similar to the karat system for gold jewelry: 18k, 14k, and 10k) (Figure 2-25).

- Porcelain fused to metal or gold is a cast crown with a porcelain cover (tooth colored) (Figure 2-26).
- Veneer crowns offer thin coverage on the facial surface with only a cast composite or resin material (Figure 2-27).
- An inlay offers partial coverage of a tooth, usually on the same surfaces as amalgam restorations. It is cast from gold or composite materials (Figure 2-28).
- An onlay offers partial coverage of a tooth, similar to the inlay, except that an onlay includes more tooth structure and a cusp is replaced. An onlay is cast from gold, porcelain, or ceramic. (Figure 2-29).

Prosthetic Procedures

Prosthetic procedures include replacing missing teeth with an artificial tooth or teeth. When a tooth is missing, it can be replaced with a removable or fixed prosthetic appliance. The construction of crowns, bridges, partials, and dentures requires more than one appointment and must be coordinated with the dental laboratory.

Fixed Prosthetics

A fixed prosthetic, or fixed partial denture, is commonly referred to as a bridge (Figure 2-30). A bridge requires that teeth on either side of the missing tooth be crowned. These teeth are called abutment teeth. Abutment teeth form the anchor for the pontic, which is the artificial replacement for the missing tooth or teeth. The pontic is soldered to the abutment teeth. When abutments are permanently cemented, the new bridge is strong and permanently in place.

Removable Prosthetics

The opposite of a permanent bridge is a removable partial. The removable partial replaces missing teeth but, unlike the bridge, can be removed and is held in place by a metal

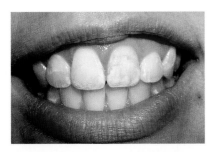

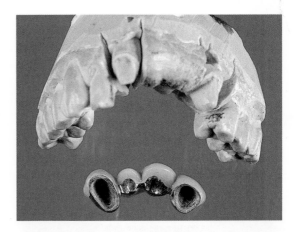

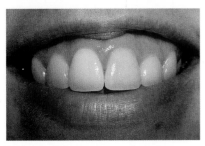

FIGURE 2-27 Porcelain veneers placed to cover hypocalcification defects. (From Heyman HO, Swift EJ, Ritter, AV: *Sturdevant's art and science of operative dentistry*, ed 6, St. Louis, 2013, Mosby.)

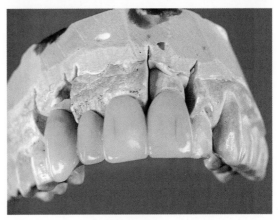

FIGURE 2-30 Four-unit porcelain-fused-to-metal (PFM) anterior fixed bridge. (From Bird DL, Robinson DS: *Modern dental assisting*, ed 11, St. Louis, 2015, Saunders.)

framework of acrylic and clasps that wrap around abutment teeth (Figure 2-31). A partial is used when several teeth are missing. The number of teeth to be replaced, the health of surrounding gingival tissue, and cost are factors to be considered when deciding whether a partial should be used instead of a bridge.

FIGURE 2-28 Inlay cast restoration fabricated from porcelain. (From Heyman HO, Swift EJ, Ritter, AV: *Sturdevant's art and science of operative dentistry*, ed 6, St. Louis, 2013, Mosby.)

Full Dentures

Full dentures replace all of the teeth in an arch. They are constructed of acrylic and are custom-fitted for each patient. Care should be taken to match the size, shape, and shade of replacement teeth as closely as possible to those of the natural teeth (Figure 2-32). It is possible to retain some or all of the natural teeth in one arch while all of the natural teeth in the opposite arch are replaced.

Surgical Procedures

Simple Extractions

Simple extractions involve the removal of one or more teeth without the need to remove bone or cut tissue.

Surgical Extractions

Surgical extractions are more involved and involve the cutting of tissue and the possible removal of bone to facilitate the removal of a tooth. Besides extractions, several

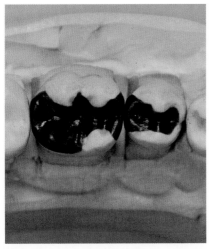

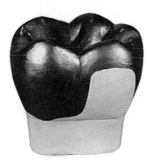

FIGURE 2-29 Onlay cast restoration fabricated from gold. (From Heyman HO, Swift EJ, Ritter, AV: *Sturdevant's art and science of operative dentistry*, ed 6, St. Louis, 2013, Mosby.)

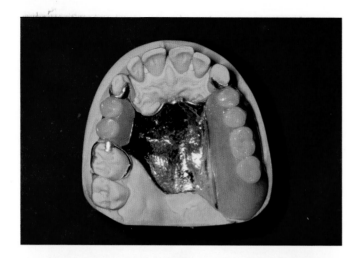

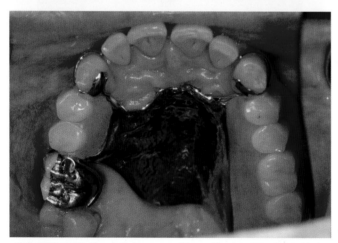

FIGURE 2-31 Partial denture. (From Hatrick CD, Eakle WS: *Dental materials: clinical applications for dental assistants and dental hygienists*, ed 3, St Louis, 2016, Elsevier.)

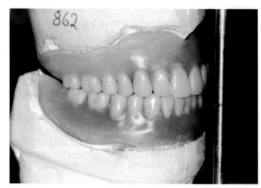

FIGURE 2-32 Components of a full denture: base, flange, post dam, and artificial teeth. (From Bird DL, Robinson DS: *Modern dental assisting*, ed 11, St. Louis, 2015, Saunders.)

other types of dental surgery may be provided. Routine extractions and surgical procedures can be performed by a general dentist. Extensive procedures that necessitate the use of general anesthesia may be referred to an oral maxillofacial surgeon.

Endodontic Procedures

Endodontic, or root canal, procedures are performed to replace the pulp. When pulp becomes diseased, it must be removed. Once pulp tissue has been removed, the tooth is no longer vital (alive) but it can remain in the dental arch and be functional. (The only other option is extraction.) The process includes removing the diseased tissue, cleaning the pulp chamber and root canal, and sealing it with a replacement material (Figure 2-33). Once a root canal procedure has been performed, the tooth may have been weakened by the loss of tooth structure and it may become necessary to reinforce the tooth with a post or build-up and place a crown to protect the tooth from the possibility of fracture.

When endodontic treatment is billed, the number of canals that have been treated determines the fee for the service. Molars have three to four canals, premolars and anterior teeth have one canal, and maxillary first premolars have two canals.

Other Common Procedures

Sealant application is a procedure that is done to cover the chewing surface of a tooth with a thin coating of resin.

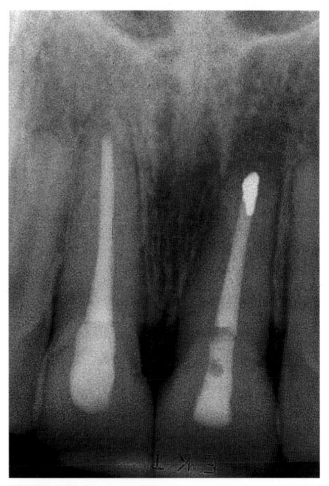

FIGURE 2-33 Root end filling is completed on a central incisor. (From Johnson W: *Color atlas of endodontics*, Philadelphia, 2002, Saunders.)

The purpose of this treatment is to seal and protect the tooth from the effects of acid attacks, which cause demineralization of enamel and lead to carious lesions. These conditions can be caused by the patient not following good oral hygiene habits and poor nutritional choices. This procedure is performed on newly erupted permanent teeth and the effects will last until a child reaches the late teens or early adulthood (Figure 2-34). Sealants, regular dental check-ups, and the use of fluorides reduce the number of cavities.

As an administrative dental assistant, you must know about the different types of dental procedures and be able to determine the amount of time each will take and the number of appointments that will be needed for their completion. This information is essential for effective scheduling and for correct coding of insurance claim forms to optimize the benefits of patients' insurance coverage. Each procedure has a specific code and fee that is based on the number of surfaces involved and the material used. It is the responsibility of the administrative dental assistant to ensure that the correct procedures have been billed to the patient and the insurance company. It is easy to forget or to overlook procedures, especially if you do not understand the language used in patients' charts. It is up to you to learn the dental language. Never be afraid to ask questions when it is not clear which procedures have been completed.

BASIC CHAIRSIDE DENTAL-ASSISTING DUTIES

In the everyday operation of a dental practice, it may be an assigned or occasional duty of the administrative dental assistant to help fellow team members in performing the functions of the back office. Current trends in dentistry and other businesses require that employees must be able to perform multiple tasks. In the dental profession, this means that dental auxiliaries must be trained in more than one aspect of assisting. With cross-training, the administrative dental assistant can, when needed, perform basic chairside

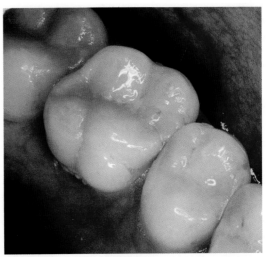

FIGURE 2-34 Enamel without significant fissures (well coalesced). (From Hatrick CD, Eakle WS: *Dental materials: clinical applications for dental assistants and dental hygienists*, ed 3, St Louis, 2016, Elsevier.)

duties and the chairside assistant can perform common functions in the front office. Multitasking also helps to increase career opportunities.

Seating and Dismissing a Patient

A basic procedure that may be asked of the administrative assistant is to seat or dismiss a dental patient (Figure 2-35). It is not necessary for the assistant to put on gloves before performing this task.

If the dentist requires the administrative dental assistant to perform functions of the chairside assistant, the assistant must be properly trained and must have been given the option of obtaining the hepatitis B vaccination series. The value of administrative dental assistants to the dentist increases if they are able to perform other duties but they must fulfill all of the same licensure and training requirements of the chairside assistant, even if they perform the tasks only occasionally.

PROCEDURES

Procedure to Seat a Patient in the Treatment Room

1. Check the room to see that it has been properly cleaned (cleaning the room requires knowledge of infection control).
2. Prepare the dental chair for the patient:
   - Cover the chair with a protective barrier.
   - Place the back of the chair in an upright position.
   - Lift the armrest on the side of the chair on which the patient will be entering.
   - Move the tray table, light, and other equipment away from the chair (to provide easy entry for the patient).
3. Check the pathway from the door to the chair and make sure that all hoses and equipment have been moved (to ensure patient safety).

4. Place the patient's chart on the counter, open the chart to the treatment page, and place any radiographs on the view box. add the following text. When using an electronic dental record, locate the patient record and have it open on the computer monitor.
5. Place a patient napkin and napkin chain on the counter for draping the patient.
6. Go to the reception area and greet the patient. Ask the patient to follow you to the treatment area. A special area should be provided for the patient to hang a coat or place other items.
7. Instruct the patient to be seated. (Ensure that the patient is seated all the way back in the chair.)

Continued

PROCEDURES

Procedure to Seat a Patient in the Treatment Room—cont'd

8. Place the napkin on the patient. (During some procedures, long plastic drapes also may be used to protect the patient's clothing.)
9. Ask the patient to remove any lipstick (provide a tissue) and jewelry that may interfere with the treatment. (A small container can be used to store jewelry safely.) Remind the patient to ask for the jewelry before leaving the office.

10. After the patient has been seated, advise the patient when the dentist will be entering the room, ask if there are any questions, and provide a magazine or turn on the television. (It is at this point that the patient can view educational videos.)
11. Notify the dental assistant or the dentist that the patient has been seated.

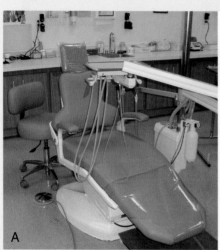

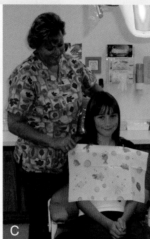

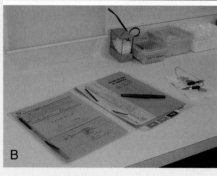

FIGURE 2-35 Seating a patient. **A,** Check the room to ensure that it has been properly cleaned and set up for the next patient. **B,** Place the patient chart on the counter along with the patient napkin. **C,** Seat the patient.

! REMEMBER

This procedure does not include setting up the room for the treatment. This is the job of the dental assistant. Unless you are trained in chairside assisting and have received OSHA training in the safe handling of equipment and instruments, you should not proceed beyond simply seating the patient.

Digital Images and Radiographs

Most states regulate the taking of dental radiographs by requiring a certificate, license, or passage of an examination. No national license is available; therefore it is necessary for interested individuals to check their state's Dental Practice Act to find out the requirements that must be met in the state in which they work.

Occupational Safety and Health Administration (OSHA)

OSHA is a national government agency that was created to protect workers from workplace injury. OSHA regulates all areas of employment. Most states also have their own version of OSHA, which in some cases is stricter than the federal agency. It is the function of OSHA to develop specific guidelines for specific occupations. Dentistry has very specific regulations concerning the safety of dental employees.

It is the legal responsibility of the dentist to inform each and every employee of all safety hazards. New employees must receive training within 10 days of hire. All employees must receive training and testing yearly.

OSHA has established categories that outline an employee's potential for exposure to toxic or hazardous materials or blood-borne pathogens. Dental office employees may be classified as Category I or Category II according to their job descriptions. An administrative dental assistant who will *never* be assigned to work in the clinical area may fall into Category III.

Most of the tasks performed by a dentist, dental assistant, hygienist, and laboratory technician fall into Category I. Administrative dental assistants who may assist in the clinical area by cleaning treatment rooms, handling contaminated instruments, and preparing laboratory cases are assigned to Category II. Both Category I and Category II classifications require that the employer provide proper training, protection, and immunization (against hepatitis B) to employees who fall into these categories.

> **! REMEMBER**
>
> Laws and regulations change periodically and it is the responsibility of healthcare workers to ensure that they are up-to-date on the latest policies and procedures for their own safety and the protection of others.

Infection Control

Infection control measures are taken to protect patients from contracting an infectious disease in the dental office. It is the duty and obligation of the dental healthcare team to protect patients at all times.

Protection from disease is ensured with proper cleaning and sterilization of instruments and equipment. It is essential that the patient be protected from cross-contamination by other patients or by members of the dental healthcare team. Proper infection control protocol must be followed at all times. If administrative dental assistants accept the responsibility of helping dental assistants in the clinical area, they must take it upon themselves to be fully trained in the proper infection control protocol. It is not a valid excuse to be negligent in this area just because someone told you to do a job that you have not been trained to perform. Each and every member of the dental healthcare team has the moral, legal, and ethical responsibility to be fully trained before performing assigned duties.

KEY POINTS

- Basic dental office design divides the dental office into two main areas. Nonclinical areas are where most of the duties assigned to the administrative dental assistant take place:
  - Reception area
  - Business and administrative offices
  - Consultation area
  - Private offices
  - Staff room
- Clinical areas are used by the dentist, dental assistant, and hygienist for tasks related to patient treatment:
  - Treatment rooms
  - Sterilization area
  - Laboratory
  - Digital images and radiology room
  - Darkroom

- Administrative dental assistants must know basic dental anatomy and terms so they can communicate effectively with patients and dental professionals about aspects of dental treatment.
- By interpreting dental charts and charting symbols, the administrative dental assistant translates information from the clinical chart for use in daily tasks.
- All assistants who wish to be cross-trained in other aspects of dental assisting require additional knowledge and must be trained in OSHA standards and infection control protocol. Other duties that may be asked of an administrative dental assistant include:
  - Seating and dismissing a patient
  - Processing radiographs
  - Setting up and cleaning treatment rooms

CAREER-READY PRACTICES

Career-Ready Practices activities are designed to provide students with experiences that can be "practiced" in preparation for skills needed on the job. In each of the following exercises, a variety of approaches may be used to address the problem, rather than "right" or "wrong" answers. Below each exercise, next to the compass icon, is a listing of suggested Career-Ready Practice numbers that correspond to the listing of 12 practices in the front of the text (see p. viii-ix); these practices provide suggestions for approaches to complete the exercise.

1. It is your first day as an administrative dental assistant. All of the dental assistants are busy and the dentist asks you to

step in and help by cleaning the room and seating the next patient.
   a. You want to make a good impression but you have not been trained to perform this task. What are you going to say and do?

✳ Career-Ready Practices
   1 *Act as a responsible and contributing citizen and employee.*
   2 *Apply appropriate academic and technical skills.*
   4 *Communicate clearly, effectively, and with reason.*

CAREER-READY PRACTICES—cont'd

2. In a small group, compare your answers and discuss if they were good choices.
   a. Were they ethical and legal choices?
   b. Develop a detailed plan that will help the assistant to be ready when asked the next time.
   c. Prepare a presentation for the class outlining your plan and describing what it takes to be a valued team member.

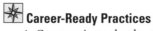 **Career-Ready Practices**

4 *Communicate clearly, effectively, and with reason.*
8 *Utilize critical thinking to make sense of problems and persevere in solving them.*
9 *Model integrity, ethical leadership, and effective management.*

PART II

Communication Skills: Principles and Practices

3 Communication Skills and Telephone Techniques, 42

4 Written Correspondence and Digital Communication, 53

5 Patient Relations, 71

6 Dental Healthcare Team Communications, 82

Communication Skills and Telephone Techniques

INTRODUCTION

Communication is a two-way process in which information is transferred and shared between a sender and a receiver. Communication can occur between individuals or groups. During the communication process, information is transferred from one person or group to another through a system of symbols (written and spoken language), behaviors (tone of voice), and actions (nonverbal gestures). Transfer is effective only when information is shared and understood. Communication may seem like a very natural and simple task but during transfer of information, several barriers can interfere with it. It is important for the dental healthcare team to understand and practice effective communication skills.

ELEMENTS OF THE COMMUNICATION PROCESS

The process of communication includes reading, writing, speaking, and listening. During the process, five elements link together to complete the exchange of information between the sender and the receiver:

- The **sender** has an idea that must be shared with another person or group.
- The idea is translated into a **message.**
- The message is placed on a **medium** or **channel.**
- The medium is sent by various channels and is received by the **receiver.**
- The receiver reacts to the message and provides **feedback.**

Transfer of information begins with the sender. The sender has an idea that must be sent and shared. The sender formulates the idea in the form of a message. The message may consist of information, directions, questions, or statements.

The message must be placed on a medium and transferred to the receiver. The medium can be verbal (oral or written words) or nonverbal (symbols, gestures, facial expressions, body language, and proximity). The receiver reacts to the message by following instructions, answering questions, or asking questions. This reaction, called feedback, is the method used by the sender to determine whether the message the sender sent was received and understood by the receiver. When the receiver reacts to the message, he or she becomes the sender, sending verbal or nonverbal cues; thus the process goes back and forth until the message or series of messages is sent and received and understanding is established and agreed upon (Figure 3-1).

MEDIUMS OF COMMUNICATION

When the message is sent, it must be placed on or in a format that can be understood by the receiver. The medium can be verbal, nonverbal, or a combination of the two.

Verbal Communication

Verbal messages (messages using words) can be divided into two categories: spoken and written. Spoken verbal messages may be delivered face to face or transferred electronically (by telephone, voice mail, or video conferencing). Written communication includes letters, memos, faxes, e-mails, newsletters, and several other forms of printed information.

The need for feedback determines the type of medium that will be used to send a message. When the sender needs immediate feedback, the message will be sent via a spoken medium. The spoken medium allows for real-time feedback and the exchange of ideas. When the message includes information and directions (postoperative instructions, consent

Elements of Communication

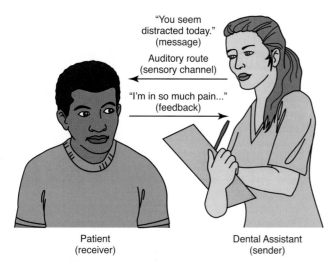

"You seem distracted today." (message)

Auditory route (sensory channel)

"I'm in so much pain..." (feedback)

Patient (receiver)

Dental Assistant (sender)

FIGURE 3-1 The communication process.

for treatment, treatment plans, financial plans), written communication can be used.

Nonverbal Communication

Nonverbal messages (body language) communicate many things without the use of words. Facial expressions can express different emotions (happiness, sadness, puzzlement, pain). Body gestures (pointing, hand signals) can indicate direction. Tone of voice can give added meaning to a message (anger, joy, importance). Proximity to the receiver and eye contact also add meaning to a message.

Imagine a patient who has left work, spent 20 minutes in heavy traffic, and rushed for a dental appointment, only to find that the dentist is running about 30 minutes behind schedule. The patient's tone of voice, along with crossed arms and frown, indicates irritation when he responds, "I understand." He has just told you he understands verbally but you know by his nonverbal message that he is very irritated.

Learning to read a nonverbal communication aids in interpreting messages. During a visit to the dentist's office, patients often communicate several different nonverbal messages: tenseness, embarrassment, anger, and fearfulness.

WHAT WOULD YOU DO?

It is a busy day in the office and the dental team is running about 30 minutes behind schedule. You hear the door to the office open and your next patient has arrived, early. There is no place to sit and he doesn't look happy. What will you do and say?

Tenseness

Tenseness can be expressed nonverbally in the way a patient sits. Tenseness can be seen in the reception area, where patients anxiously wait to be called. They may sit with their legs tightly crossed and ankles wrapped. Their hands may tightly clutch the arms of the chair. As a member of the dental healthcare team, you should try to relax the patient when you see this message. This effort may be as simple as saying a few kind words of understanding. You can also ask patients how their vacation was, offer them refreshment while they wait, or share a new magazine to provide subtle diversion.

Embarrassment

Embarrassment can cause patients to cover their mouths. This may be because they have anterior teeth that are less than perfect (caries, missing teeth, malocclusion, or poorly constructed dentures). Patients may try to conceal an imperfection by tightly closing their lips or by placing a hand or tissue over their mouths.

Anger

Anger, disapproval, and defensiveness can be deduced when patients cross their arms, clench their fists, and sit in a very tight manner (legs tightly crossed, arms crossed). This may happen when patients feel they are not being taken care of properly or if they have to wait for the dentist, are being ignored by members of the dental healthcare team, or are unhappy with the treatment they have just received. It is the responsibility of team members when they receive these nonverbal cues to identify the problem and correct it as quickly as possible.

Patients may feel ignored when they are not recognized as they enter the office, when conversations are taking place between team members while they wait, and when team members are talking on the telephone (even when it is with another patient). Care should be taken to address problems quickly and to identify areas that need attention. A simple smile as a patient enters the reception area acknowledges that the patient has been recognized. When talking on the phone, you should complete the call as soon as possible.

Nonverbal Cues from the Dental Healthcare Team

Members of the dental healthcare team also send nonverbal messages. Caution should be taken to send only positive cues.

Smiles

Smiles always communicate a positive thought. They can be used to ease a patient's apprehension, send a warm greeting to a child, or acknowledge the arrival of a patient. Smiles can even be "seen" over the telephone because they change the tone of your voice. When you are busy on the telephone or are involved in a professional conversation with another team member, a quick wave or smile acknowledges that you will be with the patient as soon as possible.

Touch

Touch can convey a message of warmth, reassurance, understanding, and caring. Patients will recognize the message when they are lightly touched or patted on the shoulder, back of the hand, or arm. Although some patients will welcome the gesture, others will not. Use this method cautiously.

Sincerity

Patients can recognize sincerity when members of the dental healthcare team remove barriers. Barriers can take the form of desks and other objects that come between the team member and the patient. For example, during a consultation, when the dentist sits behind a desk, he or she is unable to convey openness. If the desk is removed, patients may feel as though they are on the same level as the dentist and that one is not superior to the other. This allows patients to participate in the conversation on an equal status with the dentist.

INTERPERSONAL COMMUNICATION

Interpersonal communication takes place when the sender and the receiver exchange information in real time. This includes face-to-face, telephone, and video conferencing conversations. Interpersonal communication is the method most often used to communicate in the dental office. The telephone is used by patients and assistants. Face-to-face conversations take place in the dental office during scheduling procedures, treatment planning, and setting up financial arrangements. During interpersonal communication, the flow of information is transferred from one person to another.

The direction of communication varies depending on the type of transfer and the intended receiver. In the dental office, this process can be divided into four broad categories.

The first type of communication transfer occurs when a patient transfers (sends) information to a member of the dental healthcare team. Typically, this is a request for information about the dental practice, fees, the type of treatment offered by the dental practice, availability of appointments, and the type of dental insurance accepted. The patient will ask the team member questions and will expect answers in return (discussed further in Chapter 5).

PATIENT TO DENTAL HEALTHCARE TEAM

- Information seeking
- Questions
- Directions
- Telephone conversations
- Appointment scheduling

The second type of communication transfer is passed from the dental healthcare team (sender) to the patient (receiver). This information commonly takes the form of spoken directions and written communications. The information transferred may relate to treatment planning, financial arrangements, appointment scheduling, postoperative care, motivation, and education. When important information is shared with a patient, the dental healthcare team will follow the spoken word with the written word. The medium changes to facilitate the message. Patients who have just undergone extensive dental treatment may not remember or think to ask questions about the postoperative instructions they have just received. The dental assistant will follow the oral instructions with written instructions, thereby increasing the chance that the patient will remember and follow postoperative instructions (a note should be made in the patient's clinical chart to document that written instructions were also given to the patient).

DENTAL HEALTHCARE TEAM TO PATIENT

- Planning treatment
- Making financial arrangements
- Scheduling appointments
- Giving oral instructions
- Answering questions
- Sharing information
- Motivating
- Informing

The third type of communication transfer takes place between members of the dental healthcare team. This communication is necessary in the everyday operation of the dental practice and is discussed further in Chapter 6.

TEAM MEMBER TO TEAM MEMBER

- Directional
- Organizational
- Informational
- Professional
- Personal

The fourth type of communication transfer takes place between professional members of the healthcare system, dental specialists, medical doctors, laboratory technicians, and pharmacists. Members of the dental healthcare team transfer information via interpersonal communications and written communications (discussed in Chapter 4).

PROFESSIONAL TO PROFESSIONAL

- Referral
- Inquiry
- Consultation
- Direction

BARRIERS TO EFFECTIVE COMMUNICATION

We cannot communicate effectively if the receiver is not receiving the message that is sent. It is like speaking two different languages; we may be saying what we want to say but the receiver is not hearing and understanding the message as it is intended. It is necessary that the sender and receiver both speak the same language. This includes not only the same vernacular but also the same terminology, lingo, and dialect.

Semantics

Semantics is a change in the meaning of a word. For example, a word used in the context of dentistry may not have the same meaning when it is used outside of the dental field (see the box titled "Positive versus Negative Dental Terms" later in this chapter). For example, when dental personnel use the word *drill,* they mean a very small instrument used to remove tooth decay or shape tooth structure. A drill is a very important instrument in the everyday operation of dentistry. When patients hear the word *drill,* the first thing they picture is the drill that is used in construction work. This drill is large; its use in the mouth is an unpleasant thought. By exchanging the word *handpiece* for *drill,* dental personnel do not trigger the preconceived mental picture of a large drill because the word *handpiece* is less threatening. Therefore it is important for the dental professional to select words carefully when communicating with patients. When semantics enters into the communication process, the meaning according to the sender may not be the same as that interpreted by the receiver.

Jargon

Each profession and specialty group has its own jargon. Jargon refers to specialized words, acronyms (groups of initials), and other sayings that are unique to the profession. The meaning of the message is lost when the sender uses jargon that is unfamiliar to the receiver.

Credibility

Credibility is the weight that is put on a message according to the status, or qualifications, of the person who is sending the message. For example, the dentist who tells a patient what type of treatment is planned has greater credibility than a dental assistant who conveys the same information. Barriers to the message can be created when the receiver believes that the sender does not have the credibility needed to send the message. Levels of credibility also can change the meaning of the message. For example, a patient with periodontal disease is told by his wife that if he does not floss and brush his teeth, he will lose them. Although the message is understood, the receiver doubts the severity of the problem. When the dental assistant sends the same message, it is received and carries greater impact but still not enough for the patient to make changes. When the dentist sends the same message, the patient believes the message because the dentist has sufficient credibility. The patient receives the message in the context in which it was intended.

Preconceived Ideas

A major barrier to communication arises when preconceived ideas change or block the way a message is received. Information that has already been received and is considered true can block a message. For example, the patient with periodontal disease has come to believe that all adults will lose teeth and will have to wear dentures. This assumption is based on past experiences and information. When he is told about the need for brushing and flossing, he doubts the credibility of the message. Once the message has been established as truthful, the patient's idea is changed and the new information is considered factual.

Nonverbal information may lead to preconceived ideas about people. Consider, for example, the patient who is presented with a treatment plan that is costly. When presenting the information, the dentist notices that the patient is wearing inexpensive, outdated clothes. He hesitates to mention the ideal treatment because he is not sure that the patient will be able to afford the fee or will want the treatment. However, because the dentist believes that all treatment options should be presented without regard to the ability to pay, he presents all of them. As it happens, the patient is not only willing to have the work done but also wants to pay cash in advance to take advantage of the pretreatment discount given by the dentist. Because the patient wears outdated, inexpensive clothing, it was presumed that he did not have money. In fact, he was very wealthy and simply was not concerned about his outward appearance.

Other Barriers
Emotions

Emotions play an important role as barriers to communication. When people are upset, angry, or even happy, they sometimes do not hear the message. The ability to interpret nonverbal cues will help dental healthcare team members to adjust the message according to the needs of the patient, thereby avoiding negative response.

Stereotyping

Stereotyping blocks effective communication because assumptions are made on the basis of nonfactual information or preconceived ideas about a person, idea, or procedure.

Noise

Noise may alter the message if the sender and the receiver cannot hear the message. When conversations take place around machinery or large, noisy groups of people, the message that is being sent may not be received completely. When the receiver reacts to the message, the sender may not hear the feedback.

> **! REMEMBER**
>
> Dental offices have areas that are very noisy, such as treatment rooms, the area near the laboratory, and the business office area, where several activities could be occurring at once.

Conflicting Interpretation

Conflicting interpretations of nonverbal communications can alter or change the meaning of a message. People from different cultures and backgrounds will interpret nonverbal signals in different ways. Care should be taken to avoid these types of signals in the dental office.

How meaning is communicated is an important cornerstone of effective communication. We can choose the message carefully, but the true meaning may be lost in the tone of voice we use or in other nonverbal cues. In a recent study, tone of voice accounted for 38% of the interpretation of a message and body language or nonverbal communication accounted for 55%.

BARRIERS TO COMMUNICATION

- Semantics
- Jargon
- Credibility
- Preconceived ideas
- Emotions
- Stereotyping
- Noise
- Conflicting nonverbal communication

IMPROVING COMMUNICATION

Communication can be improved when the sender and the receiver follow a few basic rules of communications.

Responsibilities of the Sender

The sender has the responsibility to ensure that the proper message is sent and that the receiver understands the content of the message. This can be accomplished when the sender formulates the message in such a way that the true meaning or intent is not lost in the translation. This is a simple task when all barriers have been removed. Unfortunately, the sender may not be aware of all of the various barriers that can prevent the receiver from understanding the message. However, we can be prepared to listen to the responses of the receiver and to interpret the feedback (verbal and nonverbal).

Selecting the Medium

Selecting the proper medium for the message is the responsibility of the sender. Predetermine the type of message to be sent and the type of medium that will help to minimize misunderstanding. For example, patients who have just spent 3 hours in the dental chair undergoing extensive dental treatment are not likely to remember everything they are told. Following spoken instructions with written instructions provides confirmation for the patient.

❗ REMEMBER

To document transfer of information to the patient, give the patient a copy of the instructions and make an entry in the patient's clinical chart.

Timing

Timing the transfer of information, which is the responsibility of the sender, is a key component of effective communication. Not all messages are received and understood when the receiver is angry, busy, tired, preoccupied with others, or in pain. This does not mean that the sender does not send the message unless the conditions are just right; what it does mean is that it is important for the sender to understand the receiver and to know how the receiver reacts under less than ideal conditions. When conditions are such that the receiver will not respond to the message, the sender may consider waiting, rephrasing the message, or selecting a different medium.

Checking for Understanding

Check for understanding by listening to the questions and responses of patients and interpreting nonverbal cues. If the meaning of the message is not understood in the context in which it was sent, it is the responsibility of the sender to rephrase or change the message and to work with the receiver until the message is understood. Most often, during poor communication, this step is not followed. Sometimes, the sender believes that the message is so simple that it will be easily understood and that there is no need to check for understanding. For example, when patients are given instructions on how to brush their teeth, it is often forgotten that they may have been doing the process incorrectly. They in turn realize that they should know how to brush their teeth and are too embarrassed to ask for clearer instructions. It is the responsibility of the sender to check for understanding and to work with the receiver until the message is understood in the context that the sender has in mind.

RESPONSIBILITIES OF THE SENDER

- Formulate a message (clear, concise, complete).
- Select the proper type of medium (verbal, nonverbal).
- Use an appropriate transfer method (interpersonal, written).
- Understand the receiver (interpret possible barriers).
- Listen to feedback to ensure that the message was received and understood.

Responsibilities of the Receiver

Responsibility is shared by the sender and the receiver. The receiver has the responsibility to be attentive during the transfer of information. The receiver should block outside and internal distractions.

Listen to the Complete Message

One of the greatest barriers to effective communication occurs when the receiver evaluates the message before it is completed. When the receiver hears only a portion of the message and then begins to formulate a response or make a judgment, the remainder of the message is not heard. In addition, the receiver will sometimes try to guess what the remainder of the message is before the entire message is delivered. When the receiver does not listen attentively to the complete message, a portion or the entire message will not be heard or understood.

Characteristics of a poor listener.
- Interrupts the sender
- Comes to a conclusion before the complete message is sent
- Finishes sentences for the speaker
- Maintains poor posture
- Changes to a different subject
- Shows negative nonverbal signals (eyes wander, arms are crossed)
- Gives poor feedback ("uh huh," "okay," "mmm")
- Tells the sender to "get on with it" (verbal and nonverbal messages)
- Loses emotional control
- Shows distraction physically (taps fingers or feet, paces)

Qualities of a good listener.
- Maintains good posture; stands or sits upright
- Maintains eye contact with the sender
- Listens to the complete message (without external or internal distractions)
- Provides feedback (asks complete questions, summarizes the message, follows directions)
- Completes a message transfer before changing the subject (message sent, received, and understood)

Be sensitive to the sender. Place value and importance on the message. Help to make the message clear if the sender is having difficulty understanding it. Indicate an appropriate medium and state preferences for how to receive messages.

Initiate feedback. It is the responsibility of the receiver to initiate feedback. Feedback can be provided through verbal and nonverbal cues. Ask questions if the message is not clear, state your interpretation of the message, or summarize.

RESPONSIBILITIES OF THE RECEIVER

- Be a good listener.
- Be sensitive to the sender.
- Indicate an appropriate medium.
- Initiate feedback.

In later chapters, communication skills are applied to written communications, patient relations, and dental health-care team communications.

TELEPHONE TECHNIQUES

Communication over the telephone requires a different technique and strategy than those used in face-to-face communications. The ability to read nonverbal cues visually is replaced with listening for nonverbal cues. Developing a pleasing telephone voice is necessary if the correct message is to be conveyed.

People cannot see the person with whom they are speaking on the telephone. Therefore they formulate impressions that are based on the tone of voice and the mannerisms of the person on the other end of the line. This image is a combination of several cues that are projected during the conversation.

+ HIPAA

Privacy Rule

- Take appropriate and reasonable steps to keep a patient's personal health information (PHI) private.
  - Do not discuss PHI with anyone other than the patient (unless authorization has been given by the patient and is on file in the patient record).
  - Share PHI only with authorized healthcare providers.
- Follow the patient's request for notification.
  - Does the patient wish to be called somewhere other than at home?
  - Has the patient requested that information be sent in an envelope and not on a postcard?

WHAT WOULD YOU DO?

Mr. Alvarez has just completed extensive dental treatment. His sister is there to take him home and she has some questions about the type of dental treatment he has just received. She would also like to know the charges for the day and what type of financial arrangements can be made. Is it appropriate for you to discuss this with her? Support your answer. What would you tell her?

Developing a Positive Telephone Image

Developing a positive speaking image requires a pleasing tone of voice. Physical voice includes loudness, speed of speech, and pitch. Physical and psychological conditions combined create a negative or positive image that is based on the tone of voice. The same words can be used to send either a positive or a negative message. The receiver will interpret the meaning of the message according to the tone of voice.

Loudness

Loudness is the volume of the voice. During normal conversation, the volume goes up and down slightly, reflecting on different words. It is when the volume is either too loud or too soft that a negative impression is formed. The volume of the voice can become so uncomfortably loud that the listener has to hold the receiver of the telephone away from the ear. This distraction creates a negative image and may result in misinterpretation of the context of the message.

Many things can cause an increase in the volume of the voice. Physically, the volume may increase because of a hearing problem. When senders have a cold or permanent hearing loss or are working in a noisy environment, they may increase the loudness of their voice because they are unable to hear themselves clearly. The volume can also increase for psychological reasons, when emotions (anger, agitation, and excitement) play into the message. Some people assume (falsely) that a person who has a disability or poor speech pattern cannot hear and they raise the volume of their voice when speaking with them.

Conversely, a person who speaks in a very low voice also creates a negative image. The person who is often asked to repeat statements or who does not receive the correct responses from patients should consider whether the listener is hearing the full message. One reason why people speak in a low voice is lack of self-confidence. If this is a problem, a person needs to work on improving his or her self-image; in turn, his or her telephone image will improve.

Speed

The speed, or rate, of speech refers to the quickness with which a message is spoken. When the speaker speaks quickly, the receiver may not understand a portion of the message. Several of the types of telephone calls the administrative dental assistant makes are repetitive in nature.

When the same message is given several times in a row, the message begins to sound mechanical. Patients, however, are hearing the technical information for the first time; therefore the rate at which the message is transmitted must be slow, so that the receiver can understand the full message.

When developing your rate of speech, consider the person who is receiving the message. During a normal conversation, speech should sound natural and should be easily understood by the receiver. If your voice becomes too mechanical or your speech is too fast, you will send a negative image.

Pitch

Tone, or pitch, refers to the sound of your voice. Those who speak in a low pitch have a deep, gravelly voice, whereas those who have a high-pitched voice speak in a high, squeaky tone. Although it may be very difficult to fully change the pitch of your voice, you should be able to control the sound. Developing a pleasing tone in your voice is key. This may take time and practice.

In addition to the physical voice (volume, speed, and pitch), you also must develop the psychological voice. The psychological voice refers to the quality of what you say and how you choose the message you send. Although you do not intend to convey nonverbal messages such as depression, anger, agitation, or excitement, these emotions can be seen in the way you phrase your words, the tone of your voice, the rate at which you speak, and the loudness of your voice.

Vocabulary

Proper word usage adds to the quality of a message. Often patients develop a mental picture on the basis of the words we use. These words or phrases may be very common to the dental profession but may represent something different to the patient.

POSITIVE VERSUS NEGATIVE DENTAL TERMS

Positive	Negative	Positive	Negative
Dentures	False teeth	Injection	Shot
Reception area	Waiting room	Empty your mouth	Spit
Remove	Pull	Prepare your tooth	Drill your tooth
Treatment area	Operatory	Examination	Check-up
Instrument	Tool	Consultation	Case presentation
Dentistry	Work	Continued education	Convention
Discomfort	Pain	Change in schedule	Cancellation
Statement	Bill	Investment	Cost
Confirm	Remind	Condition	Acid etch
Fee	Price		

WHAT PATIENTS MAY VISUALIZE WITH NEGATIVE TERMS

Shot

Waiting room

Drill your tooth

Pull

False teeth/plates

Check-up

POSITIVE VERSUS NEGATIVE DENTAL TERMS—cont'd

WHAT PATIENTS MAY VISUALIZE WITH NEGATIVE TERMS

Spit   Operatory   Tool

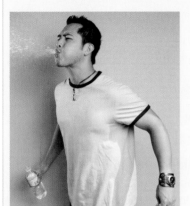   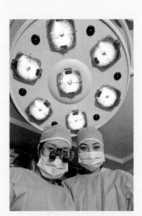   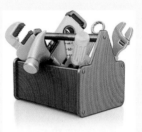

All images from www.iStock.com. *Shot:* Copyright © 2014 hatchapong, iStock.com. All rights reserved. *Waiting room:* Copyright © 2014 skynesher, iStock.com. All rights reserved. *Drill your tooth:* Copyright © 2009 Lisa Thornberg, iStock.com. All rights reserved. *Pull:* Copyright © 2011 dnberty, iStock.com. All rights reserved. *False teeth/plates:* Copyright © 2010 stocksnapper, iStock.com. All rights reserved. *Check-up:* Copyright © 2015 Minerva Studio, iStock.com. All rights reserved. *Spit:* Copyright © 2007 claudiahung, iStock.com. All rights reserved. *Operatory:* Copyright © 2009 btrenkel, iStock.com. All rights reserved. *Tool:* Copyright © 2012 pagadesign, iStock.com. All rights reserved.

Active Scripts

It is necessary for dental personnel to develop an active script that creates a positive image and avoids misunderstandings. Practice some of the phrases listed in the box titled "Developing an Active Script" and develop them into normal conversations that take place in the dental office. Practice is the only way that correct phraseology can be incorporated on a daily basis. When developing a professional voice, you will need to learn new phrases, words, and ways in which to communicate. As you grow in your profession, you will develop your own voice and apply it to the workplace. At first, some of the terms and phrases will seem unnatural but as you practice them, they will begin to sound natural and you will become an effective communicator.

DEVELOPING AN ACTIVE SCRIPT

Instead of saying...	Practice saying...
Are you a new patient?	When was your last visit to our office?
I don't know the answer; I am just the receptionist.	Sharon processes all of our insurance claims and she will be able to answer that question for you. Would you like to hold while I transfer your call?
We don't do that in this office.	In this office, we see patients for general dentistry. Would you like the telephone number of the dental society that has a list of dentists in the area who perform that procedure?
I don't know where he is.	He is unavailable at this time.
It's crazy here today.	It seems that several of our patients need us today.
I can't.	I won't be able to because _____.
You're wrong.	Let me see if I can clarify this situation.
I have to check on that.	I will be happy to check on that.
What is this in regard to?	Is there any information that would be helpful for Dr. Edwards to have before she returns your call?
I don't know.	May I check on that for you and call you back?
We can see you today but you will have to be here by 3:30.	Yes, we can see you today. Can you be here by 3:30?
No, we cannot see you at 5:30.	Mr. Smith, I wish we could see you at 5:30 but our time to see emergency patients today is at 3:30. If you like, we could see you tomorrow at 10:00 AM or 4:00 PM. Which day and time is convenient for you? (Paraphrase. Tell what you can do and why.)
There is no way. We cannot do that for you.	I'm sorry but we are unable to _____. (If conceivable, give more than one option. This returns control to the patient. If you are unable to offer solutions, ask the patient if you can call back later. Research the problem, develop a plan, and return the call as soon as possible.)

In addition to the telephone script, several dental practice management consultants suggest that scripts should be used in different areas of the dental practice. For example, they should be used with new patients to ensure that all necessary information is collected. Scripting helps the dental healthcare team to ask questions that will elicit the answers they are seeking. As discussed in Chapter 5, each patient is different and has different thoughts and opinions about dentistry. Scripting helps staff to obtain answers to many questions by asking them in a logical, concise, and well-organized sequence.

Before a script is used, whether for telephone conversations, appointment scheduling, financial arrangements, or case presentation, it is necessary that it be practiced until it becomes a natural and normal procedure. To help facilitate the outcome, practice sessions are scheduled. In these sessions, a variety of techniques are used, including role playing and audio and video recording. These techniques are numerous and all sessions should be perceived as learning experiences. Even assistants and dentists with several successful years of experience are finding the use of scripts helpful and rewarding. Once scripts are developed for an office, they should be monitored for effectiveness and adjusted when needed.

Answering the Telephone

When the telephone rings, you may have no idea who is on the other end of the line. It could be a prospective patient looking for information, a personal friend of the dentist, another dental professional, an angry patient, an emergency caller, and so forth. Each call must be answered in the same professional manner. A few simple rules should be followed for all telephone calls. Once the caller has been identified, proper responses can be provided.

It may be necessary from time to time for you to take a message for the dentist or for another team member. Be prepared to take a message by having a message pad and pencil next to all telephones used for incoming calls. Message pads come in a variety of sizes and formats. Each has space in which the same basic information can be inserted: the name of the caller, who the message is for, the telephone number to call, the time and date of the message, and a space for notes. Message pads that make a duplicate copy are preferred because a record of the original message is kept (which can save time used looking for lost messages).

When you take a message, make sure that all information is recorded, the names are spelled correctly, and the return telephone number is correct. Record any additional information if necessary and note the type of response that is requested (return the call, wait for a call back, none because the purpose was only to convey information). Once the message has been taken, the next step is to deliver the message to the correct person. This can be accomplished in several ways; a preset protocol must be established and followed. (Is there a central location for all messages? Are they delivered personally to the individual? Are they placed on the dentist's desk? Are they left with the receptionist and picked up later?)

PROFESSIONAL TELEPHONE MANNERS

- Answer the telephone within three rings.
- Identify the dental practice by name.
- Identify yourself by name.
- Speak in a clear, distinct voice that conveys a smile.
- Use appropriate terminology (no slang).
- Give your full attention to the caller.
- Use good listening skills.
- Do not place the caller on hold (if necessary to do so, thank the caller).
- Speak directly into the telephone receiver.
- Thank the caller.
- Hang up after the caller does.

Placing Outgoing Telephone Calls

During the course of a business day, the telephone is used to receive and place calls. Outgoing telephone calls may involve confirming scheduled dental appointments, scheduling recall appointments, speaking with insurance companies and other dental professionals, or ordering supplies. Several steps should be followed when a telephone call is placed:

✚ HIPAA

Privacy Rule

- Place calls in a private area if a call contains the private health information (PHI) of a patient.
- Do not leave PHI in a voice mail message.
- You can leave a message as long as it does not contain PHI.

1. Gather all necessary documents (patient chart, recall list, referral forms, order forms) to which you will need to refer.
2. Plan the call so that you will not be interrupted. Provide privacy if the call will require discussion of confidential information.
3. When using a multiline telephone system, select an open line before you pick up the receiver.
4. Before dialing, check for a dial tone.
5. Take care to dial the telephone number correctly.
6. Know the extension number of the person you are calling.
7. When the phone is answered, identify yourself and the dental office: "Hello, this is Diane from Canyon View Dental." Briefly state the reason you are calling: "I am calling regarding a mutual patient, Rose Budd." Stop at this point and wait for the response of the answering party; he or she may transfer you to a different department.
8. At the end of the conversation, summarize the outcome of the call: "I will send you a release of information form and you will then send Dr. Edwards a report. We can expect the report to be in our office next Friday, is that correct?" If the answer is yes, say, "Thank you. Goodbye."
9. Make sure that the conversation has ended before you hang up. This is usually signaled with a simple "goodbye."

10. If you call the wrong number, apologize for the error and verify the number. Never ask receiving parties their telephone numbers; instead, you should repeat the number you called.

Conference Calls

Occasionally, it may be necessary for the dentist to receive or place a conference call. Conference calls, including videoconferencing, allow several people to be present at one time. The purpose of a conference call is to hold a meeting without having everyone in the same location. Video conferencing is especially effective when there is a need for the sharing of visual information. Like other meetings, video and audio conferencing is scheduled at a predetermined date and time. Anyone who is expecting a conference call should notify the administrative dental assistant as soon as possible. Once the date and time have been set, the appointment schedule needs to be adjusted to ensure that scheduled parties will be available.

A third-party conference call is initiated and managed by a service other than the dental office. The call is arranged with the service, contact information is given for each party joining the call, and at the time of the prearranged conference the call is placed by the service. When all parties have been contacted, they are connected to a single line and can begin their conference. If a party is not available at the time the operator calls, the operator will leave a telephone number and a conference number to be used when the party does call in, at which time the party will be connected to the conference call.

Another type of third-party conference call gives each conference attendee a telephone number and access code. When it is time for the conference to begin, each attendee personally initiates the call. This type of call is usually less expensive and can be accessed by the attendee from any telephone (eliminating the need for the attendee to be at a given number at the arranged time). Some telephone equipment also allows for conference calling that can be initiated without the assistance of a third party.

Videoconferencing uses a different type of technology. Typically you will need a computer, broadband Internet connection, Voice over Internet Protocol (VoIP), desktop videoconferencing software, and a webcam. If you have all of the proper equipment and are familiar with the technology, placing and receiving calls are very similar to the audio conference call. The advantages of videoconferencing will depend on the need to have a face-to-face conversation, share visual information, or other specialized needs. As the technology improves, the use of videoconferencing will become more commonplace.

✚ HIPAA

Privacy Rule

Take appropriate and reasonable steps to keep a patient's protected health information (PHI) private.

Voice Mail

When you place calls to patients and others, it may be necessary to leave a message on their voice mail. The person called can access the mailbox at a later time and retrieve the message. When you leave a message, be sure to identify yourself and the dental office, speak slowly, keep the message brief, leave a return number (given in a slow, distinct, clear voice), and specify the type of response you want:

"Hello. This is Diane from Canyon View Dental. I would like to place an order for dental supplies. Please return my call before 5:30 today. The office number is 909-555-2345. (Give the number slowly so that the receiver can write it down as you speak.) Talk to you later, thanks."

Personal Calls

Personal calls and the use of cellphones are never appropriate during working hours. From time to time, it may be necessary to place a personal call during working hours. When this happens, make the call during your break or lunch time. The policy for the use of cellphones in a dental office will vary. Some offices may request that you do not carry your phone with you during working hours; others may request that you have it set on a quiet mode. Whatever the policy, always follow the office protocol. If absolutely no personal phone calls are allowed, abide by the rule. If an emergency arises and you have to place a call, notify the dentist or the office manager first and ask permission. Receiving personal calls during the day is also not acceptable. If an emergency arises, callers should identify themselves and state that it is an emergency call.

▊ KEY POINTS

- Communication is a two-way process in which information is transferred between a sender and a receiver. The five elements of the communication process are:
  - Sender
  - Message
  - Medium or channel
  - Receiver
  - Feedback
- Verbal communication occurs through words, both spoken and written. Nonverbal communication does not use words. Messages are sent through facial expressions and body gestures. The administrative dental assistant uses verbal and nonverbal communication on a daily basis to communicate with patients, dental healthcare team members, and other professionals.
- Telephone communication requires a set of skills needed to convey a positive image. These skills include:
  - Developing a pleasing tone of voice
  - Using positive dental terms
  - Referring to an active script
  - Speaking with professional telephone manners
  - Taking appropriate and reasonable steps to keep a patient's protected health information (PHI) private

CAREER-READY PRACTICES

Career-Ready Practices activities are designed to provide students with experiences that can be "practiced" in preparation for skills needed on the job. In each of the following exercises, a variety of approaches may be used to address the problem, rather than "right" or "wrong" answers. Below each exercise, next to the compass icon, is a listing of suggested Career-Ready Practice numbers that correspond to the listing of 12 practices in the front of the text (see p. viii-ix); these practices provide suggestions for approaches to complete the exercise.

1. At your last staff meeting it was discussed that patients have a difficult time finding the dental office and you volunteered to write up directions to the office. These directions will be posted on the website and written directions will be included in information sent to patients as well as placed near the phone so they can be easily given by any member of the team. You need to consider that people are coming from different directions and determine how to modify directions for the different types of application (website, written, and verbal).
   a. Write the directions for your website. For this exercise, choose an address in your local area.
   b. Write the directions to be included in patient information.

   c. Write directions that can be given to your patients over the phone.

 Career-Ready Practices
   2 *Apply appropriate academic and technical skills.*
   4 *Communicate clearly, effectively, and with reason.*
   6 *Demonstrate creativity and innovation.*

2. In the exercise above, you have written your directions and feel that you have done a good job. The first time you give the directions over the phone, the patient tells you he or she is really bad at directions and not sure he or she understands how to get to the office.
   a. How can you modify the directions to help the patient understand?
   b. How will you know if the patient truly understands? What are some clues?

 Career-Ready Practices
   4 *Communicate clearly, effectively, and with reason.*
   8 *Utilize critical thinking to make sense of problems and persevere in solving them.*

Written Correspondence and Digital Communication

LEARNING OBJECTIVES

1. Discuss the four elements of letter writing style.
2. Describe letter style appearance as it applies to a finished business letter.
3. Identify the five basic letter styles and recognize the different parts of a business letter.
4. Evaluate a completed business letter by judging letter style appearance, identifying letter style format, and assessing punctuation style.
5. Describe the types of correspondence used in dentistry.
6. Compare and contrast the various forms of writing resources, including digital communications, and the application and function of each.
7. Identify when Health Insurance Portability and Accountability Act (HIPAA) Privacy and Security Rules apply to written communications.
8. Discuss the various types of mail and determine how each type should be handled.

INTRODUCTION

Written correspondence is no longer limited to letters sent to patients and other professionals. Today, the progressive dental practice uses written communication to perform a wide variety of tasks, both paper based and digitally. Computers are useful in a dental practice because they can be used to create printed and digital communication. They can be used to develop patient brochures and monthly newsletters, create office manuals for employees, store databases and sample letters, and perform merge techniques to mass mail an assortment of letters and notices. In addition, computers are used to create and distribute web-based communications. Even with all of the available resources for producing communications, you must still understand the basic letter styles that are used in the business world. This chapter reviews the basic letter writing skills necessary to create a well-organized, appealing, and effective business letter and electronic communication.

LETTER WRITING STYLE

Writing style is a combination of elements that, when arranged properly, help to communicate a message. The style selected to communicate the message varies according to the type of message and the receiver.

Tone

Tone is very similar to "tone of voice" in spoken communication. It is intended to clarify meaning. When people speak, they change the tone of the message by adjusting their voice.

TYPES OF WRITTEN CORRESPONDENCE

- Letters
- Insurance company correspondence
- Laboratory instructions
- Prescription orders
- Newsletters
- New patient information letters
- Continuing care notices
- Collection letters
- Thank-you and referral letters
- Inactive patient letters
- Birthday cards
- Special recognitions
- Employee manuals
- Office policy
- Office philosophy

In written communications, the tone can be changed through the selection of words and phrases. Tone should set the mood of the letter and should sound natural.

As per your request, please find enclosed herewith the radiographs of Traci Collins.

Unnecessary phrases such as *as per* and *herewith* do not add to the message. The writer sounds forced and unnatural. Include words that are natural and that fit the intended tone of the letter (formal or informal).

As you requested, I am enclosing the radiographs for Traci Collins.

The above statement sounds natural and is easy to read.

PHRASES TO AVOID IN LETTER WRITING

- According to our records
- Acknowledge receipt of
- As to, with reference to, with regard to, with respect to
- At hand, on hand
- Attached please find, attached hereto, enclosed herewith, enclosed please find
- Beg to inform, beg to tell
- Duly
- For your information
- Hereby, heretofore, herewith
- I have your letter
- I wish to thank, may I ask
- In due time, in due course of time
- In receipt of
- In the near future
- In view of
- Our girls
- Permit me to say
- Thank you again
- Thank you in advance
- Thereon

Outlook

Another important element in business communication is outlook. **Outlook** refers to presentation of information in a positive form, even when the letter contains unpleasant subject material. Because patients are customers and we should strive for customer satisfaction, it is important to remain diplomatic and considerate. The objective is to convey to readers that they are your first priority. Simple terms like *please* and *thank you* help to project a positive image.

Instead of:

We have received your payment of $100.00.

Try:

Thank you for your payment of $100.00. (positive)

Instead of:

We have not received your payment of $100.00.

Try:

Please send your payment of $100.00.

Avoid being impersonal:

A check of our records confirms that an error was made on your March statement.

Add a positive personal statement, which will help to smooth any negative feelings the patient may have developed because of an error in the March billing:

We hope that you have not been seriously inconvenienced by the error in your March statement.

Letters that deal with unpleasant subject matter should be checked carefully to ensure that the correct message is being

sent. You may want to say *pay now*, but you will not get results if you sound as if you are attacking an individual. For example, avoid:

Because you have been delinquent in paying your account, it is necessary to report your delinquency to a credit reporting agency.

Try a more positive approach:

Because the balance on your account is now over 90 days past due, your credit rating may be at risk.

Because the second statement is not a personal attack on the reader, it will probably be read and accepted as information.

PHRASES TO USE IN LETTER WRITING

Instead of...	Use...
Advise, inform	Say, tell, let us know
Along these lines, on the order of	Like, similar to
As per	As, according to
At an early date, at your earliest convenience	Soon, today, next week
At this writing	A specific date
Check to cover	Check for
Deem	Believe, consider
Due to the fact that, because of the fact that	Because
Favor, communication	Letter, memo
For the purpose of	For
Forward	Send
Free of charge	Free
In accordance with	According to
In advance of, prior to	Before
In compliance with	As you requested
In re, re	Regarding, concerning
In the amount of	For
In the event that	If, in case
Kindly	Please
Of recent date	Recent
Party	Person (a specific name)
Said	(Not to be used as an adjective)
Same	(Not to be used as a noun)
Subsequent to	After, since
The writer, the undersigned	I, me
Up to this writing	Until now

Modified from Geffner A: *Business letters, the easy way,* ed 3, New York, 1998, Barron's Educational Series, pp 1–2.

Personalizing Letters

It is important to use the "you" technique. This technique, which personalizes the letter for the reader by using the word *you*, conveys courtesy and concern for patients and gains their attention. Care should be taken not to overuse the reader's name in the body of the letter; this tactic, when overdone, may make the message sound condescending.

Instead of:

Please accept our apologies for the error on your March statement.

Try:

We hope that you have not been seriously inconvenienced by the error in your March statement.

This statement lets the patient know that you care.

The "you" technique does not eliminate the need to use *I* and *we* in letters. When you use these pronouns, remember some key points in their proper use:

- *I* refers to the person who is signing the letter.
- *We* refers to the company (dental practice) that is sending the letter.

> **! REMEMBER**
>
> Do not use the company name or the doctor's name in the body of a letter signed by the company or the doctor. This is the same as using your name instead of *I* or *me* in a letter you sign. You can refer to the doctor by name in a letter that you sign (because the doctor is not sending it).

Organization

The final element in letter writing style is organization. Organization is a process through which you identify what you want to say and the results you hope to attain. The end product must be logical (make sense), complete (state everything you want to say), and concise (not say too much).

Logical

Before you write the letter, make a list of the information you wish to convey to the reader. Start with the reason, list the facts, and give any explanations that may be needed. Next, arrange the list in a logical order. This will help the reader to understand the message you are sending.

Complete

Always check for completeness. This step is completed in the organizational stage. When checking, make sure that you have included all of the information, facts, and explanations that the reader needs. You will want to say everything you can to obtain the desired response from the reader. It is not uncommon to include a phrase that appeals to the reader's emotions or understanding.

Concise

The final consideration in organization is being concise. You want to say just the right amount without overusing words and phrases. Developing this skill takes practice. We often think that we need to say more than is necessary to convey the idea to the reader. One way that letters are overwritten is the reiteration of points. One example is ending a letter with:

Thank you once again.

If you have thanked the reader once, it is not necessary to thank him or her again. This type of statement breaks the logical flow of the letter and distracts the reader.

Adding information at the close of a letter that is not related to the main point of the letter lessens the desired effect. Consider how you would feel if you received a collection letter from a dental office that concludes as follows:

Just a friendly reminder that you are due for your 6-month appointment. Please call our office today to schedule your appointment.

Do not give readers more information than they need. Unnecessary information only confuses readers and dilutes the desired effect.

Redundancy is another block to effective letter writing. Redundant words and phrases distract from the correspondence:

Dr. Jones and Dr. Smith will cooperate together in the treatment of their mutual patient, Patty Payne.

Cooperate means *working together*; drop *together*. Because we know that they are working together, drop the phrase *of their mutual patient*:

Drs. Jones and Smith will cooperate in the treatment of Patty Payne.

> **DEVELOPING LETTER WRITING STYLE**
>
> - Tone: Select pleasant, natural-sounding words and phrases.
> - Outlook: Be courteous and polite (use *please* and *thank you*).
> - Positive approach: Use words that emphasize good points instead of bad.
> - "You technique": Use the word *you* and direct information to the reader personally.
> - Organization: Be logical, complete, and concise.
> - Plan, plan, plan.

LETTER STYLE (APPEARANCE)

The appearance of correspondence is as important as the writing style. It is necessary to gain the attention of the reader before the letter is read. If the letter is neat, well formatted, and written on appealing stationery, it has a better chance of being read.

Appearance

The first impression of your correspondence will be formulated by its physical appearance. Factors that contribute to the first impression are the type of paper, color, font (print style), placement of type, and use of a logo.

Stationery

Stationery is a collection of similar-looking paper products that are used in a variety of correspondence. Effective professional communication is a combination of selected stationery and the message. Stationery comes in a variety of sizes and styles (Figure 4-1). Letterheads are placed at the top of the paper and include the name of the dentist or dental practice and the address. Additional information may include the telephone number, fax number, and e-mail address.

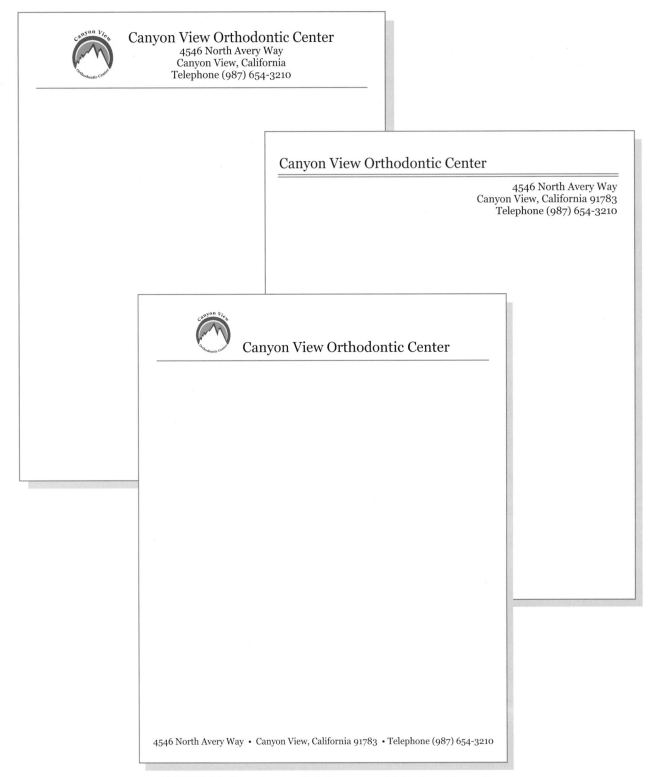

FIGURE 4-1 Assortment of stationery and letterhead formats.

Although the letterhead is typically centered at the top of the paper, it can be attractively placed in other locations at the top. In addition to names and addresses, it may include a logo. Occasionally, the information is divided between the top and bottom of the page: the logo and the practice name are at the top and the address and telephone number are at the bottom. Once the dentist has selected a style and a logo, these will be used on all corresponding stationery. The key to the placement of information included in the letterhead is appearance. The letterhead should be attractive and balanced on the page.

Stationery is made in papers of different weights (thickness), color, and style. Professional stationery is made from a combination of different natural products, such as cotton, linen, and flax. Each material or combination of material adds to the appearance of the paper. The paper may be lightly textured and may contain a watermark (a light mark on the paper that identifies the type or manufacturer of the paper).

Stationery is available in a variety of colors. The color selected should project a professional image. Common colors available for stationery are beige, ivory, white, blue, and other subtle tones. The style and color of the print should harmonize with the overall desired appearance of the letterhead. Type used in the letterhead will be of one or two colors and can be raised or flat.

TYPES OF STATIONERY

- Standard paper (8½ × 11 inches)
- Note-sized paper (6¼ × 9¼ inches)
- Appointment cards
- Standard #10 envelopes (standard paper)
- Note envelopes (note-sized paper)

! REMEMBER

The finished product will be used for communicating with patients and professionals.

Lettering

The lettering is single spaced in the body of the letter, with double spacing between paragraphs. The font should match the style of the letter and be easy to read. A good rule is to use a traditional style such as Times New Roman, Helvetica, or Garamond. A casual font may include Arial, Trebuchet, or Lucinda Handwriting. The size of font should be 12 point (can be scaled down to 11 or even 10 to keep the letter to one page) and black in color. The document must be checked carefully for mistakes before it is printed. If an error is discovered after the letter has been printed, return to the original document, make the correction, and reprint the letter.

Paragraphing

Paragraphing is the method used to insert natural breaks in the flow of information. Care should be taken to create paragraphs of equal lengths. When a short paragraph is followed by a very long paragraph, the document appears to be unbalanced and this distracts from the appearance of the letter.

White Space

White space is the empty areas surrounding the text of the letter. This surrounding space should be uniform and balanced. A short letter should be started farther down on the paper than usual so that there is approximately the

same amount of white space above and below the text. Longer letters may require the addition of a second page. When a second page is started, it is always started at the top of a blank page (no letterhead) and is not centered down on the page (Figure 4-2). When a second page is used, care should be taken to include one full paragraph or several lines. It is poor style to end a letter on a second page with just one line.

Line Spacing

Line spacing is the number of empty lines between the different elements of a letter. Typically, a line, or space, is created when the return key is struck. For example, if you wanted to create a double space, you would strike the return key twice; for a single space, you would strike it once.

LINE SPACING

Date line	Below the letterhead, 2 to 6 inches (adjust for the length of the letter)
Inside address	Three lines below the date line
Attention line	Two lines below the inside address (optional)
Salutation line	Two lines below the inside address (or attention line when used)
Reference line	Two lines below the salutation line (optional)
Body of the letter	Two lines below the salutation line or reference line (when used). Text is single spaced; a double space is used between paragraphs
Complimentary	Two lines below the last line of text closing
Company signature	Two lines below the complimentary closing (optional)
Signature	Four lines below the complimentary closing or company signature (allows space identification for signature)
Reference initials	Two lines below the signature identification
Enclosure reminder	One line below the signature identification
Notation line	One line below the enclosure reminder

LETTER STYLE (FORMAT)

Five basic letter styles are used in business correspondence:
1. Full-blocked
2. Blocked
3. Semi-blocked or modified blocked
4. Square-blocked
5. Simplified or AMS (Administrative Management Society)

Style is selected according to the type of letter and the preference of the dentist. (The two types of punctuation that can be used, open and standard, are explained later.) Within

Canyon View Orthodontic Center

4546 North Avery Way
Canyon View, CA 91783
Telephone (987) 654-3210

September 27, 2016

Michael James, D.D.S.
11765 Oak Drive
Canyon View, CA 91783

Dear Dr. James:

Thank you for the opportunity to evaluate Jason William

I appreciate the difficulty of this case. Not having the op
you in person, I hope you will take into consideration m
to Jason's case.

Two issues come to mind when considering the final res
Jason has a very strong chin in profile, which seems to b
amount of upper anterior segment retraction could result
facial appearance; (2) Closing space in a Class II Divisio
be extremely difficult. With both of these issues in mind
comfortable if you were to level, align and rotate as nece
prior to any extractions, another set of records for reeval
prudent.

The final results are my greatest concern. I have talked v
profile and what "could happen". We have also discusse
degree of overjet.

Jason takes great pride in his appearance. I feel he may l
accept an orthodontic compromise, i.e., some overjet or

September 27, 2016
Page 2

a stronger chin and nose. I think he would greatly appreciate the opportunity
to evaluate his preextraction profile.

Thank you for the opportunity to consult with you on this case. If you would
like to discuss it further, please give me a call.

Sincerely,

Jon Lamoure, D.D.S.

JJL/lg

Enclosure

FIGURE 4-2 The second page starts at the top of a blank page and is not centered down on the page.

each style, spacing and margins can be adjusted to allow for flexibility in producing a visually appealing letter.

In the **full-blocked** format, all letter sections begin at the left margin. The spacing outlined earlier is applied between sections (Figure 4-3).

In the **blocked** format, all sections begin at the left margin, except the date line, **complimentary closing,** company signature, and writer's identification, which all begin at the horizontal center of the page (Figure 4-4, *bottom*). Variations can be used. The date line can be justified right (end at the right margin) and the attention and subject lines can be centered or indented 5 or 10 spaces.

The **semi-blocked** or **modified blocked** format is the same as the blocked format with one change. Paragraph beginnings are indented five spaces (Figure 4-4, *top*).

The **square-blocked** format is very similar to the full-blocked format. The date line is on the same line as the first line of the inside address and is justified right. Reference initials and enclosure reminder are typed on the same line as the signature and signer's identification and are justified right. This style allows for squaring of the letter and is used when space is needed (Figure 4-5, *bottom*).

The **simplified** or **Administrative Management Society (AMS)** style is fast and efficient. The style is the same as full-blocked, with the following changes:
- Open punctuation is used.
- No salutation or complimentary closing is included.
- A subject line must be used, in all capital letters, with the word *subject* omitted.
- The signer's identification is provided in all capital letters.

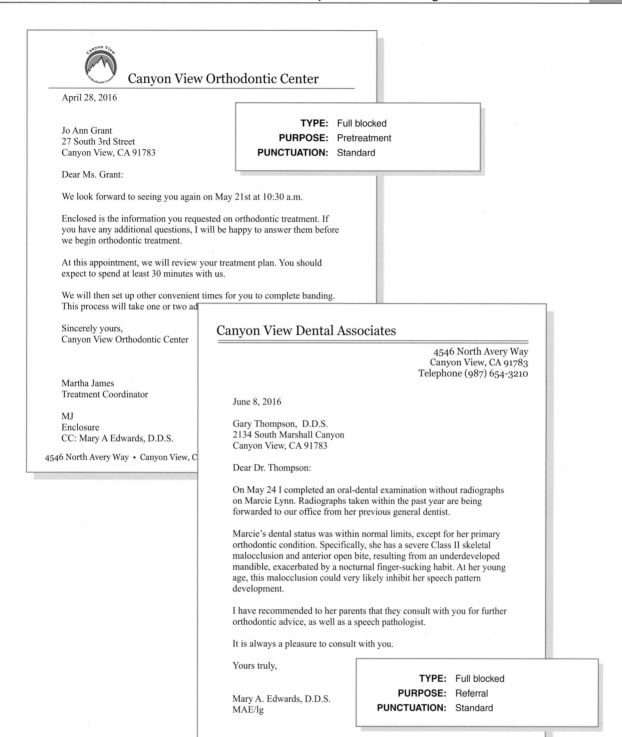

FIGURE 4-3 Full-blocked style. *Top,* Pretreatment letter. *Bottom,* Referral letter.

Lists are indented five spaces. If a numbered list is used, the period is omitted and the list is not indented.

The simplified or AMS style does not include personal identification of the reader. It is therefore recommended that the reader's name be mentioned at least one time in the body of the letter (Figure 4-5, *top*).

PUNCTUATION STYLES

Punctuation marks within the body of the letter are used according to the same rules in any formal document. The punctuation style used in the salutation and complimentary closing can be either open or standard. In **open punctuation,** no punctuation is used in the salutation and complimentary

Canyon View Dental Associates

April 28, 2016

Mr. and Mrs. Fred Collins
35901 E. 10th Street
Flora, CA 91782

Dear New Neighbors:

WELCOME GIFT

We have a gift for each member of your family. We would be delighted to have you stop by our office between 9:00 a.m. and 5:00 p.m., Monday through Thursday to pick up your complimentary dental kits.

All of us at Canyon View Dental Associates really take pride in our friendly, gentle atmosphere. We listen and are sensitive to your dental needs. If you have any dental need or emergency, we'll be available to help.

Welcome to the community! It will be great to meet you and your family.

Sincerely yours,
Canyon View Dental Associates

MAE/lg
Enclosure

4546 North Avery Way • Canyon View

TYPE:	Semi-blocked/Modified block
PURPOSE:	Welcome to the Community (Direct Mail)
PUNCTUATION:	Standard

Canyon View Dental Associates

September 7, 2016

Blue Cross of California
P.O. Box 3254
Flora, CA 91783

To Whom It May Concern:

Re: Rose Budd, Group 8476, ID# 123-45-6789

Ms. Rose Budd's tooth #3 was extracted on 7-23-09 because of prior unsuccessful endodontic treatment, which caused chronic periapical and intraradicular infection. The endodontic procedure was not done in my office and I have no prior radiograph of the tooth.

To prevent mesial drift and occlusal trauma, I am recommending a permanent three-unit porcelain bridge from tooth #2 to #4 for Ms. Budd. I am enclosing a preextraction periapical radiograph and a post-extraction panograph for your review.

Thank you.

Sincerely yours,
Canyon View Dental Associates

MAE/lg
Enc. 2

TYPE:	Blocked (dateline and attention line options)
PURPOSE:	Insurance correspondence
PUNCTUATION:	Standard

4546 North Avery Way • Canyon View, California 91783 • Telephone (987) 654-3210

FIGURE 4-4 *Top,* Semi-blocked or modified block "welcome to the community" letter (direct mail). *Bottom,* Blocked insurance correspondence.

Canyon View Dental Associates

4546 North Avery Way
Canyon View, California 91783
Telephone (987) 654-3210

Ms. Johanna Nolan
14678 East Nogales Way
Canyon View, CA 91782

CONGRATULATIONS

Your promotion to vice-president of BRVO is great news! I read about
you and your company in the paper. Under your capable leadership,
BRVO will certainly develop and flourish in the consulting business.

Congratulations, Johanna, and best wishes for your continued success!
Canyon View Dental Associates

SHARON WILL~~~~
OFFICE MANA~~~~

SAW: lg

TYPE:	Simplified or AMS
PURPOSE:	Congratulatory
PUNCTUATION:	Open

Canyon View Dental Associates
4546 North Avery Way
Canyon View, California
Telephone (987) 654-3210

Mr. William Smith   April 26, 2016
1277 South Spring Street
Flora, CA 91723

Dear Bill,

We are delighted to announce our exciting news. Our office has moved to
a new, more convenient location.

We have relocated our practice into the attractive dental suites at 4546
North Avery Way, Canyon View. We hope you will enjoy our new
"home" as much as we do. We are enclosing a couple of our new
business cards with a map printed on the back. Perhaps you might like to
pass one of these cards on to a neighbor or friend. Our phone number is
still the same: 987-654-3210.

We are now offering extended office hours to accommodate our patients'
busy schedules. When you call for your next appointment, ask us about
evening hours.

We're also sending you a refrigerator magnet with our new address and
phone number for your convenience. Thank you for letting us be your
dental professionals.

Yours in Health,

Mary A. Edwards, D.D.S.   MAE/lg
                                           Enclosure

TYPE:	Square-blocked
PURPOSE:	New location (mass mail)
PUNCTUATION:	Standard

FIGURE 4-5 *Top,* Simplified or Administrative Management Society (AMS) congratulatory
letter. *Bottom,* Square-blocked "new location" letter (mass mail).

closing (punctuation *is* used in the body of the letter) (see Figure 4-5, *top*). In standard punctuation, the salutation is followed by a colon (:) and the complimentary closing is followed by a comma (,) (see Figures 4-2, 4-3, and 4-4).

> **! REMEMBER**
>
> Be consistent in the use of open and standard punctuation. If the salutation is punctuated with a colon, the complimentary closing must be followed by a comma. The salutation is never followed by a comma in business letter writing; this is used only in personal correspondence.

PUNCTUATION AND GRAMMAR BASICS

- Start every sentence with a capital letter.
- Make sure every sentence has a subject and a verb.
- Use commas to separate three or more words or phrases in a series.
- Use commas to separate two or more adjectives in a description.
- Use a comma between city and state names.
- Do not use contractions (e.g., don't) in formal business writing.
- Put commas and periods within quotation marks at the end of a quotation.
- Do not put colons or semicolons within quotation marks at the end of a quotation.
- Use quotation marks to set off exact quotations from other sources. Do not use quotation marks when you paraphrase.
- Spell out numbers from one to nine and use numerals for numbers 10 and above.

TYPES OF CORRESPONDENCE USED IN DENTISTRY

Dental professionals use a number of different types of letters in their correspondence with patients and other professionals. Letters are used for marketing and public relations, patient continuing care, professional correspondence (referring patients to specialists), and prescriptions for laboratory work. Often these types of communications will contain protected health information (PHI) that must be kept confidential. A key to following the Health Insurance Portability and Accountability Act (HIPAA) Privacy and Security Rules is to ask the following questions when processing written communications:

- Does the communication contain PHI?
- What is the office policy for handling PHI?
- Which office personnel have been identified in the office policy as "needs to know"?
- How do you alert the addressee that the communication contains PHI?
- Has the patient requested that PHI not be shared with others?

 HIPAA

Privacy Rule

> Protected patient health information is anything that ties a patient's name or Social Security number to that person's health, healthcare, or payment for healthcare, such as x-rays, charts, laboratory reports, or invoices.

Letters to Patients

Welcome to Our Practice

Welcome letters are used effectively to communicate a variety of items to new patients. The practice philosophy is stated, office hours are listed, and what to expect at the first visit to the dental practice is described briefly. A simpler form of the welcome letter simply thanks the patient for making the appointment, restates the day and time of the appointment, and briefly states the office philosophy. This letter can be adjusted for adults and children. Follow-up letters can be sent after the first visit to thank the patient.

Thank You

Thank-you letters are used to thank patients for referring new patients, family, and friends. A thank-you card shows appreciation.

> **! REMEMBER**
>
> Most patients choose a new dentist on the basis of word-of-mouth information (talking with other patients). A card or letter of thanks encourages patients to continue referring others.

Direct Mail Promotion

Direct mail promotions are sometimes used to introduce a dental practice to a large number of potential patients. A letter of introduction sent along with a practice brochure or newsletter is an excellent way to build a practice. This method is used in rapidly growing communities and by the new dentist who is just starting a practice (see Figure 4-4, *top*). Before sending out direct mail, you should check with the state dental board and the American Dental Association to ensure that your letter and brochure conform to all legal and ethical regulations.

Introduction of a New Associate or Other Team Member

A letter can be sent to all patients to introduce a new dentist, associate, or other team member. This letter is intended to give background information about the new member and serves as a formal introduction.

Birthday and Holiday Greetings

Letters and cards can be sent to patients to acknowledge birthdays and to send holiday greetings. Holiday greeting cards must be appropriate to the holiday that the patient celebrates (for example, Easter or Passover, Christmas or Hanukkah). It is easy to generate mailing labels, lists of birthdays, and even personalized cards with computers and databases.

ANATOMY OF A BUSINESS LETTER

① **Canyon View Dental Associates**
4546 North Avery Way
Canyon View, California
Telephone (987) 654-3210

② April 28, 2016

③ Canyon View Medical Group
2908 Circle Drive
Canyon View, CA 91783
④ Lynn Saunders, M.D.
Director of Pediatric Medicine

⑤ Dear Dr. Saunders:

⑥ Subject: NURSING BOTTLE SYNDROME

⑦ₐ Keeping smiles is our business and recently we have treated several young children with rampant decay. We are treating cavities caused by nursing bottle syndrome.

⑦ᵦ As you know, this is caused by giving a baby a bottle with milk, formula, or juice at bedtime. The sugars in these liquids feed the mouth bacteria-producing acids that dissolve tooth enamel in a relatively short period of time.

Babies and young children should be given only water at bedtime or before a nap. If a child falls asleep with a bottle containing anything else, the potential for nursing bottle syndrome increases.

⑦꜀ Thanks for passing this information to the parents of your young patients. If you need more information or pamphlets, please call us at 987-654-3210.

⑦ BODY OF THE LETTER

⑧ Sincerely,

⑨ Canyon View Dental Associates

⑩ Mary A. Edwards, D.D.S.

⑪ MAE/lg
Enclosure **⑫**

⑬ CC:

① LETTERHEAD

Identifies the company or dental practice sending the letter. The letterhead style will vary in color, font style, and size. The name and address of the dental practice (company) are included, but telephone number, fax number, e-mail address, web address, or company logo are optional. Traditionally the letterhead is placed at the top of the paper, but this may vary. Letterheads are used only on the first page.

② DATELINE

The date the letter was written is placed a few lines below the letterhead (if the letterhead is at the top of the page). Rules for spacing the dateline are flexible, to allow for a well-balanced, appealing letter.

③ INSIDE ADDRESS

The same as the address on the outside of the envelope. When addressing the letter to an individual, several different methods can be used:

1) The name of the intended reader is listed, followed by the company name and address.
2) The company name and address is listed, followed by an attention line to identify the intended reader.

These styles vary and may be determined by the type of computer software being used. Most software packages can print envelopes with information from the inside address.

④ ATTENTION LINES

Used to draw attention to the person you wish to read the letter. The full name should be typed and underlined, or typed in all capital letters. Do not include redundant titles such as Dr. Mary A. Edwards, DDS. A person's company title can be placed on a second line, for example:

Lynn Saunders, M.D.
Director of Pediatric Medicine
2908 Circle Drive
Canyon View, CA 91783

⑤ SALUTATION

Greets the reader. When the reader's name is known, it is best to use the name: Dear Ms. Jones, Dear Tom Smith. If the reader is familiar with you and this is a less formal letter, Dear Tom is appropriate. If the reader is unknown, general titles may be used: Dear Sir, Dear Madam, Dear Sir or Madam, Dear Ladies and Gentlemen, Gentleman, To Whom It May Concern.

⑥ SUBJECT LINE

Draws attention to the subject of the letter. Its use is optional. It can be underlined or typed in all capital letters.

⑦ BODY OF THE LETTER

Within the body of the letter there are three sections, the introduction, the main body, and the closing. The introduction is the first paragraph and states the reason you are writing. This section is one paragraph long and should contain a brief list of the important points you will cover in the main body of the letter. The main body gives details of the points that you stated in the introduction. This section is one or two paragraphs long, depending on the number of points that you cover. This section should be concise and to the point.

⑦ₐ **The introduction** is the first paragraph and states the reason you are writing. This section is one paragraph long and should contain a brief list of the important points you will cover in the main body of the letter.

⑦ᵦ **The main body** gives details of the points that you stated in the introduction. This section is one or two paragraphs long, depending on the number of points that you cover. This section should be concise and to the point.

⑦꜀ **The closing paragraph** describes the next step or expected outcome. Clearly state what action will be taken. For example, if you are sending a letter of referral to a specialist introducing a patient, inform the dentist what the patient will do next (call for an appointment, wait for the dental office to call and set up an appointment, or explore options and then decide what to do). The closing paragraph should enable the reader to determine what to do next.

⑧ COMPLIMENTARY CLOSING

Closes the letter courteously. Typical complimentary closings are Yours truly, Truly yours, Sincerely yours, and so on. The type of complimentary closing should follow the overall intent of the correspondence. For example, you would not close a collection letter with Best wishes.

⑨ COMPANY SIGNATURE

Identifies the company of the person who is sending the letter and is optional. It is used when the sender of the letter represents the company.

⑩ SIGNER'S IDENTIFICATION

Occurs four lines below the previous item (complimentary close or company signature) to allow room for a signature. Type the signer's name and appropriate title (if needed).

⑪ REFERENCE INITIALS

Identify the sender and the typist of the letter. Type the sender's initials in capital letters, followed by a slash (/) or a colon (:) and the typist's initials in lower case. The purpose is to identify the preparer.

⑫ ENCLOSURE REMINDER

Alerts the reader that there is more to the letter. Use a reminder line when attachments or enclosures are included with the letter.

⑬ COPY NOTATION

Notifies the reader that a copy of the document is being forwarded to another party. CC is the notation used. It stands for "carbon copy" or "computer copy" and states that a copy of the letter has been forwarded to the recipient whose name follows the CC notation.

Congratulatory Occasions

Congratulatory letters are a wonderful way to acknowledge the accomplishments of patients, both young and old (see Figure 4-5, *top*). The newspaper serves as a resource tool. Articles about patients can be clipped from the paper and enclosed with a brief message.

OTHER TYPES OF LETTERS TO PATIENTS

- Abandonment of patient
- Advertisements
- Bills and collection
- Consent
- Expanded hours
- Financial arrangement letter
- Financial policy
- Newsletters
- Postexamination information
- Post-treatment information
- Continuing care (recall)

Letters between Professionals

Referral letters are used to send information about patients to other professionals (see Figure 4-3, *bottom*). The purposes of the referral letter are to introduce the patient and state the reason for the referral. When the dental practice refers patients on a regular basis, a template can be designed that will facilitate the writing of referral letters.

Several different types of letters may result from one referral letter. These include letters to specialists to refer a patient and letters to patients to confirm referrals. In addition, the specialist may write to acknowledge the referral or to present clinical information. As you can see, there are several different types of correspondence just between a dentist, specialist, and patient.

! REMEMBER

The dentist and the dental specialist work together as a team when they have mutual patients. This is accomplished by following ethical and professional standards. Written correspondence plays a key role in communication between the general dentist and the dental specialist.

Other areas of the dental practice also require written correspondence. These areas are discussed in greater detail throughout this text.

OTHER TYPES OF LETTERS TO DENTAL PROFESSIONALS

- Consent forms to obtain records
- Insurance correspondence
- Specialist referrals
- Thank you to a specialist
- Personal, professional, dental society, and other professional organization correspondence

---

Correspondence between Staff Members

Different types and formats of written correspondence are used between dental healthcare team members (see Chapter 6).

CORRESPONDENCE BETWEEN STAFF MEMBERS

- Interoffice memo
- Office policy and procedures
- Performance reviews
- Professional goals

WRITING RESOURCES

Today, it is possible for you to access a multitude of resources to help you perfect your letter writing skills. Those who may lack the skills or knowledge to write a flawless letter can consult specific resources that may help. The first step is to identify what type of letter will be generated and then check for appropriate resources. Several publications furnish different form letters that can be copied and customized. In this case, you simply retype the letter on the dentist's letterhead, change the name and the date (given in the example), and customize the letter for your needs. Other resources include electronic versions of the letters that you download to your computer, customize, print, and save.

Newsletters can be produced with the help of public relations firms and other publishers. Information supplied to the publisher is formatted and printed as a newsletter. With the help of desktop publishing software, some offices publish their own newsletters. These newsletters are sent to patients and other members of the community.

RESOURCES FOR LETTER WRITING

- Publications of sample letters
- Practice Management Software
- Public relations firms
- Online resources

LETTER TEMPLATES

Dental Practice Software systems can be preloaded with sample letters and notices that can be adapted and customized to the dental practice. Most systems will interface with word processing software, such as Microsoft Word, that will allow the user to create and upload customized letters. Once the desired letters are loaded into the system, the administrative dental assistant will be able to produce quality letters quickly and efficiently. This type of system provides a smooth interface with the patient database and the word processing software. For example, if you want to send a birthday greeting to all patients within a range of birth dates, you would select the type of letter, identify the date range, and merge the letters. From there, you will be able to direct how you would like the letters to be printed and mailed (letters, postcards, e-mail, or text message).

DIGITAL COMMUNICATIONS

Digital communications is the electronic exchange of information such as e-mail, instant messaging, social media, video conferencing, blogs, web pages, and online meetings. The technology and uses of digital communications are rapidly expanding with new hardware, software, and communication applications being introduced to the market at an ever-increasing rate. In the business community, these new modes of communication have many applications.

Digital communication has many functions that will help to communicate information, confirm appointments, market the dental practice, and provide a forum for professional networking (more detail is provided in later chapters). The same basic communication foundations apply to digital communications. Whether you are writing a letter, communicating via e-mail, maintaining a website, or instant messaging, you need to be clear, concise, complete, and correct.

Electronic Mail (E-mail)

E-mail is intended for use in sending brief messages quickly. E-mail can be used to communicate within an organization or to communicate with others who have e-mail accounts. A few things need to be remembered when e-mail is used. First, e-mail is not a secured method of transferring information; therefore any document that needs to be kept confidential should not be sent via e-mail. Second, if you send a personal message, make sure it does not contain information that would embarrass you if someone else reads it.

Sending PHI electronically through e-mail or online storage sites such as Dropbox is not HIPAA compliant. Even if your computer is secure, the message passes through dozens of unknown servers en route to its destination. Even if these servers are secure, privacy legislation requires the ability to audit systems for a detailed log of who is able to view PHI along the way, complete with times and dates.

Besides lacking security, e-mail systems typically do not meet the needs of the dental practice to transmit files between practices or between a practice and a dental lab. High-resolution digital images and other documents far exceed the typical 15 to 20 MB e-mail limitations. Systems that offer large-file storage, such as Dropbox and ShareFile, as an alternative to e-mail may not be compliant because the documents are stored unsecured and unorganized. New technology has made it possible for vendors to offer secure and compliant options. Before using a service, ensure that the company is in compliance with HIPAA and the Health Information Technology for Economic and Clinical Health (HITECH) Act.

GUIDELINES FOR SENDING E-MAIL

- Use business letter format.
- Use a tone that is appropriate to your message.
- Keep sentences short.
- Keep the length of the letter to one page (screen).
- Use professional or trade jargon (if appropriate).
- Use abbreviations (if appropriate).
- Include only questions that can be answered in one or two words.
- Let your reader know from the beginning the subject of the message and what you want done.
- Let your reader know if you are sending an attachment.

! REMEMBER

Avoid overuse of e-mail. Stop to think whether a phone call would be more productive.

✚ HIPAA

Privacy Rule: Confidential Communications

- Do not send PHI via digital media (unless the site is HIPAA and HITECH Act compliant).
- Do not reference patients (in text or photo) without their permission.

MAIL

Mail is classified into several categories, each requiring a special handling process. Mail to a dental office is delivered by a postal worker and is placed in a mailbox or is picked up at the post office by the dentist or the dentist's employee. Once the mail has been received, it is sorted according to the correct protocol and distributed to appropriate persons for further processing. In addition to the paper version of mail, there is also electronic mail (e-mail). Although mail may arrive in different formats, it still requires careful consideration in how it is handled.

✚ HIPAA

Privacy Rule: Confidential Communications

- If a letter arrives and is marked *confidential,* do not open it; deliver the sealed envelope to the addressee.
- All mail should be removed quickly from the sight of patients or unauthorized personnel to protect patient confidentiality.
- Open mail may need to be placed in a file folder to protect confidential information in laboratory reports or other correspondence.

Incoming Mail

Incoming mail (paper and electronic) must be sorted. It is separated according to category and routed to the correct person or department. Mail can be separated into the following categories:

- Payments (insurance and patient)
- Requests for information, insurance company correspondence, transfer of records, referrals
- Professional journals (for example, *The Journal of the American Dental Association*), new product information, articles, state and local dental society publications
- Personal mail, investment reports, accounting information, professional correspondence
- Laboratory cases
- Requests for payment, invoices, billing statements
- Magazines, newsletters, and publications for the reception room

- Catalogs, ordering information, advertisements (dental)
- Junk mail

Each of these categories when delivered in paper format requires special handling to ensure that the correct party receives the correct mail. Not all mail should be opened before it is delivered. It may be the protocol to stamp the mail with the date on which it was received and then route it unopened to the correct person. If the mail is to be opened before it is stamped, carefully open the letter with a letter opener (an instrument used to cut an envelope by placing the blade under the flap of the envelope and slicing) and deliver it without taking the letter out of the envelope.

E-mail may or may not be delivered directly to the intended person. You must determine the correct action for each incoming message. E-mail, like paper mail, will have to be sorted and handled according to the protocol of the office.

When mail that contains payments is handled, care should be taken to route the mail to the correct party as quickly as possible; checks should never be left lying on a countertop or desk. When you separate the check from the envelope, make sure that all documentation is removed, including the top portion of a statement that contains accounting information about the patient or the Explanation of Benefits (EOB) from insurance companies. This saves time when payments are made and ensures that payments will be credited to the correct account.

Quick and efficient handling of the mail helps to eliminate the possibility that mail will be lost or misplaced. Efficiency will be measured by how quickly and accurately the mail is routed, how efficiently payments are processed, and how soon mail is answered.

> ### ! REMEMBER
>
> Procedures for handling incoming mail vary from office to office. Care should be taken to respect the privacy of all mail to ensure that the HIPAA Privacy Rule is applied; any information seen should be held in strictest confidence.

Outgoing Mail

A variety of items will require the administrative dental assistant to send outgoing mail. Types of outgoing mail include the following:

- Insurance claims
- Patient statements (bills)
- Professional correspondence, referral letters, transfer of records, professional letters, letters to patients, promotional letters
- Continuing care notices
- Mass mailings of newsletters and promotional items
- Laboratory cases
- Sharps containers

The type of mail determines the method needed to deliver the mail in the fastest, most economical way. General

categories of delivery are overnight delivery, priority mail, bulk mailing, and e-mail. Each service is designed for different special handling requirements. A number of private companies provide mailing services. For bulk mailings and special handling needs, obtain specific instructions from the company you will be using.

The United States Postal Service (USPS) also offers a wide variety of services (www.usps.com) for mailing paper mail (Table 4-1).

> ### WHAT WOULD YOU DO?
>
> You have just received a telephone call from a patient who has moved to a different state. The patient would like you to send his records to his new dentist (he has an appointment in 1 week). What information do you need? How will you ensure that the patient's records will arrive in time?

Postage

Postage is the amount of money required to mail an item. Postage can be purchased in several different ways. One way is to buy postage stamps. Stamps can be purchased at the local post office or over the Internet and printed to your desktop printer. Postage meters are another way to purchase postage. Various companies, in cooperation with USPS, provide a technology that allows the user to download postage into these meters via the Internet. The meter weighs the item and prints the correct amount of postage on a label or directly onto an envelope. The use of a postage meter expedites the stamping process and eliminates the need to weigh each item manually and affix a postage stamp. These various ways of purchasing postage are possible because of the different types of payment methods accepted by USPS, such as checks, credit cards, and electronic transfer through an Automated Clearing House (ACH) account.

The size and weight of the item being mailed determine the postage. First-class postage is used for standard envelopes and business envelopes that do not weigh more than 1 ounce. Additional postage is required when items do not meet standard size and weight. Pieces of mail will be returned if they do not meet the following requirements:

Shape		Length	Height
Postcards	minimum	5 inches	3½ inches
	maximum	6 inches	4¼ inches
Letters	minimum	5 inches	3½ inches
	maximum	11½ inches	6⅛ inches
Large envelopes	minimum	11½ inches	6⅛ inches
	maximum	15 inches	12 inches
Packages	maximum length plus girth of 108 inches (130 inches for Standard Post)		

Mail that does not fall within the standards listed above will be assessed a surcharge for special handling because it cannot be read electronically. The purposes of the

TABLE 4-1   Choosing a Service for Mailing

Shape	Speed	Cost	Service
70 lbs or less	**1-2 days** money-back guarantee	**$$$** based on weight and distance	**Priority Mail Express®** Letters, large or thick envelopes, tubes, and packages containing mailable items can be sent using Priority Mail Express. This money-back guaranteed service includes tracking and insurance up to $100. Additional insurance up to $5,000 may be purchased. Sunday, holiday, as well as early in the day delivery is available to many destinations for an additional fee. Select Priority Mail Express envelopes and boxes are available at the Post Office. All packaging can be ordered free of charge online at www.usps.com/store.
70 lbs or less	**1, 2, 3 days** on average	**$$** based on weight, shape, and distance	**Priority Mail®** Large or thick envelopes, tubes, and packages containing mailable items can be sent using Priority Mail. This service is typically used to send documents, gifts, and merchandise. Select Priority Mail envelopes and boxes are available at the Post Office. All packaging can be ordered online at www.usps.com/store.
13 oz or less	**1-3 days**	**$** based on weight and shape	**First-Class Mail®** Postcards, letters, large envelopes, and small packages can be sent using First-Class Mail. This service is typically used for personal and business correspondence and bills.
70 lbs or less	**2-8 days***	**$** based on weight, shape, and distance	**Standard Post®†** Small and large packages, thick envelopes, and tubes containing gifts and merchandise can be sent domestically using Standard Post.
70 lbs or less	**2-8 days***	**$** based on weight	**Media Mail™†** Small and large packages and thick envelopes can be sent domestically using Media Mail. Contents are limited to books, manuscripts, sound recordings, and certain other educational materials. Formerly called "Book Rate," Media Mail cannot contain advertising, except eligible books may contain incidental announcements of books.

Speed depends on distance. Mail takes longer to travel across the country than to travel across town.
Flat Rate packaging is available in many convenient sizes for Priority Mail Express and Priority Mail, and can be used for domestic and international mailings. Flat Rate shipping lets you send your items for a low Flat Rate.
*Except off-shore locations
†Not available for international shipping

surcharge are to cover the added expense of hand processing the item and to encourage the use of standard or business-sized envelopes.

Preparing an Envelope for Mailing

Special instructions are available for addressing an envelope. The use of abbreviations is emphasized in the USPS Guidelines (Table 4-2). Mail is processed at large processing centers by electronic readers that have a difficult time reading script. The use of bar codes and zip codes expedites processing. When mail has to be read by a person, the processing time is longer.

Use the following formatting guidelines:

- Capitalize all letters. Use plain block (UPPERCASE) letters and place the address information in a block format (Figure 4-6).
- Do not use punctuation (except for the hyphen in the ZIP+4 code).

- Use the abbreviations listed in Table 4-2.
- Use correct zip codes.
- Place special delivery information, such as ATTENTION or CONFIDENTIAL, below the return address or above the delivery address only (see Figure 4-6).

The delivery address is formatted as follows:

- Line 1: Recipient's name
- Line 2: Name of company, if applicable
- Line 3: Street address, post office box, rural route number and box number, or highway contract route number and box number
- Line 4: City, state (see Table 4-2), zip code

Dual addressing is use of a post office box and a street address in the same destination address. The address listed directly above the city, state, and zip code line is where the mail will be delivered.

The return address is placed in the upper left corner of the envelope. The same type of information is included as in

TABLE 4-2   Official Postal Service Abbreviations

AL	Alabama	MS	Mississippi	WA	Washington	Jct	Junction
AK	Alaska	MO	Missouri	WV	West Virginia	Lk	Lake
AS	American Samoa	MT	Montana	WI	Wisconsin	Ln	Lane
AZ	Arizona	NE	Nebraska	WY	Wyoming	Mtn	Mountain
CA	California	NV	Nevada	AA	Armed Forces the	Pky	Parkway
CO	Colorado	NH	New Hampshire		Americas (not	Pl	Place
CT	Connecticut	NJ	New Jersey		including	Plz	Plaza
DE	Delaware	NM	New Mexico		Canada)	Rdg	Ridge
DC	District of Columbia	NY	New York	AE	Armed Forces	Rd	Road
FM	Federated States of	NC	North Carolina		Africa	Sq	Square
	Micronesia	ND	North Dakota	AE	Armed Forces	Sta	Station
FL	Florida	MP	Northern Mariana		Canada	St	Street
GA	Georgia		Islands	AE	Armed Forces	Ter	Terrace
GU	Guam	OH	Ohio		Europe	Trl	Trail
HI	Hawaii	OK	Oklahoma	AE	Armed Forces	Tpke	Turnpike
ID	Idaho	OR	Oregon		Middle East	Vly	Valley
IL	Illinois	PW	Palau	AP	Armed Forces	Way	Way
IN	Indiana	PA	Pennsylvania		Pacific	Apt	Apartment
IA	Iowa	PR	Puerto Rico	Ave	Avenue	Rm	Room
KS	Kansas	RI	Rhode Island	Blvd	Boulevard	Ste	Suite
KY	Kentucky	SC	South Carolina	Ctr	Center	N	North
LA	Louisiana	SD	South Dakota	Cir	Circle	E	East
ME	Maine	TN	Tennessee	Ct	Court	S	South
MH	Marshall Islands	TX	Texas	Dr	Drive	W	West
MD	Maryland	UT	Utah	Expy	Expressway	NE	Northeast
MA	Massachusetts	VT	Vermont	Hts	Heights	NW	Northwest
MI	Michigan	VA	Virginia	Hwy	Highway	SE	Southeast
MN	Minnesota	VI	Virgin Islands, U.S.	Is	Island	SW	Southwest

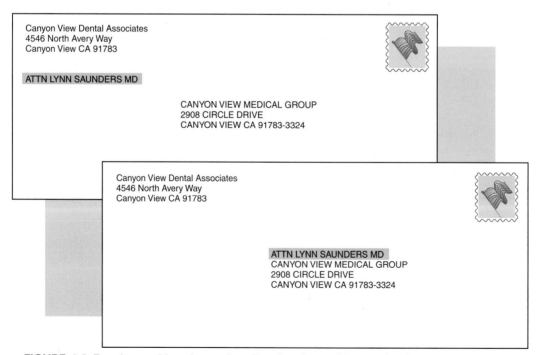

FIGURE 4-6 Envelope addressing styles. *Top,* Envelope with attention line below the return address. *Bottom,* Envelope with attention line above the delivery address.

the destination address. The return address can be pre-printed, printed on a label, or placed with a stamp.

> **! REMEMBER**
>
> The zip code of the street address may be different from the zip code of the post office box.

Folding the Letter

A correctly folded letter adds professionalism. A standard business letter (8½ × 11 inches) is folded in thirds. The bottom of the paper is brought up one third (minus ¼ inch) of the way and creased. The middle and bottom thirds are then folded up over the top one third of the letter, leaving a ¼-inch tab. When a letter is correctly folded, the letterhead and inside address are on the third of the page that the reader lifts and looks at first. The letter is inserted into the envelope in such a way that when it is removed by pulling on the ¼-inch tab, it will unfold and be ready to read (Figure 4-7). The same method can be used with a smaller envelope and paper. It is never good business practice to place a full-sized sheet of paper into a small envelope. If this must be done, the letter is folded in half, from top to bottom, and then folded into thirds, side to side, and placed in the small envelope.

Postal Cards (Postcards)

Postal cards (postcards) are used to send short messages. Continuing care (recall) cards and appointment reminders are commonly used in the dental profession. When correspondences such as birthday greetings; thank-you notes; and congratulatory, welcome, and get-well messages are sent to patients, preprinted postal cards can be used instead of letters. Simply order several cards of each type. Cards can be customized to fit the needs and style of the dental practice.

Keep a supply on hand and ready to use when the need arises.

> **! REMEMBER**
>
> Follow all HIPAA regulations:
> - Don't disclose PHI on a postcard.
> - Don't send a card to a patient who has requested not to receive this type of notification.

A postcard comes in two different formats. The first is a colorful card with a picture on one side and the address and message on the other side. This type of card is used effectively to remind patients that it is time to return to the dental practice for an examination and cleaning (prophylaxis). The message and address side of the card is divided vertically. The right side of the card is used for the address and the left side is used for the message. The size of the card is 3½ × 5 inches. Another style of postcard has the address on one side and the message on the other. Advantages of using postcards instead of letters include their size, the cost of postage, and the colorful graphics, which attract the attention of the person receiving the card.

DICTATION

Some reports and correspondence may require the use of dictation machines. These machines are recorders into which the originator of the message dictates (speaks). The machine may be physically present or can be accessed by telephone. The recording is then given to a transcriber, who translates the spoken message into a report or letter. This method is used for lengthy medical and dental reports. Typically, the transcription is done by an outside service and the transcriber works in another office or at home. Once the message has been transcribed, the finished report is sent to the doctor to be proofread and signed.

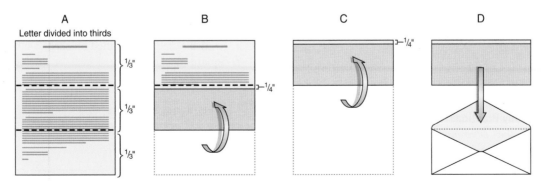

FIGURE 4-7 Folding a business letter. A, Divide the letter visually into thirds. **B,** Fold the bottom third up over the middle third (minus ¼ inch). **C,** Fold the middle and bottom thirds up over the top third of the letter, leaving a ¼-inch tab. **D,** Insert the letter into the envelope so it can be removed by pulling the ¼-inch tab at the top of the letter.

KEY POINTS

- Written forms of communication are used for a variety of tasks in the dental office. The creation of business letters requires basic letter writing skills to produce a well-organized, appealing, and effective letter.
- **Letter writing style** includes the following elements:
  - **Tone:** The way words and phrases are used to convey a message
  - **Outlook:** Presentation of information in a positive form
  - **Personalizing letters:** A means of gaining the reader's attention by conveying courtesy and concern (e.g., use of the pronoun *you*)
  - **Organization:** A process used to identify what you want to say and the results you hope to achieve in a logical, complete, and concise manner
- **Letter writing, appearance:** To make a positive impression on the reader, the letter must be neat, well formatted, and written on appealing stationery
- **Letter style, format:** Following a specific format helps to make the letter look neat:
  - Full-blocked

- Blocked
- Semi-blocked or modified blocked
- Square-blocked
- Simplified or AMS
- Digital communications is the electronic exchange of information such as e-mail, instant messaging, social media, video conferencing, blogs, web pages, and online meetings. Digital communications in the dental practice has many functions that will help to communicate information, confirm appointments, market the dental practice, and provide a forum for professional networking
- Processing of mail consists of receiving and sending mail (paper and electronic). Mail received at the office must be classified and delivered to the correct department or person in accordance with the office protocol for protection of PHI. Considerations for outgoing mail are delivery time and which company to use (USPS, FedEx, UPS, e-mail, and so forth). Correct postage is also important for expediting delivery.

CAREER-READY PRACTICES

Career-Ready Practices activities are designed to provide students with experiences that can be "practiced" in preparation for skills needed on the job. In each of the following exercises, a variety of approaches may be used to address the problem, rather than "right" or "wrong" answers. Below each exercise, next to the compass icon, is a listing of suggested Career-Ready Practice numbers that correspond to the listing of 12 practices in the front of the text (see p. viii-ix); these practices provide suggestions for approaches to complete the exercise.

1. You have been assigned the task of researching and comparing at least three third-party vendors that offer dental file storage services that comply with HIPAA and HITECH Act guidelines.
   a. What features are required to comply with HIPAA and the HITECH Act?
   b. What are the common features among all three vendors?
   c. What are the features you consider to be important?

 Career-Ready Practices
   5 *Consider the environmental, social, and economic impacts of decisions.*

   7 *Employ valid and reliable research strategies.*
   8 *Utilize critical thinking to make sense of problems and persevere in solving them.*

2. Prepare a letter to your dental office business manager outlining your findings from the exercise above. Compare each vendor and conclude with your recommendation, explaining why the vendor is your choice.

 Career-Ready Practices
   2 *Apply appropriate academic and technical skills.*
   6 *Demonstrate creativity and innovation.*
   11 *Use technology to enhance productivity.*

3. Using word processing, create a sample letter for each of the letter styles.
   a. Full-blocked
   b. Semi-blocked or modified blocked
   c. Square-blocked
   d. Simplified or AMS

 Career-Ready Practices
   11 *Use technology to enhance productivity.*

Patient Relations

INTRODUCTION

Patient relations involve empathy, understanding, concern, and warmth for each patient. These emotions can be demonstrated in the way we communicate with patients, in the type of service we provide, in how members of the dental health-care team relate to each other, and in how problems are solved. Every aspect of the dental practice should be conducted with the understanding that the patient is "number one."

> **! REMEMBER**
>
> Most patients have a choice of when and where they will seek dental treatment.

Dentistry is considered a service-based business (a business that provides a service to customers). All service-based businesses have the same common element: They provide a direct service to customers (patients). Customers, in turn, can usually choose the providers of these services. Customers, when given a choice, will select a business that meets their personal needs. Conditions that contribute to a positive image include the attitude of team members, professionalism, friendliness, and so forth.

PSYCHOLOGY: HUMANISTIC THEORY

Numerous articles and books have been written about and research conducted to study the psychology of human beings—what they want, why they react, what makes them happy, and how they relate to others. Theories are interpretations and observations that provide a framework of general principles. The works of Abraham Maslow (1908–1970) and Carl Rogers (1902–1987) have contributed to the humanistic theory.

Maslow: Hierarchy of Needs

Maslow believed that each individual has to reach a level of physiologic need before he or she is motivated to seek the next level. These levels range from the basic needs of life (food, shelter, safety) to the higher needs of love, belonging, and self-esteem to the highest need of self-actualization. For example, homeless people living on the street have to struggle to meet their daily needs of food and shelter. It takes all of their energy to fulfill those needs. Homeless people are not motivated to seek safety, love, or self-esteem until they are assured that their basic needs have been met (Figure 5-1).

According to Maslow, people who have grown up well fed, loved, and respected are more likely than those who have not done so to reach the self-actualization or self-fulfilled stage. This stage is normally achieved in later life and can be seen in those persons who devote time and energy to discovering the meaning of life and to understanding their unique purpose.

Rogers: Fully Functioning Human Beings

Rogers concurred with Maslow that all healthy people are constantly trying to obtain their potential. Rogers termed the concept *"fully functioning human beings"* (Rogers: *On becoming a person: a therapist's view of psychotherapy,* Boston, 1961, Houghton-Mifflin). Rogers theorized that each healthy individual believes in an ideal self and that he or she is constantly trying to achieve the ideal self as much as possible. Working toward the ideal self is a two-step process. The first step is to improve the real self and the second step is to modify the concept of the ideal self to be realistic. By adjusting the concept of the ideal self, a person can assume a wider variety of emotions and behaviors that fit into real life.

People need the help of those around them to become fully functional human beings. These people around them are considered "significant others"—parents, marital partners, and close friends. They offer unconditional positive regard, which is perceived to be total love and respect, no matter what the problem. For example, consider the child who complains that he or she did poorly on a test. Parents express unconditional

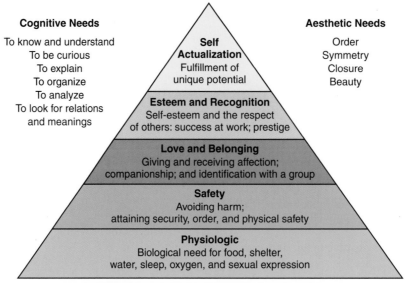

Cognitive Needs

To know and understand
To be curious
To explain
To organize
To analyze
To look for relations
and meanings

Aesthetic Needs

Order
Symmetry
Closure
Beauty

Self Actualization
Fulfillment of
unique potential

Esteem and Recognition
Self-esteem and the respect
of others: success at work; prestige

Love and Belonging
Giving and receiving affection;
companionship; and identification with a group

Safety
Avoiding harm;
attaining security, order, and physical safety

Physiologic
Biological need for food, shelter,
water, sleep, oxygen, and sexual expression

FIGURE 5-1 Maslow's hierarchy of needs.

positive regard when, instead of becoming angry and criticizing, they help the child to understand why he or she did poorly and then help to correct the problem. Rogers states that unconditional positive regard is simplified by a **phenomenological** approach to others, which is the ability to view a situation from the other person's point of view. Rogers' humanistic approach of unconditional positive regard is founded on the theory that we must respect each person's human worth and dignity.

Humanistic Theory in the Dental Office

In the dental office, we can use **humanistic theories** to help us understand the needs of our patients and team members. Young parents who are struggling to provide food and shelter for their children may not see the need for extensive orthodontic care. Their motivation may change once they have provided for the basic needs of their family. Instead of becoming angry and disapproving of patients' decisions regarding healthcare, the dental healthcare team should provide unconditional positive regard, with respect for their decisions and dignity.

Meeting the needs of patients and understanding their motivation are not always easy. It is difficult to understand the motivation of a patient who has money, status in the community, and knowledge of good oral health but refuses treatment. Once the dental healthcare team has informed the patient of a dental need, answered all questions, and educated the patient, it becomes the choice of the patient to continue treatment; this decision must be respected, even when we do not agree.

PRACTICE BRANDING: CREATING A POSITIVE IMAGE

Have you ever wondered how a person selects a dentist, manicurist, or hairdresser, or a particular store in which to

shop? What images, logos, taglines, and practice names create a positive emotional response? These questions have long been the basis for countless seminars and workshops. A basic understanding of the needs of people tells us that all people want is to feel safe and to feel that they are important. We are all individuals and will make selections according to our own needs, goals, and objectives. Individuals pass through several stages when they are formulating an impression of a dental practice.

Investigation Stage: Where Should I Go?
Name of the Dental Practice

What is in a name? If the dental practice is a group, the selection of the name can be very important. Things to consider in the selection of a name are the message it conveys, where it will be located in the telephone book (alphabetically), and whether the name has been used before. With the rise of electronic media, the name of the dental practice becomes less important for its placement in a telephone book but takes on new meaning when searched on the Internet. What information will be posted to a website; how do others describe the practice in online reviews; what do they see when they check out the practice on Facebook? No matter what type of medium is being used, names and logos need to connect to the targeted audience, not only for the purpose of attracting new patients, but also for the retention of current patients. Names and images that may have a negative connotation should not be used. For example, two brothers with the last name of Payne who want to open a dental practice should not name it "Payne Dentistry." They may be proud of their accomplishments and name, but the name also has an unpleasant association.

ELEMENTS THAT CONTRIBUTE TO A PROSPECTIVE PATIENT'S IMPRESSION

Investigation Stage: Where Should I Go?
- Is the name of the dental practice pleasing and memorable?
- Do logos and other images connect emotionally with the targeted audience?
- What insurance plans are accepted?
- Are the advertisements (websites, telephone directory, mailings, signage) appealing?
- What do others say about the dental practice?

Initial Contact Stage: What Are They Like?
- How is the telephone answered? What does the website look like?
- How are questions answered?
- Is a sufficient amount of information given?
- Do the answers to questions match the individual's needs?

Confirmation of Initial Impression Stage: What Are They Really Like?
- Is the office easy to find?
- How does the outside of the office appear?
- Is there a sign on the door?
- How does the reception area appear?
- What is the greeting by the administrative dental assistant like?
- How much time is spent waiting?

Final Decision Stage: Am I Going to Become a Regular Patient?
- How did the first appointment go?
- Did the financial arrangements meet the patient's needs?
- Was the patient's insurance plan accepted?
- What types of communication skills do the staff and dentist have?
- Did the dental team's attitudes and professionalism meet the patient's expectations?

Generic names should also be avoided. "Family Dentistry," "Gentle Dental Care," and so forth can easily be confused with other practices and may not connect emotionally with the patient.

Insurance Plans

Patients may base their decision to visit a new dentist on the type of dental insurance the practice accepts. A list of plans with specific information should be kept near the telephone to help the administrative dental assistant answer questions about insurance policies.

Advertisements

Some dental practices want to let others know about their practice. Advertisements can take the form of websites, print ads (telephone directories, magazines, newspapers), mass mailings, a sign on a building, or graphics on an office window (Figure 5-2). According to the American Dental Association (ADA) Code of Ethics, advertisements must present realistic statements and slogans. Whenever electronic or print media is used to advertise to the public, care should be taken to check Federal Trade Commission regulations, state Dental Practice Acts, and the ADA for specific guidelines.

Asking Others about the Dental Practice

How do other patients describe their experience with your dental practice? If you want your patients to refer others and to speak highly of you, it is necessary to develop and maintain the image you wish to convey, not just during the first visit but during all visits. The patient has to feel that he or she is "number one." Patients want schedules to be kept and staff to be friendly, and they want to feel that the staff is working together for the benefit of patients (not themselves).

Initial Contact Stage: What Are They Like?

Once prospective patients decide whom they are going to contact, the next step is to place the call (or send an e-mail) and ask questions. If successful communications have taken place, the patient will decide to make an appointment.

The first few seconds that prospective patients are in contact with the dental practice can determine whether they will make an appointment. Patients have several different concerns, from infection control to the types of insurance plans accepted. Assistants who answer the telephone must be skilled in communication. They must be ready to answer questions and to tell why their dental practice is unique.

Whether the conversation will continue is based in part on the tone of voice and the greeting used when the telephone is answered. The tone of voice should be friendly and light.

The greeting should contain a welcome, identify the dental practice, and identify the person answering the telephone: "Thank you for calling Canyon View Dental. This is Diane. How may I help you?" The script selected can vary but the three main ingredients—welcome, practice identification, and assistant identification—remain the same. Some practices prefer that assistants identify themselves with their full name while others are comfortable with just the first name. If two assistants or staff members have the same first name, it is advisable to use the first and last name. Practice the script until you are comfortable with it. It may take some adjustment to fit your tone and presentation. Each person who answers the telephone should use the same or a similar script.

> **! REMEMBER**
>
> Smile. It can be heard.

A script can also be developed to maintain constancy in dealing with several different situations. The use of telephone information forms helps to maintain consistency in answering questions and obtaining necessary information.

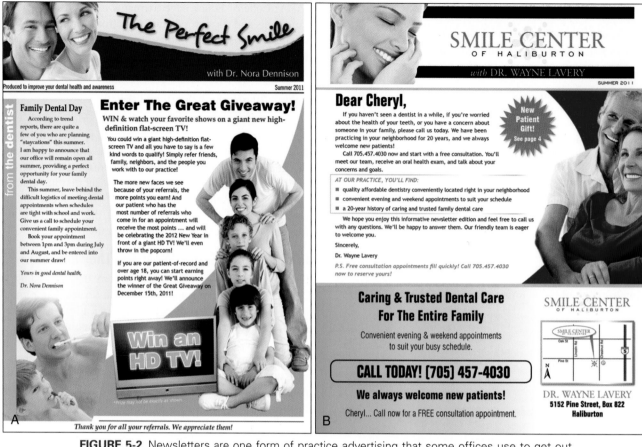

FIGURE 5-2 Newsletters are one form of practice advertising that some offices use to get out the word about their practice to potential new patients and to inform and educate current patients. **A,** Sample patient newsletter (internal marketing). **B,** Sample neighborhood newsletter (external marketing). (Courtesy Patient News, Niagara Falls, NY.)

FACTORS THAT INFLUENCE A PATIENT'S IMPRESSION

- Was the telephone answered quickly (within three rings)?
- Did the patient receive the full attention of the assistant during the conversation?
- Was the voice of the person answering the phone pleasant?
- Were questions answered with ease?
- Was the patient's name used correctly during the conversation?
- Were the patient's needs identified and met?

How Long it Takes to Answer the Phone

Telephones must be answered within three rings. If the assistant is on the telephone and receives a second call, it may be necessary to place the first caller on hold. When this happens, follow the correct protocol; ask permission and thank the patient. When answering the second call, open with the correct script and obtain the following information: name of the person calling, the reason for the call, and whether you can put the caller on hold. You may find at this time that the patient simply wants to know if his or her appointment was at 10:00 or 10:30. It will take only a few seconds to answer the

question and return to your first call. When you anticipate having to place patients on hold for more than 1 minute, ask if they would prefer if you returned the call as soon as possible.

Attention to the Patient during the Conversation

Patients and others will not feel that they are receiving the attention they deserve if they are not given full attention during a conversation. Patients on the telephone should not be placed on hold unless it is absolutely necessary. The advancement in telephone systems is changing rapidly. Large practices may use telephone systems that incorporate an automatic answering system that gives the patient a menu (choice) of what department or person he or she wishes to contact. No matter what system is used, it is important to remember that a calling patient wants to speak with a "real" person. Patients who are not able to speak with an assistant and have to call back or leave a message may feel that they have not been given full attention.

Telephone Voice

Smile and never seem rushed. Patients like to have your full attention when they are calling. If they feel rushed, they may perceive that their dentistry will be handled in the same manner. Conversely, do not take more time than necessary. Be efficient.

> **! REMEMBER**
>
> A script or telephone log can help you to organize your thoughts and maintain speed and efficiency.

Questions Answered with Ease

Be prepared to answer common questions such as the hours that the dentist sees patients, directions to the office, types of insurance plans accepted by the dentist, different types of payment plans available, and infection control protocol followed (Figure 5-3). When you are not familiar with a question, tell callers that you will find out the answer and get back to them or that you will have another team member who can answer the question take the call. Rehearsing scripts will help you to answer questions with speed and ease.

It is a good idea to write scripts for commonly asked questions and place them in a notebook near the telephone. When a patient calls and asks questions, the assistant can refer to the answers in the script book to ensure speed and ease in answering the question. (Caution: Do not sound like you are reading from a book.) This works well for training a new assistant or using temporary help or when an assistant who normally does not answer the phone is helping in the business office. Patients may never suspect that the assistant they are speaking with is not the assistant who usually answers the phone.

Patient's Name Used Correctly during the Conversation

When you address patients, it is vital that you give them the courtesy of addressing them properly. Unless otherwise instructed, address all adults using the correct form: Mr., Mrs., Ms., or Miss. For example, a new patient calls and tells you her name is Rose Budd. When ending the call, thank Ms. Budd for calling (you have not been instructed to refer to her by her first name). Once a patient relationship has been established, the patient may request that you use his or her first name.

> **! REMEMBER**
>
> Members of different cultures and generations have very strict rules on how they are addressed. Using the incorrect name may be interpreted as disrespect for the patient. When dealing with a culturally diverse patient population, it may be wise to seek the assistance of an expert in cultural relations before you establish office protocol.

Patient's Needs Identified and Met

How will you know when patients have identified their needs and you have answered their questions? Communication is key and you must be a good listener. Research has shown that you cannot be an effective communicator if you do not listen. When you listen, you must give full attention to the speaker. Look at the person (when on the telephone, do not work on other tasks) and concentrate on what is being said. Do not start to formulate an opinion or try to answer the question while someone is still speaking. As soon as you start to think about an answer, you will not hear the remainder of the conversation. Patients expect to know what fee is going to be charged, if they will be required to pay at the time of service, what treatment will be performed, and approximately how long they will be in the office.

Patients will make an appointment only if they believe that their needs will be met.

Confirmation of Initial Impression Stage: What Are They Really Like?

After patients arrive for their appointment, they continue to take into account several factors that will confirm or change their first impression.

Office Location

Patients do not want to drive around for a long time trying to find the dental office. If the office is difficult to find, give clear directions and describe the area. For example, if the office is located behind a fast-food restaurant or another identifiable landmark, let the patient know this.

Outside Appearance

The appearance of the dental practice is very important. Think about going to a restaurant for the first time. Your friends tell you about a wonderful new restaurant where the food is good and the service is outstanding. You decide that you want to try the new restaurant and ask your friend for directions. On your way to the restaurant, you have a difficult time finding the correct building (it is behind another and is not seen easily from the street). Once you locate the building,

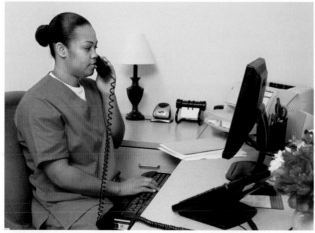

FIGURE 5-3 Patients form first impressions of a dental practice during the initial contact stage, which is often via telephone. Calls should be answered within three rings and the staff answering calls should be prepared to answer a variety of common practice-related questions in a pleasant and unrushed voice. (From Young-Adams AP: *Kinn's the administrative medical assistant: an applied learning approach,* ed 8, St. Louis, 2014, Saunders.)

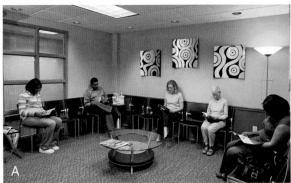
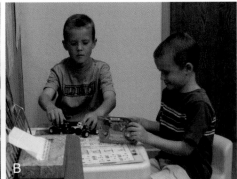

FIGURE 5-4 A, The reception area should create a positive image. Patients appreciate cleanliness, restful colors, good ventilation, reading material, and adequate light by which to read when they wait in the reception room. **B,** Many reception areas offer special areas with activities for young children. (**A,** From Young-Adams AP: *Kinn's the administrative medical assistant: an applied learning approach,* ed 8, St. Louis, 2014, Saunders.)

you notice that it is not maintained well. As you walk to the door, you look inside and see only one other couple seated for dinner. At this time, you are going to make a choice about whether to enter or find another restaurant where you would feel more comfortable. Most people at this point will make a decision to find another restaurant based only on the fact that they do not feel comfortable. The situation is the same for dental offices. If the office is difficult to locate and does not send out a warm welcome, patients may choose to seek care elsewhere.

Sign on the Door

It confuses patients when they arrive for an appointment and the dentist they have an appointment with is not listed on the front door. When only the name of the dental practice is listed—for example, Canyon View Dental Associates—the names of individual dentists should be attractively posted in the reception area.

Appearance of the Reception Area

After the patient enters the office for the first time, the condition of the reception area is the next most influential factor. A positive image will be formulated when the reception area is clean and organized and provides current reading material (Figure 5-4). Once a negative factor is discovered, such as a stain on the carpet, patients will look for other negatives.

Greeting

The administrative dental assistant should identify patients as soon as they enter the reception area (Figure 5-5). Plan to spend the first 60 seconds giving a new patient your undivided attention. Reconfirm the reason for the visit (emergency, examination, consultation). Explain what the patient can expect: "Mrs. Potter, this is your first visit to our office. I have forms for you to complete. Dr. Edwards will examine the area where you are having discomfort. Once a diagnosis is made, she will discuss treatment options. Our goal today is to relieve your discomfort."

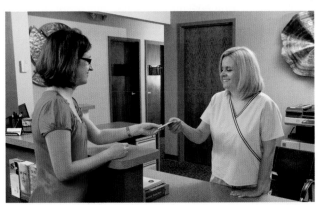

FIGURE 5-5 Greet all patients with a warm smile and give them your undivided attention, confirming the reason for their visit and assisting them with any questions or forms. (From Young-Adams AP: *Kinn's the administrative medical assistant: an applied learning approach,* ed 8, St. Louis, 2014, Saunders.)

Time Spent Waiting

Many dental practices are judged by the amounts of time patients spend waiting. New patients should not have to wait for longer than a few minutes. There are always ways to fill time before a patient sees the dentist for the first time. Forms can be reviewed or a tour of the office can be conducted. Patients who must wait longer than 10 minutes during a subsequent visit should be given options: "Mrs. Potter, Dr. Edwards will be ready for you in about 20 minutes. If you would like, there is a coffee house around the corner where you could wait or you are more than welcome to stay here. We have water or coffee available for you." When you give patients options, they accept the wait more easily. You have made it clear that their time is valuable.

Final Decision Stage

The First Visit: Will I Become a Regular Patient? Or Is It "One and Done"?

Allow ample time for the dental healthcare team to meet the new patient. The appointment should never be rushed and the patient should have the opportunity to get to know the dental healthcare team.

Financial policies should be explained to patients and a written copy of these policies given to them for review when they get home. A consultation should take between 20 and 30 minutes.

Communication Skills

The skills of the staff and dentist are important elements in creating a positive first impression. Effectively communicating with patients to better understand their needs involves asking questions and transmitting the objectives of the dental healthcare team.

Attitude and Professionalism

Patients must leave the office after their first appointment honestly believing that the dental healthcare team cares about them as individuals, understands their needs, and is willing to work with them to improve their dental health. This will lead to mutual trust.

Managing Patient Expectations

When patients decide to make an appointment with a dentist, they have certain expectations. These expectations are formed during their initial investigation of the dental practice. During their investigation, they obtain information from several different sources: friends, advertisements or marketing campaigns, websites, insurance companies, and professional referrals. In addition, they often will call a dental office, ask questions, formulate an opinion, and, if satisfied, make an appointment. It is at this point in the process that the expectations that patients have may not be fulfilled by the dental

office staff. This discrepancy will occur if communications have been inadequate.

It is important to answer the question: What can we, as a dental healthcare team, do to ensure that we are meeting the expectations of our patients?

Create the image that you want your patients to see. This applies to everything from websites to the location of the office.

- Inform your patients about the vision and mission of the dental practice. Communicate this information in all media (websites, letters, pamphlets, brochures, newsletters, and so forth). The information should clearly outline the mission of the practice, office hours, types of insurance accepted, types of financial plans available, and types of patients seen (if a specialty office), along with an introduction of the dental healthcare team (Figure 5-6). Include answers to often-asked questions. List the procedure that will be followed at the first visit. Provide office hours and emergency telephone numbers.
- Provide all patients with a standard financial policy. Provide this for patients before they have to ask for the information.
- Clarify insurance information before dental treatment is begun. Ask patients to bring you a summary of their policy.
- Inform patients of the treatment process before treatment is begun, keep them informed of each step, and inform them as changes occur. Do not promise unrealistic results and do find out (through feedback) what results the patient hopes to accomplish. If the expected results are not the same, this must be worked out before treatment is begun. Patients often share this information with an

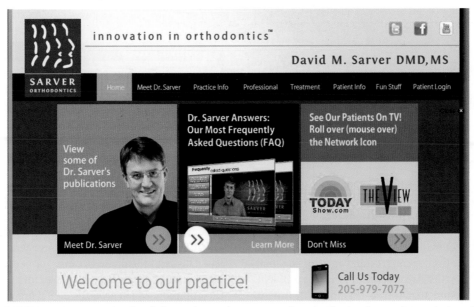

FIGURE 5-6 An example of an informative and easy-to-navigate orthodontic practice website with links to necessary patient information. (Courtesy David M. Sarver, DMD, MS, Sarver Orthodontics, Birmingham, Ala.)

assistant instead of the dentist. It is important that each member of the team understand the intended treatment and be able to communicate with the patient. Assistants should ask for clarification of any information they do not understand before they speak with patients.

- Infection control or standard precautions are anticipated by all patients. Inform your patient of the process and steps you take in the office. Be prepared to answer questions about the procedures used in the office to protect patients and team members.
- Be prepared to interpret patients' messages by reading body language. What they are saying may not be what they actually mean.
- Patients want to be treated as special individuals. Keep notes about patient preferences, activities, special events, likes, and dislikes: "Mr. Perez, how did your granddaughter like the playhouse you built for her?" "Jennifer, I understand your wedding was picture perfect." Such statements send a message of caring for the patient as an individual. In addition, they open dialogue to help relieve anxiety about the pending dental treatment.

PROBLEM SOLVING

Good patient relations require that the dental healthcare team have effective problem-solving skills. Patients who choose not to follow instructions require special attention. The problem must first be identified and then it must be solved. Some patients complain about everything. Some of their complaints will be justified and others will not. Pressures inside and outside the dental practice will affect patients and how they cope. Dealing with angry patients requires skill and tact.

> **! REMEMBER**
> Patients whose expectations are realistic (created through effective communications) will be happy patients.

Noncompliance

Successful dental treatment requires the combined effort of the dental healthcare team and the patient. Frustration results when a patient chooses not to follow the dentist's instruction.

Identify the Problem

Each patient is an individual with different goals and ideals. As Maslow points out, motivation is not the same for each person and we must discover what motivates our patients (see Figure 5-1).

Treatment that requires patients to change their habits, such as increasing the time spent brushing and flossing, may cause them to abandon these regimens. To solve this problem, it is necessary to ensure that before beginning treatment, patients understand what will be expected of them. When patients understand and accept a treatment, they will be more likely to follow the instructions. When noncompliance

is discovered, explain to patients what will happen if they do not follow the recommended treatment:

> *John, I can understand your reluctance to stop jogging, but for a week after surgery it is advised because of the possible complications, such as prolonged bleeding.*

Ask open-ended questions (which require the patient to explain). Begin with "what," "why," "how," or "tell me":

> *Why do you feel that way?*
> *Tell me why you don't think it is necessary.*

Closed-ended questions require a simple answer—"yes" or "no"—and are used to confirm information:

> *Can you come next Tuesday?*

Describe the outcome when the patient follows instructions:

> *Judy, I understand your teeth are sensitive and your gums bleed easily. If you brush and floss daily, within a few days you will experience less sensitivity and bleeding.*

Give positive instead of negative information:

> *Jeff, 85% of our patients have reported whiter teeth within the first week of treatment.*

Contrast the positive statement above with this negative statement:

> *It does not work in 15% of our patients.*

Take time to demonstrate techniques to patients. Show a patient correct brushing and flossing techniques, have them demonstrate back to you, and correct them when needed. Send patients home with instructions so that they can review the techniques at home. When patients understand how and why, they will be more likely to follow instructions.

A final technique is to ask the patient for help in solving the problem:

> *If we changed places, how would you help to solve this problem?*

> **! REMEMBER**
> All detection of noncompliance must be entered in the patient's clinical record. State the problem and document the action taken by both the dental healthcare team and the patient.

Complaints

When patients have a complaint, they will react in one of three ways: stop using the dental practice, voice their concern, or ignore the problem. Exiting the practice occurs when a patient chooses to leave instead of confronting the issue. Often dental practices do not understand why a patient has left. This is unfortunate because the underlying issue is not discovered or corrected. Some patients will choose to voice their opinion, which gives the dental practice the opportunity to identify and solve the problem. A few patients are "loyal" to the practice and therefore choose to ignore the problem instead of creating an unpleasant situation.

PROCEDURES

Steps in Identifying and Solving Complaints

1. Watch for changes in attitudes and nonverbal cues.
2. Consider both sides of the issue; the patient could be right.
3. Consider each complaint as an opportunity to improve patient services. "Thank you for bringing this to our attention; we will try to improve."
4. Listen to the full complaint without interrupting before suggesting a solution to the problem.
5. Show empathy for the complainer by restating the issue in an empathetic tone of voice.
   - "In other words, you are concerned with the way you will feel after the extraction."
   - "You feel it is unfair that the insurance company will not cover sealants."
   - "It sounds as though you might not have understood the extent of the treatment."
   - "As you see it, it is upsetting when Dr. Edwards leaves you during treatment to see another patient."
6. Proceed only when the patient agrees that you understand the nature of the complaint.
7. Avoid phrases and words that put the complainer on the defensive.
   - "You are the only person who has complained about..."
   - "We have other patients who need our attention."
   - "These are our rules; everyone has to follow them."
8. State what you will do next.
9. Assure the patient that you want him or her to continue using the services of the dental practice.

Angry Patients

Some patients bring with them outside issues that cause them to become angry easily. Some believe that the only way a problem will be solved is if they become angry. This gives them a feeling of power and control. Never assume that such a person is angry with you. If you look closely at the causes of their anger, you will discover that they are usually not angry with you personally. They are angry because of circumstances; most often, these circumstances are out of your control.

WHAT WOULD YOU DO?

Mrs. Page has just completed a series of dental appointments. Typically Mrs. Page is positive and very complimentary of the dental healthcare team. However, today you notice that she is very quiet and not positive. As she leaves your desk, she turns and begins to tell you how upset she is with how she has been treated today.
- How will you react? What are you going to do?
- What clues did you have that something was wrong?
- How could you have avoided the "meltdown"?

Dealing with angry patients requires a special talent to separate the issue from the person. Becoming personally involved and reacting negatively makes you the loser and gives control to the angry patient. Remaining professional is the key to successful resolution of the problem.

PROCEDURES

Steps to Consider When Dealing with an Angry Patient

1. Listen to the whole story. Do not interrupt the patient, even if the accusations seem ridiculous.
2. Do not pass judgment before you understand the reason for the anger.
3. Change the environment. Take the patient to another area and offer water or a cup of coffee. Remove all barriers and sit down. (Sit at the same level, not behind a desk.)
4. Use humor but be careful not to ridicule.
5. Do not involve others in the dispute. This will make it appear that you are "ganging up" on the patient. Listen to the full story and then suggest involving another person to help solve the problem. (If you add others, which is sometimes advisable, ask permission first.)
6. Do not pass the patient off to another team member without explaining that the other person can help.
7. Do not become angry yourself. This will only increase the tension. Add a tone of empathy and understanding.
8. Try to find a positive aspect of the problem.
9. Ask the patient: "If you were in my shoes, how would you handle the situation?" or "How would you handle this situation?"
10. Above all else, *do not become defensive*. Always remain positive and professional.

PROVIDING OUTSTANDING CUSTOMER SERVICE

Some who are able to provide outstanding customer service have shared their successes with others. A composite of several different resources includes the following elements.

Team Strategies

- **Be available.** Adjust appointment hours to meet the needs of the patients you serve. Rotate the schedule to provide for both early morning and evening appointments. Provide for continued telephone coverage during lunch hours.
- **Have a unique image.** Develop an image that you want to be known for (you cannot be everything to everybody). Become the best at what you do well.
- **Show appreciation.** Show appreciation by thanking patients for their referrals. Become a kind and caring team, placing the needs of your patients above your own.
- **Personalize.** Keep in touch with patients; call them after treatment and inquire how they are doing. Personally call each patient to schedule recall appointments. Send birthday cards and holiday greetings.

- **Listen.** Develop listening skills. Be able to recognize concerns and address them. Identify individual patient needs.
- **Set goals.** Set practice goals. Measure your goals by industry standards and continually modify them to meet the needs of your patients.
- **Understand value.** Understand the value of a long-term patient, and constantly strive to provide quality care.

Personal Strategies for Providing Exceptional Patient Care

- Acknowledge patients when they arrive for an appointment. Greet them with a warm smile and a sincere "Hello."
- Answer the telephone within three rings and greet the caller with a smile.

- Use the patient's name at least once during a conversation.
- Explain to the patient what will happen next.
- Identify verbal and nonverbal signals. Become aware of the warning signs that indicate that a patient is dissatisfied or concerned. Respond to the concern and be willing to work with the patient until the problem is solved.
- Become an active listener.
- Observe confidentiality at all times. Safeguard the integrity of clinical records and do not discuss patients with persons who are not team members.
- Do what you say you will do, when you say you will, 100% of the time.
- When patients leave, thank them for coming, bid them goodbye, wish them well, and tell them you are looking forward to seeing them the next time.

KEY POINTS

- **Good patient relations** include empathy, understanding, concern, and warmth for each patient.
- **Humanistic theory** is based on the works of Maslow and Rogers. Maslow identified a hierarchy of needs. This hierarchy can be applied to a patient's motivation and desire to receive dental treatment. Rogers theorized that all healthy individuals believe in an ideal self and that they are constantly trying to achieve the ideal self as much as possible. Applying humanistic theories helps us to understand the needs of our patients and fellow team members.
- **Practice branding: Creating a positive image** is necessary to attract and keep patients. Patients will go through several stages before they select a dentist:
  - Investigation stage: Where should I go?
  - Initial contact stage: What are they like?
  - Confirmation of initial impression stage: What are they really like?

- Final decision stage: Am I going to become a regular patient? Or is it "one and done"?
- **Managing patient expectations** is a process of communication. What image is being sent and will the dental healthcare team live up to the expectations of the patient?
- **Problem solving** requires that the dental healthcare team develop skills that identify and solve problems of
  - Noncompliance
  - Complaints
  - Anger
- **Providing outstanding patient care** requires a team strategy as well as personal characteristics:
  - Team strategies: availability, image, appreciation, personalization, goals, and values
  - Personal characteristics: care for the patient as an individual, development of good listening and communications skills

CAREER-READY PRACTICES

Career-Ready Practices activities are designed to provide students with experiences that can be "practiced" in preparation for skills needed on the job. In each of the following exercises, a variety of approaches may be used to address the problem, rather than "right" or "wrong" answers. Below each exercise, next to the compass icon, is a listing of suggested Career-Ready Practice numbers that correspond to the listing of 12 practices in the front of the text (see p. viii-ix); these practices provide suggestions for approaches to complete the exercise.

1. Research a minimum of three dental practice websites.
   a. What is the name of each dental practice?
   b. Describe each practice's website graphics. What does it tell you (how does it make you feel)? Can you identify if there is a targeted audience? Is the site appealing?
   c. What elements and information are included? Do the practices identify the types of insurance plans they accept?

Do they have a financial policy? Do you know the practice philosophy? Can you make appointments online? Do they introduce the staff? Are the sites just for information or can you communicate with the dental office?
   d. Do they have patient reviews? What are the patients saying? Do you think this is staged?
   e. Which office would you call to get further information or make an appointment (if you were a patient looking for a new dentist)? Explain why.

Career-Ready Practices
   5 *Consider the environmental, social, and economic impacts of decisions.*
   7 *Employ valid and reliable research strategies.*
   8 *Utilize critical thinking to make sense of problems and persevere in solving them.*

2. In a small group, compare your research results.
   a. Make a list of the qualities that everyone thought were the most important.
   b. As a group, prioritize the list, from the most important qualities to those just nice to have.
   c. Review the list and select the items that you would include if you were developing a website. Add to the list if you feel something additional is needed.
   d. Prepare a presentation for the dentist that outlines what needs to be on the website, what group of patients you hope to attract, and the purpose of the site.

 Career-Ready Practices

   4 *Communicate clearly, effectively, and with reason.*
   6 *Demonstrate creativity and innovation.*
   8 *Utilize critical thinking to make sense of problems and persevere in solving them.*
   12 *Work productively in teams while using cultural/global competence.*

3. In your journal, reflect on a time at a dental or medical office (or a store or restaurant) when you did not receive the best customer service.
   a. Describe the situation.
   b. How did it make you feel?
   c. What could have been done (by you and the other persons involved) to prevent the event?
   d. What recommendations would you make to help the practice improve its service?

 Career-Ready Practices

   1 *Act as a responsible and contributing citizen and employee.*
   4 *Communicate clearly, effectively, and with reason.*
   9 *Model integrity, ethical leadership, and effective management.*

6

Dental Healthcare Team Communications

LEARNING OBJECTIVES

1. Discuss the purpose of a dental practice procedural manual and identify the different elements of the manual.
2. Categorize the various channels of organizational communication and identify the types of communication that are used in each channel.
3. Identify and discuss barriers to organizational communications.
4. Describe different types of organizational conflict and select the appropriate style for resolution.
5. Explain the purpose of staff meetings.

INTRODUCTION

A team can be described as a group of two or more persons who work toward a common goal. Similar to those on a sports team, all members must understand and practice established rules and have a common goal. An effective healthcare team requires a shared philosophy, excellent communication skills, the desire to grow and change, and the ability to be flexible while providing quality care for all patients.

DENTAL PRACTICE PROCEDURAL MANUAL

The dental practice procedural manual is a detailed manual that is used as a form of written communication. The objective of the manual is to provide a reference for all team members. This resource provides each team member with specific details on practice goals, personnel procedures, business office procedures, and clinical procedures. The manual should be developed as a team project, with each team member contributing in his or her specific area of expertise. As procedures change, it is the team members' responsibility to update the manual. To be effective, the manual must be updated at regular intervals and all team members must be given updated manuals.

The key to developing a good procedural manual is to include as much information as possible without making the manual cumbersome. The idea is for the manual to be a resource for all team members. It will not be used on a daily basis by experienced team members but it will be used to help train new team members and will serve as a guide for substitute team members or, when necessary, for a team member who fills in for another. The purposes of the manual are to provide written documentation of and to eliminate inconsistency in policies. Such inconsistencies are a common cause of conflict among members of the dental healthcare team.

The initial writing of the manual can be overwhelming if it is done without guidance. Several resources, including established manuals and workbooks, can be purchased through professional organizations, supply catalogues, and consulting services.

One of the most important sections of the procedural manual is the practice philosophy. This statement tells the reader the purpose of the dental practice, how the practice will meet the needs of its dental patients, and the core values of the practice. In addition to it serving as the introduction to the dental procedural manual, the mission statement will be communicated to the public in several different ways such as in newsletters, welcome letters, websites, and practice brochures.

! REMEMBER

The practice philosophy should answer the following three questions:
1. What is the purpose of the dental practice?
2. What type of services do we (the members of the dental practice) provide to our patients?
3. What are the core values that guide our work?

EXAMPLE OF HOW THE THREE QUESTIONS CAN BE ANSWERED

American Dental Association (ADA) Mission Statement: The ADA is the professional association of dentists committed to the public's oral health, ethics, science and professional advancement; leading a unified professional through initiatives in advocacy, education, research and the development of standards.

1. Purpose: leading a unified professional through initiatives in advocacy, education, research and the development of standards
2. Service: a professional association
3. Core value: dentists committed to the public's oral health, ethics, science and professional advancement

ELEMENTS OF A PROCEDURAL MANUAL

Practice Philosophy
- Mission Statement
- Vision Statement
- Goals and Objectives

General Instructions
- Mission Statement for the Manual (team mission statement)
- How to Use the Manual
- Responsibility for Updating and Revising

Personnel Procedures
- Hiring
- Work Schedules
- Job Descriptions
- Benefits
- Dress Codes
- Code of Conduct
- Grievance Procedures
- Reviews and Evaluations
- Termination Procedures

Health Insurance Portability and Accountability Act (HIPAA) Procedures
- Identify Who Manages HIPAA Compliance
- Establish a Plan for Compliance
- Identify the Components of HIPAA
- Describe the Roles and Responsibilities of Various Members of the Dental Healthcare Team

Mandated State and Federal Requirements
- Health and Safety
- Federally Mandated Employment Laws
- Federal Healthcare Reform
- Electronic Health Records

Business Office Procedures
- Specific Duties and Job Descriptions (detailed descriptions of each procedure and duty performed in the business office)
- Records Management Protocol (detailed information for each type of record)
- Ordering Information for All Supplies and Equipment

Clinical Area Procedures
- Specific Duties and Job Descriptions (detailed description of each procedure and duty performed in the clinical area, including identification of team member responsibilities)
- Description of the Inventory Procedure
- Description of the Hazardous Material Program
- Outline of Emergency Procedures

COMMUNICATIONS

Personal Communications

The basic rules of communication are outlined in Chapter 3. These rules and concepts apply to communication in general and can be used to enhance communication among members of the dental healthcare team.

Barriers to communication listed in Chapter 3 (semantics, jargon, credibility, preconceived ideas, emotions, stereotyping, noise, conflicting nonverbal communications) can be expanded and applied to communications among team members. It is an ongoing task to evaluate the communication skills of the team and to identify barriers that exist.

Organizational Communications

One of the most important elements of creating a dental healthcare team is the establishment and practice of effective communications. Similar to communications with patients, communications between team members must be effective. A team cannot perform at its highest potential if it has no communication skills. Communication includes the spoken word, the written word, and body language (see Chapter 3). Effective communication can be accomplished when there is a policy of open communication. This allows for identification of problems and provides a means for conflict resolution without the stress and anger that can occur with ineffective communications.

Channels

Information is transferred through a variety of different channels (directions): formal downward channels, horizontal channels, upward channels, and informal channels. The method or medium of communication is referred to as the *communication network*. Channels and networks are necessary means of facilitating organizational communication. Improper use of channels and networks is a characteristic of an ineffective dental healthcare team.

Formal Downward Channels

A formal downward channel of communication can best be described as communication that originates at the top of the organizational structure and moves downward. Several different types of organizational structure may be used (Figure 6-1). One common element within all structures is that one person or group is at the top of the structure. This can be the chief executive officer (CEO), the president, a board of directors, the manager, or the dentist.

TYPES OF COMMUNICATIONS SENT THROUGH A FORMAL DOWNWARD CHANNEL

- Policies
- Vision
- Goals
- Changes in rules and procedures
- Job designs
- Performance appraisals

Although several people or groups may participate in designing, writing, and implementing ideas and functions, ultimate responsibility rests at the top of the organization and is formally communicated downward to others (Figure 6-2).

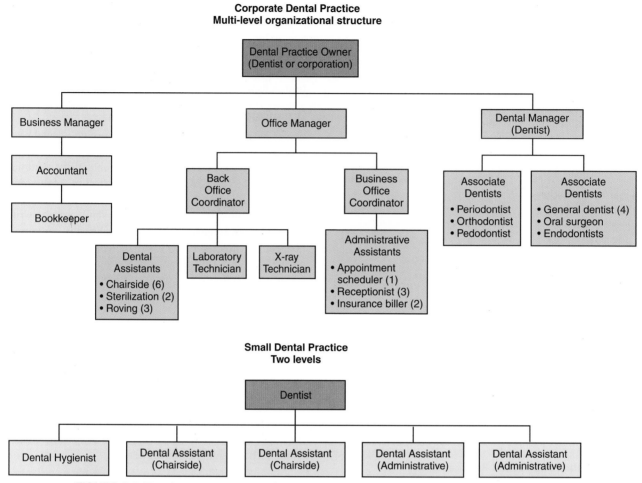

**Corporate Dental Practice
Multi-level organizational structure**

FIGURE 6-1 *Top,* Organizational chart of a business that is structured in several levels, typical of a large or corporate dental practice. *Bottom,* Organizational chart of a business consisting of two levels, typical of a small dental practice.

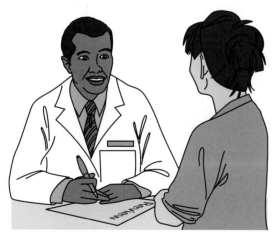

FIGURE 6-2 Example of a downward communications channel.

Horizontal Channel

When communication goes across (horizontally) the organizational structure, it is transmitted between the members. The horizontal channel of communication is used primarily by members at the same level.

Upward Channel

For the dental healthcare team to work well together, there must be a means by which those at the lower level of the organizational structure can communicate with those at higher levels of the structure. An upward channel of communication is the flow of information from one level to a higher level. This can take place between two layers or can move upward through all layers. In most cases, this communication must move sequentially through all levels.

TYPES OF COMMUNICATIONS SENT THROUGH AN UPWARD COMMUNICATION CHANNEL

- Feedback
- Requests for assistance
- Problem solving
- Conflict resolution

TYPES OF COMMUNICATIONS SENT THROUGH A HORIZONTAL CHANNEL

- Goal setting
- Defining of goals and roles
- Improving methods of maintaining working relations
- Gathering and processing of information
- Sharing of day-to-day information

In a dental office, horizontal communications can and will include all members of the team and will affect how they relate to patients and how well they work together on a daily basis (Figure 6-3).

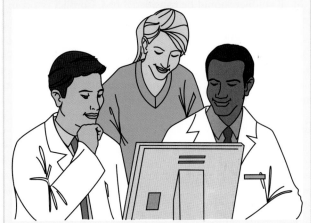

FIGURE 6-3 Example of a horizontal communications channel.

A typical dental practice will have only two or three layers of organizational structure. It is vital for a successful team to be able to communicate in an upward direction, as well as downward and horizontally (Figure 6-4).

► WHAT WOULD YOU DO?

There are three administrative dental assistants responsible for updating patient information (change in billing address, change in insurance coverage, or change in the patient's health). You have noticed that there has been inconsistency in when and how patient information is updated. Sometimes information is updated when the patient first arrives, other times not until they check out, and more often lately is forgotten completely. The dentist has asked you to develop a plan to improve the process. Describe your plan. How will you communicate the information to the other two assistants?

Informal Channel

Informal channels of communication are often referred to as "the grapevine." This type of communication takes place in an informal setting and does not include the official communications of the organization. Informal communications can be accurate or inaccurate. A good manager listens carefully to informal communications because they are a good indicator of the mood of staff members and reveal how they

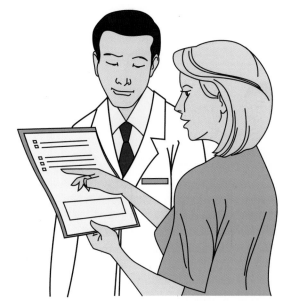

FIGURE 6-4 Example of an upward communications channel.

perceive formal communications. When questions are asked in an informal setting, this may be an indication that the communication process is not effective and that employees do not understand the messages. Additionally, if there is an atmosphere of mistrust, informal communication may be the only way that employees have to state their position. Informal communications can be very destructive when employees use their time to repeat gossip and rumors about patients, fellow employees, or the management staff.

✚ HIPAA

Privacy Rule: Protecting Personal Health Information (PHI)

- Do not discuss a patient's PHI if it may be overheard by other patients

TYPES OF COMMUNICATIONS SENT THROUGH AN INFORMAL COMMUNICATION CHANNEL

- Rumors
- Gossip
- Accurate information
- Inaccurate information
- Sharing and helping (informal)

Members of the dental healthcare team must be very careful about how they use informal communications. Patients have the right of confidentiality and this can be broken by gossip and rumors (in many cases, information is communicated without the knowledge of other team members). The layout of a dental practice is such that patients can overhear informal conversations between members of the dental

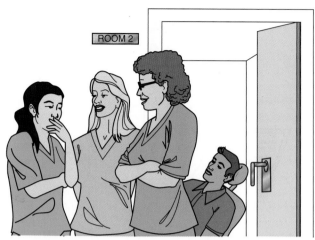

FIGURE 6-5 Example of an informal communications channel.

healthcare team; therefore it is vital that informal conversations be limited (Figure 6-5).

Organizational Barriers to Communication

Organizational barriers to communication create an undesirable environment for members of the dental healthcare team and the patients they serve. Stress due to poor communication is easily perceived by patients. Patients can feel the tension and may begin to question the motives of the dental healthcare team. Some communication barriers encountered in the dental office are the following:

- Work overload: Any amount or type of work that adds to daily stress. When employees feel the stress of work overload, they do not take the time to communicate effectively. In a dental practice, work overload can be caused by the volume of work or by performing more than one job, filling in for an absent employee, accommodating emergency patients, constantly answering the telephone, and not managing time effectively.
- Filtering by level: Information sent is not received because it has been changed or stopped at some level. If, as an administrative dental assistant, you send a message or idea to the dentist and it is stopped or changed by the office manager, there is a breakdown in the upward flow of the message.
- Timing: A good idea not presented at the right time or in the right manner will not be accepted.
- Lack of trust and openness: When feedback is not accepted, it is very difficult to communicate effectively. This can occur at all levels of the organization and leads to conflict.
- Inappropriate span of control: This leads to lack of trust and fuels resentment. It may be the result of poor communication, lack of direction, or poor or nonexistent policies and procedures.
- Change: When not accepted or understood, change places a barrier on communication. For some people, change is perceived as a negative. Good communication provides a means of discussing the need for change and how it will improve the organization.

- Rank and status: Some people use position (rank) as a form of power over others, which closes channels of communication.
- Electronic noise: In a dental office, it is common to encounter electronic noise from high-speed handpieces and other electronic equipment. This hinders communication of the full message (message sent is not heard and feedback is incomplete).

ORGANIZATIONAL CONFLICTS

Not all conflict should be considered bad. Conflict is a common experience in any relationship. How we use conflict determines its benefit. If conflict is used as a weapon and is destructive, it is considered to be nonfunctional. If conflict is used as a means to identify a problem and improve a situation, it can be viewed as a valuable tool for change and improvement.

Constructive

Conflict can be constructive if:
- Team members improve their decision-making skills
- Different solutions to a problem are identified
- New solutions are developed
- Group solutions are devised for shared problems
- Team members find new ways to state their problems
- Team members are stimulated to become more creative, resulting in growth
- Individual and team performance is improved

Destructive

Conflict can be destructive if it:
- Causes unhealthy stress, leading to job burnout
- Reduces communications
- Produces an atmosphere of cynicism and mistrust
- Reduces job performance
- Increases resistance to change
- Affects quality of patient care

Classifying Conflict

Conflict has many different meanings and sources. Organizational conflict can be described as intraorganizational conflict (within the organization) and interorganizational conflict (between two or more organizations). Intraorganizational conflict can also be divided into levels between groups, departments, and individuals. There are four types of intraorganizational conflict:

- Intrapersonal conflict: Intrapersonal conflict (within oneself) occurs when an individual is expected to perform a task that does not meet his or her personal goals, values, beliefs, or expertise. For example, the dental hygienist who has to clean the darkroom may feel that this is not in her job description and is below her level of training.
- Interpersonal conflict: Interpersonal conflict (between two team members) occurs when members of the team at the same level (assistant and assistant) or different levels (hygienist and assistant) disagree about a given matter.

This can occur between any two or more members of the dental healthcare team.

- **Intragroup conflict:** Intragroup conflict (within the group) occurs among members at the same level (assistant and assistant, dentist and dentist). This conflict usually occurs when there are differences in goals, tasks, and procedures.
- **Intergroup conflict:** Intergroup conflict (between two or more groups) occurs when members of one group are in disagreement with members of another group. For example, dental assistants may be in conflict with the management staff if the vacation schedule is set without personal consultation with each staff member. Conflict can also occur when dentists and hygienists do not agree with the Dental Practice Act.

Conflict-Handling Styles

The type of conflict, who is involved, and the amount of time that has elapsed before the problem is addressed determine which conflict style should be used to address the problem. There are appropriate and inappropriate situations for each style. Not every problem can be solved in the same manner and the manner chosen may determine whether resolution is successful. Conflict resolution is a complex process that takes time, knowledge, and understanding. The following are some suggestions for selecting the appropriate resolution style:

CONFLICT-HANDLING STYLES

Ways of handling conflict have been studied and identified by many researchers. Rahim describes the following styles:

- **Integrating style:** High concern for self and others (also known as *problem solving*). This style is collaborative because both parties work together in openness, exchanging information to achieve an equitable solution.
- **Obliging style:** Low concern for self and high concern for others (also known as *accommodating*). This style is one of self-sacrifice and giving to others.
- **Dominating style:** High concern for self and low concern for others (also known as *competing*). This type of person has a win–lose mentality and goes out to win with little regard for others. This person is usually very competitive.
- **Avoiding style:** Low concern for self and others (also known as *suppression*). This style is associated with side-stepping and buck passing. People who use this style avoid issues so as not to be in conflict with themselves and others and appear not to be aware of conflicts when they occur.
- **Compromising style:** Intermediate in concern for self and others. With this style, there is a give-and-take attitude; compromise is the key and both parties are willing to give up something to arrive at a solution.

Data from Rahim MA: *Managing conflict in organizations,* ed 2, Westport, Conn, 1992, Praeger.

- **Integrating style:** This style works best when time is available to address the problem. Usually, problems are complex and their resolution requires the expertise of more than one person. The problem must be identified and then input from all members is needed to develop a solution.

Once the solution is developed, the support of the full team is needed to implement the changes. Good communication is essential when this style is used. It is inappropriate to use this style when the problem is simple, when a decision is needed at once, or when other parties are unwilling to contribute or do not have the necessary problem-solving skills.

- **Obliging style:** This style is used when the issue is unimportant and someone is willing to defer to the other party to preserve a relationship. It is sometimes used by people who are unsure about whether they are correct. It would be inappropriate to use this style if you believe that the other person is wrong or is behaving unethically.
- **Dominating style:** This style is used when a decision must be made quickly and the results are trivial. It is also appropriate when an unpopular course of action is needed, when the decisions of others will be costly, or when an overly aggressive subordinate must be managed. This style is inappropriate when an issue is complex, when decisions do not have to be made quickly, or when both parties are equal in status or power.
- **Avoiding style:** This style is best used when an issue is trivial, when a cooling-off period is needed, or when the benefits do not go beyond the discord that the style will cause between the involved parties. It is inappropriate when the issue is important, when it is someone's responsibility to make a decision, or when a decision is needed quickly.
- **Compromising style:** This style is best used when both parties are equally powerful, when a consensus cannot be reached, when an integrating or dominating style is not successful, or when a temporary solution to a complex problem is needed. It is not appropriate when a problem is complex and requires problem-solving skills or when one party is more powerful than the other.

▶ WHAT WOULD YOU DO?

What did you do to solve the inconsistency in patient information recording in the previous What Would You Do box? What was your approach and how did you communicate the information? What type of conflict do you think your approach might produce? Describe how you would use the conflict to produce a constructive and positive outcome.

STAFF MEETINGS

Staff meetings serve several different functions. They can be formal, informal, social, and so forth. Staff meetings should always be constructive and never be destructive. They may serve as an effective tool for organizational communication and problem solving. The type and duration of the meeting depend on its purpose. Short meetings at the beginning of each day may be needed to prepare members of the dental healthcare team for their day (Figure 6-6). Clinical charts are reviewed and potentially difficult situations are identified. Longer staff meetings may include a week-long retreat to a resort. This type of meeting combines work and social interaction.

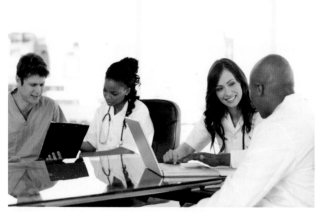

FIGURE 6-6 Morning team huddle technique to review charts and prepare for the day. (Copyright © 2012 Wavebreakmedia, iStock.com. All rights reserved.)

All types of meetings require a preset protocol. Setting of ground rules for a meeting helps to eliminate potential barriers when an unexpected gripe session evolves. Common guidelines for staff meetings are discussed in the following sections.

Before the Meeting

- Identify the type of meeting that will be held—that is, formal or informal. Describe the purpose of the meeting—that is, to share information (exchange of ideas or knowledge), to solve problems, or to set goals. Establish a protocol and set the ground rules for various types of meetings.
- Set a date and time. Establish dates well in advance so that schedules can be set and do not change the date if at all possible. Regular meetings can be set a year in advance. When meetings are scheduled weekly or even monthly, they will be viewed as normal. Try to avoid having meetings only when there is a problem.
- Develop an agenda. Appoint a team member to act as facilitator, note taker, and time keeper. Seek input from others on items they would like to include on the agenda. Agendas should include a review of minutes from the previous meeting, reports, old business, and new business. Post the agenda a few days in advance of the meeting.

During the Meeting

- Each member receives a copy of the agenda.
- The facilitator moves the meeting forward according to the agenda. It is easy for meetings to get out of hand if the protocol is not followed. The facilitator ensures that everyone follows the guidelines and keeps everyone focused.
- The note taker keeps notes. The notes are later typed; one copy is placed in a record book and other copies are given to members present at the next meeting. Notes serve as documentation and as a method of recording what was discussed, who is responsible for implementing change or following through on actions decided on, and what was decided. It is very important to keep records of meetings for future reference.
- Each team member is given an opportunity to voice opinions and to help in problem solving. It is also vital that one or two people should not be allowed to dominate the meeting. It is the duty of the facilitator to keep everything positive.
- The time keeper helps the facilitator to move the meeting along. When there is much work to be accomplished in a short time, the responsibility of the time keeper is very important.

After the Meeting

- Minutes are typed and properly distributed.
- Those who were assigned tasks must carry them out.

 WHAT WOULD YOU DO?

You have been asked to organize the next staff meeting. The topic will be to write the dress code for the procedural manual. How will you approach the topic?

KEY POINTS

- An effective dental healthcare team requires:
  - Shared philosophy
  - Excellent communication skills
  - The desire to grow and change
  - The ability to be flexible while providing quality care for all patients
- A dental practice **procedural manual** is a form of written communication. It is a reference for all team members. This resource provides each team member with specific details about practice goals, personnel procedures, business office procedures, and clinical procedures.

- Effective **organizational communications** are accomplished when the lines of communication are open. This allows for identification of problems and provides a means for conflict resolution without the stress and anger that can result from ineffective communication. The channels of organizational communications are as follows:
  - Downward
  - Horizontal
  - Upward
  - Informal

- Barriers to organizational communications include the following:
  - Work overload
  - Filtering by level
  - Timing
  - Lack of trust and openness
  - Inappropriate span of control
  - Change
  - Rank and status
  - Electronic noise
- **Organizational conflict** is common. How conflict is dealt with determines its benefit. If conflict is used as a weapon and is destructive, it is nonfunctional. If conflict is used as a means to identify a problem and improve the organization, it can be a valuable tool for change and improvement. Classifications of organizational conflict are listed here:
  - Intrapersonal conflict
  - Interpersonal conflict
  - Intragroup conflict
  - Intergroup conflict
- **Handling conflict** can be done appropriately or inappropriately. Results depend on the style used to resolve the conflict. Conflict resolution can be accomplished with use of the following styles:
  - Integrating style
  - Obliging style
  - Dominating style
  - Avoiding style
  - Compromising style
- **Staff meetings** serve various functions. They can be formal, informal, or social. They should always be constructive and never be destructive.

CAREER-READY PRACTICES

Career-Ready Practices activities are designed to provide students with experiences that can be "practiced" in preparation for skills needed on the job. In each of the following exercises, a variety of approaches may be used to address the problem, rather than "right" or "wrong" answers. Below each exercise, next to the compass icon, is a listing of suggested Career-Ready Practice numbers that correspond to the listing of 12 practices in the front of the text (see p. viii-ix); these practices provide suggestions for approaches to complete the exercise.

1. As the office manager, you have just hired a new chairside dental assistant, Greg. After the first week, you have had several patients compliment Greg on his abilities and personality. However, a few have mentioned that he must like to stay up late because it looks as if he has just jumped out of bed. His hair is messy and looks dirty and his scrubs are wrinkled. Describe how you will solve the problem.

 Career-Ready Practices
8 *Utilize critical thinking to make sense of problems and persevere in solving them.*
1 *Act as a responsible and contributing citizen and employee.*
5 *Consider the environmental, social, and economic impacts of decisions.*

2. The dentist has realized that the problem described above goes beyond Greg. In small groups, discuss how you solved the "Greg problem" and what professional standards you feel are required for the entire dental healthcare team. Draft a new section for your office procedural manual that describes the dress code for the entire office (male and female) and present your proposal at the next staff meeting. As a large group, after all of the proposals have been presented, come to a consensus on what needs to be included in the new policy.

 Career-Ready Practices
9 *Model integrity, ethical leadership, and effective management.*
8 *Utilize critical thinking to make sense of problems and persevere in solving them.*
4 *Communicate clearly, effectively, and with reason.*
3 *Attend to personal health and financial well-being.*

3. Write a short, reflective paper on why you feel it is necessary to have office policies.

 Career-Ready Practices
1 *Act as a responsible and contributing citizen and employee.*
9 *Model integrity, ethical leadership, and effective management.*
4 *Communicate clearly, effectively, and with reason.*

4. Amber is an office manager. She has worked her way up the dental assisting ladder (chairside assistant for 12 years, administrative dental assistant for 3 years, office manager for 1 year). James is a chairside assistant with 6 years of experience. He is very good with patients and his assisting skills are excellent. Amber and James disagree about patient scheduling procedures. He is concerned because patients are squeezed into the schedule when needed and dental treatment is diagnosed during their recall appointments. Treatments take about 30 minutes for the dentist to complete. Amber wants patients seen on the days they request, to save them an extra trip but most of all because this will boost daily production. James is concerned because when an extra patient is squeezed in, the following happens: Patients with scheduled appointments must wait longer because of the addition to the schedule; when the

schedule runs late, one of the assistants must stay during lunch or after work; and the dentist does not take a position because Amber has been a loyal employee for 16 years.

- What types of organizational conflict are involved?
- What style of conflict resolution would you use to solve this problem? Why?
- How would you solve the problem?

 Career-Ready Practices

5 *Consider the environmental, social, and economic impacts of decisions.*

8 *Utilize critical thinking to make sense of problems and persevere in solving them.*

4 *Communicate clearly, effectively, and with reason.*

9 *Model integrity, ethical leadership, and effective management.*

PART III

Managing Dental Office Systems

7 Computerized Dental Practice, 92

8 Patient Clinical Records, 107

9 Information Management, 136

10 Dental Patient Scheduling, 149

11 Recall Systems, 163

12 Inventory Management, 173

13 Office Equipment, 188

Computerized Dental Practice

LEARNING OBJECTIVES

1. Compare the basic and advanced functions of dental practice management software and discuss their application.
2. Explain how to select a dental practice management system and list the functions to consider during the selection process.
3. Discuss the role of the administrative dental assistant in the operation of a computerized dental practice.
4. Identify the daily computer tasks performed by the administrative dental assistant, including the importance of a computer system backup routine.

INTRODUCTION

If you are a digital native (born after 1988), you have grown up in the digital world. The use of computers, cellphones, smartphones, iPods, video games, and other digital tools has always been a part of your world. This is not the case for those of us who are considered immigrants to the digital world. We have performed many tasks in the dental office without the aid of a computer. We have manually maintained clinical records, written in an appointment book, used a one-write (pegboard) system, and manually submitted dental insurance claim forms. Although these practices are still used in many offices, the use of digital technology has become the standard in the majority of dental practices. The fully integrated digital dental practice integrates the functionality of several software systems to seamlessly gather, process, connect, and store digital information, connecting the business office with the clinical practice.

The computerized dental practice management system is an integrated system of software or application suites that are seamlessly linked to perform related functions. These powerful software suites connect the dental business office to the clinical treatment area and eliminate the need to store patient information on paper. At its basic level the software should store patient records, the practice schedule, and all business. Advanced capabilities can be added, such as digital imaging, integrated workstations, insurance processing, and patient communications. The ability to customize desired functions is a key to enhance patient care and increase the dental practice profitability.

BASIC SYSTEMS

Patient Dental Records Management

Patient records software will provide a platform for the dental office to gather patient information to build the patient's electronic health record (EHR). These data elements are the same as the information needed to create a paper patient record (see Chapter 8). Initially the patient may enter his or her personal information and medical and dental histories by completing online questionnaires. The questionnaires can be completed through a secure web-based portal or directly in the system at the dental office. Paper documents also can be scanned and entered into the system. In a basic system, the data entry task may be assigned to a member of the dental healthcare team. After the initial entry, the record becomes part of the office workflow and entries are made by various members of the dental healthcare team and through the integration of other software applications.

Basic Patient Information

- Communications with referring or referral dentist and/or physicians
- Database information, such as name, birth date, address, and contact information
- Diagnostic records, including charts and study models
- Health Insurance Portability and Accountability Act (HIPAA) documents, consent forms, waivers, and authorizations
- Medical and dental histories, notes, and updates
- Medication prescriptions, including types, dose, amount, directions for use, and number of refills
- Patient communications, including postoperative or home instructions, complaints and resolutions, conversations, and correspondence
- Place of employment and insurance plans
- Progress and treatment notes
- Proposed treatment notes, including nature of proposed treatment, potential benefits and risks associate with alternative treatment, or the risks of no treatment
- Radiographs
- Recall and reactivation recommendations
- Treatment plan notes

Basic Business Functions

The basic business functions of a computerized system streamline the business functions that take place on a daily bases and integrate the basic functions of posting dental treatment, generating insurance claim forms, electronic scheduling, and reporting. Integrating these tasks will maximize the efficiency of the dental practice and save time.

Process Insurance Information

- Accommodate multiple providers
- Database of insurance carriers, including group plans, deductibles, fee schedules, and allowable benefits
- Determine the patient portion based on information stored in the database
- Generate insurance claims
- Process claims for preauthorization
- Track unpaid claims

Perform Accounting Tasks

- Accounts receivable aging reports
- Basic credit and debit card processing
- Post transactions (payments, charges, and adjustments)
- Profit and loss statements
- Use a coding system for insurance processing and accounting reports

Perform Recall and Reactivation Procedures

- Generate notices
- Identify patients who have not completed treatment plans
- List patients who are due for recall
- Track overdue recall

Maintain an Audit Trail

- Identify patients scheduled without a charge or entry
- Identify patients with incomplete transactions
- List scheduled patients daily
- Mark entries with date of entry, time, and employee identification (hidden information)

Perform Electronic Scheduling

- Color code types of treatment
- Customize matrixing of the scheduler
- Print daily routing slips
- Produce electronic reminders for patients
- Schedule and track appointments
- Schedule by treatment room or provider
- Set production goals
- Track patients who missed or canceled appointments

Provide Software Security

- HIPAA and Health Information Technology for Economic and Clinical Health (HITECH) Act compliants
- Online backup
- Prevent unauthorized entry to the system

Provide Training and Support

- Initial systems training and transition
- On demand training and support
- Upgrades

Additional Software Suites

There are many software suites that provide additional tools and resources needed to achieve a higher level of productivity. These applications can create a seamless workflow that enhances patient care and increases profitability. Information such as patient treatment, digital imaging, treatment planning, and appointment scheduling is connected instantly to the patient record. Software suites also perform non–treatment-related tasks, such as communicating with patients, managing inventory, connecting with financial institutions, and linking to vendors and other dental professionals. Mobile access allows authorized members of the dental healthcare team to view patient information, financial information, and the practice schedule on many different devices, such as smartphones, tablets, and computers. For security reasons, information is never stored on these devices. This application is very useful when there is more than one office location, as it allows the patient to be seen at any of the practice locations by eliminating the need for multiple patient records. By incorporating these functions and services, the dental healthcare team will save time, which will allow them to concentrate on providing outstanding patient care.

Patient Communications Applications

- Dental education with images and videos that can be customized for the patient in the language of their choice.
- Integrated website
- Patient billing sent automatically
- Patient online access to their dental information: update contact and health information, review treatment, schedule appointments, and make payments 24/7
- Presentation of treatment plans incorporating digital imaging
- Send reminder e-mails, text messages, and postcards to patients automatically

Workflow Applications

- Access data from any computer or device
- Allow for real-time recording and viewing of information (when data are entered they are instantly available on the network)
- Computer-based interoffice communications
- Electronic data transfer for sharing information with vendors, ordering supplies, and lab work
- Mobile access so that information such as patient records, financial information, and the schedule can be viewed from anywhere 24/7
- Order and track patient prescriptions
- Patient checkout can take place from any workstation
- Produce tickler files to remind staff of tasks
- Submit insurance claims electronically

Integrated Clinical Workstation Applications

- Communicate treatment plans
- Digital imaging (radiographs and intraoral images)
- Periodontal charting
- Progress notes

- Treatment and tooth charting
- Update medical and dental histories

Business Tool Applications

- Automated e-mail and text messaging for appointment confirmation
- Automated patient billing
- Customized reports, including production reports and accounts payable and receivable reports

- Cyber security
- Data management, storage, and backup
- Electronic funds transfer (EFT) banking
- Electronic insurance eligibility verification
- Integrated credit and debit card processing
- Integrated third-party credit processing
- Integrated website hosting
- Marketing
- Remote appointment management

✚ HIPAA

HIPAA Standards

Practice management software programs provide the data fields needed to enter information necessary for compliance with HIPAA standards. The following screen shots are examples of how a program may address the four different HIPAA standards.

Security Rule

Password protection is one method of securing electronic protected health information (ePHI).

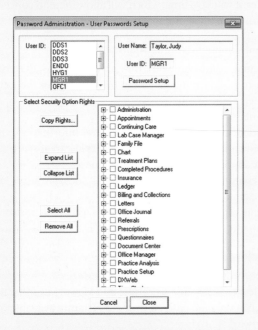

National Provider Identifier Standard

The National Provider Identifier (NPI) Standard is required on all electronic transactions.

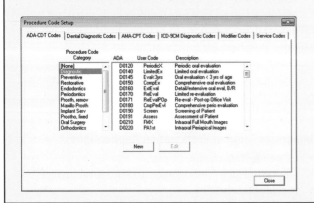

Electronic Transactions and Code Sets

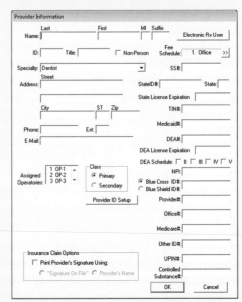

Examples of Code on Dental Procedures and Nomenclature (CDT Code) include procedure code category (standardized), American Dental Association (ADA) or current dental terminology (CDT) code (standardized), user code (unique to software program), and description (unique to software program).

Provider Specialties

Provider specialties are listed in the Provider Information window for selection. Dentrix comes with the following specialties:
1. 122300000X Dentist
2. 126800000X Dental Assistant
3. 124Q0000X Dental Hygienist
4. 1223D0001X Dental Public Health
5. 1223E0200X Endodontics
6. 1223X0400X Orthodontics
7. 1223P0106X Pathology, Oral and Maxillofacial
8. 1223P0221X Pediatric Dentistry
9. 1223P0300X Periodontics
10. 1223P0700X Prosthodontics
11. 1223S0112X Surgery, Oral and Maxillofacial
12. 126900000X Dental Laboratory Technician
13. 1223G0001X General Practice
14. 1223X0008X Oral and Maxillofacial Radiology

Examples of the Healthcare Providers Taxonomy Code list used in HIPAA transactions.

Dentrix screen shots courtesy Henry Schein Practice Solutions, American Fork, Utah.

SELECTING A PRACTICE MANAGEMENT SYSTEM

Before software suites are selected, it is necessary to assess the need for a system. Questions should be asked and careful consideration should be given before a package is selected. One way to accomplish this is to meet with all those who will have a stake in the system: dentist, business manager, accountant, associate dentists, hygienists, and administrative dental assistants. These people will provide feedback on what they consider important. Accountants and dentists may be interested in the types of reports generated. Hygienists will want to look at the recall function and administrative dental assistants will want to know how the system will help them with paperwork (maintaining patient records, posting transactions, sending statements, and completing insurance claims). Each individual will provide valuable information and identify different needs of the dental practice.

After basic needs have been determined, the next step is to assess additional services and functions that are needed. Most software vendors provide complex questionnaires to help dental personnel identify what they want and what they need in a package. Not all systems offer the same services and features. It is important for dental personnel to select a package that will meet their needs and provide them with the support they need to run the software.

FUNCTIONS TO CONSIDER WHEN SELECTING A SOFTWARE PACKAGE

Many different functions should be considered when a software package is selected: general requirements, patient information, patient billing, treatment planning, insurance processing, recall and reactivation, practice management reports, electronic scheduling, database management and word processing, clinical integration, and HIPAA requirements for system security. Not all functions will be important to all dental practices. The following questions and descriptions of common function can be used to identify what may or may not be important functions for the dental practice. Once target functions have been identified, the next step is to compare the functions of software packages and select the package that will meet the needs of the practice. Although this process is time consuming, it is essential.

Questions to consider when selecting a software vendor:
1. What type of financial functions are provided? Are they what you need? Do they provide accurate reports?
2. What is the total cost? What is the cost for additional services? What is the maintenance fee? Is there a monthly service fee?
3. Is it a complete system that meets your current needs? Can it accommodate additional software integration as the need arises?
4. Does the flow of the software match the practice workflow?
5. Will the software help to keep the schedule full? Will it predict actual income from the schedule? How does it optimize productivity?
6. What type of support and training is available? How will it support system conversation? Will the training be adequate for the staff? How are upgrades supported?

General Requirements

General requirements are those elements of the software program that permit it to perform different functions. These functions are typically not seen by the user but are necessary for the intended function and security of the program.
- Security systems protect the integrity of the information stored. Those who operate the software are given passwords and must follow established HIPAA protocol to ensure the integrity of electronic protected health information (ePHI).
- Data that are transmitted and stored on servers (in house or remote) meet the established security standards.
- Audit trails identify who entered or edited information. This is important for a paperless dental practice because it records all changes to information and identifies who made the changes and on what date; it also meets the mandates of the HIPAA Security Rule.
- Those with access to the software may be assigned different levels of access. This protects the system from unauthorized changes to system functions.
- The system can purge inactive accounts automatically.
- Some systems support clinical applications: tooth charting, periodontal charting, digital radiographs, and imaging.
- Context-sensitive help screens are useful.
- The system permits error checking to correct erroneous dates and tooth numbers, thereby preventing incorrect tooth surfaces from being entered.
- The system allows you to move between screens without returning to the main menu.
- The system allows print options, such as starting from where you left off, using preprinted forms, and creating documents with a laser printer.
- The system can track more than one provider and provide multiple fee schedules.

Patient Information

Functions that help the administrative dental assistant to organize patient information include the following.
- Locate a patient by name or number.
- Scan or directly enter information into the system, such as patient history, medical and dental histories, laboratory reports, insurance correspondence, and referral letters.
- Use two different addresses for each patient, such as home address and billing address.
- Correct errors within fields without retyping the complete field.
- Automatically capitalize names, addresses, cities, and so forth.
- Use coded information for repeated information, such as zip codes matched with cities, insurance carrier information for common carriers, and group and employer information for patients with common employers.

- Integrate patient clinical records, treatment notes, medical history, and registration information into the system to create a paperless dental practice.

Patient Billing

Patient billing should be flexible and should offer the dental practice more than one way to produce statements. Statements include monthly billing statements, budget plan statements, and walkout statements. These statements can be produced in the dental office or they can be an integrated third-party service.

Patient Checkout

- Produce walkout statements for each patient.
- Generate an insurance form.
- List the next appointment or series of appointments and state what treatments will be provided.
- Facilitate the use of credit cards, debit cards, and third-party payment options.

Patient Statements

- Produce one statement for each patient.
- Customize patient messages, such as collection notes and recall notices.
- Customize for different providers within the same dental practice.
- Print budget plans, interest charges, and truth-in-lending statements.
- Itemize insurance payments, patient portions, and calculated adjustments.

Billing Statements in Cycles

- Produce billing statements for accounts that are overdue at specific times, such as every 30 days.

Year-End Summaries

- List all treatments.
- List all payments made by the patient for tax reporting.

Treatment Planning

Treatment planning is an important component of practice management software. With several options available, the administrative dental assistant is able to efficiently develop a clear and concise plan for patients.

- Print treatment plans and options.
- Prioritize treatments for long-range planning.
- Integrate the treatment plan with insurance information to show all treatments for the year, deductibles, and patient portion.
- Provide online access for the patient to view treatment plans.

Insurance Processing

The system allows the administrative dental assistant to submit claims daily, track all claims, and print reports for follow-up. The dental practice or a third-party vendor can perform these services.

The program knows what additional information, such as a radiograph or a report, is needed for a specific procedure and prompts the user for that additional information.

- Claims can be printed a second time so that lost claims are replaced.
- The system prompts the user to submit insurance claims.
- The system prompts the user to submit secondary insurance claims after the primary insurance company pays.
- The system can separate treatment dates if the patient changes insurance carriers midway through treatment.
- The complete insurance form is filled out, including the charting of missing teeth.
- Orthodontic treatments can be billed cyclically.
- The system can generate medical claims, including correct International Classification of Diseases (ICD)-10 and diagnostic codes.
- When a procedure code is entered, the system automatically files the correct dental or medical claim form using the appropriate HIPAA transaction and code sets.
- The system stores fees reported on paid insurance claims, creating a database that is accurate when estimating the insurance company's portion.
- The system can estimate the insurance company's portion by considering deductibles and remaining insurance or unused benefits and coordinating benefits for primary and secondary insurance companies.
- Notations and procedures can be entered on the patient insurance form but not on the patient statement.
- Narratives can be added to both printed and electronic insurance forms.
- In group practices, the provider of the service can be identified on the individual claim form, even if the provider changes from visit to visit.
- The system can track patients who have not completed preauthorized dental treatment plans.
- The system can submit claims electronically with digital images.

Recall and Reactivation

In a computerized system, information stored in the database is used to generate notices automatically and produce reports that identify patients who are scheduled for recall and reactivation.

- Recall dates for an entire family are easily identified in account and patient records.
- Recall dates can be customized at various monthly intervals (1 month, 2 months, 3 months, 4 months, 5 months, 6 months, or longer).
- The system alerts the user if the recall does not meet the insurance company's standard.
- Recall notices for all patients due in a month are produced automatically.
- Selected recall letters, e-mails, text messages, or cards are produced automatically.
- Appointment notices for patients who are scheduled with the electronic scheduler are produced automatically.

- Patients are tracked for recall compliance and tracking reports and notices to patients who do not keep appointments are generated.
- The type of recall is identified and notices are customized to match the type of recall.
- Patients with incomplete treatment are tracked with lists and letters to gain compliance are generated.
- Patients who are due for recall are listed until they schedule and keep an appointment or wish to be removed from the list.

Management Reports

A number of reports can be generated, depending on the needs of the practice.

- Produce age accounts, which are customized reports showing the oldest account, past due budget plans, and the largest amount past due.
- Produce production reports according to provider (dentist, associate dentist, hygienist) and categorize by hour, day, week, and month.
- Generate reports by transaction code.
- Produce insurance reports that show the amounts billed to different carriers and then age the amount due.
- Customize reports according to the needs of the dental practice.
- Be flexible in generating the types and designs of reports required to meet the individual needs of the practice.

Electronic Scheduler

The electronic scheduler is the digital version of the appointment book. An electronic scheduler aids the administrative dental assistant in organizing and maximizing the schedule for efficiency.

- Allows the scheduling of patients 1 year in advance.
- Allows the scheduler to leave one screen and schedule an appointment for another patient on another screen.
- Keeps a list of patients who wish to come in earlier than their scheduled appointment, including their telephone numbers, the time they wish to come in, and the last time you contacted them.
- Allows the user to matrix the appointment scheduler according to production goals, preferred time of day for emergencies, and high- and low-production procedures.
- Customizes according to dental healthcare provider.
- Schedules by treatment room.
- Generates outside reminders such as meeting notices, to-do lists, and staff reminders.
- Tracks laboratory cases and alerts the staff if the patient is scheduled before the laboratory work will be returned.
- Alerts the scheduling staff if sufficient time is not scheduled between appointments.
- Prints a report of all patients due the next day.
- Runs an audit report to ensure that a charge or entry is made for every patient scheduled.
- Allows the addition of emergency and walk-in patients to the schedule (ensuring that all patients are part of the audit trail).

- Allows daily reports that will age accounts and shows outstanding treatments and medical alerts (for patients with scheduled appointments).
- Automated appointment confirmation.
- Alerts the staff in a group practice if appointments are scheduled with the hygienist when the dentist of record is not scheduled.
- Coordinates schedules when the patient sees more than one provider in the same day.
- Has a find feature for easy access to a patient's record.
- Tracks patients from the time they enter the dental practice until they have completed the checkout process.
- Prints routing slips for all scheduled patients, listing scheduled treatment, recall information, insurance information, and medical alerts.
- Allows the user to customize the routing slip to meet the needs of individual practices.

Database Management and Word Processing

Information stored in the database can be merged into word processing software to create a variety of letters, referrals, and marketing tools.

- The system, under designed conditions, automatically generates letters without staff direction.
- The system keeps track of letters sent to patients and others.
- The system automatically accesses a database to merge letters, reports, and statements by such criteria as past due account information, incomplete dentistry, and scheduling information.
- Word processing programs can be accessed without exiting the dental software.
- The word processor interacts with the scheduler so that it can generate confirmation letters automatically, such as notes confirming preappointed recall visits.
- The system stores commonly used letters and forms and merges information such as name and address to personalize each letter.

Clinical Integration

- A fully integrated system.
- Alerts clinical staff as to when patients enter the practice, what treatment rooms they are assigned to, and what treatments are scheduled for the day.
- Integrates information recorded via an intraoral camera in the patient's digital record.
- Records digital radiographs to the digital record.
- Allows scanning of traditional radiographs to the digital record.
- Uses strategically located monitors in treatment areas to directly record patient information such as clinical findings, periodontal examination results, and treatment notes.
- Allows hands-free chart entries.
- Allows scheduling from any monitor.
- Integrates with other digital devices such as periodontal probes to record the findings.

- Creates a legal paperless clinical record.
- Applies HIPAA Security Rule standards.

BASIC OPERATION OF A SOFTWARE PACKAGE

Although many software packages are available, most offer similar basic features and operations. Most updated and revised editions use a Windows format. Windows offers the ability to complete more than one task at a time. The various screens of these programs have the same basic elements: **title bars, menu bars, tool bars, power bars,** and **status bars.**

ROLES OF THE ADMINISTRATIVE DENTAL ASSISTANT

The roles of the administrative dental assistant vary, depending on the software program used by the dental practice. All programs have some common functions. These common functions include recording patient demographics, posting transactions, using a general database, processing insurance claims, scheduling electronically, and producing reports.

Recording Patient Demographics

In a basic system, patient demographic information is taken from the registration form and entered into the software database by the administrative dental assistant. In an advanced system, the information is entered directly into the system by the patient using a kiosk computer (typically located in the reception area), mobile device such as an iPad, or web-based document service (Figure 7-1).

Creating an Account

A computerized account is the same as a manual account; it identifies the person who is financially responsible for paying the account (Figure 7-2). When all fields are filled in, the system stores this information in its database and uses it to bill patients and complete insurance claim forms. The system assigns an account number that is unique to this account and used to locate the account in the computer database. In a system that uses paperless clinical charts, this information is entered directly into the system once and the database automatically fills in all necessary fields.

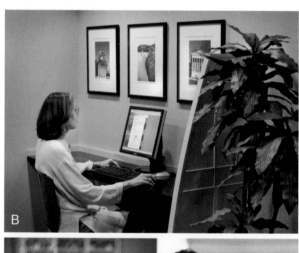

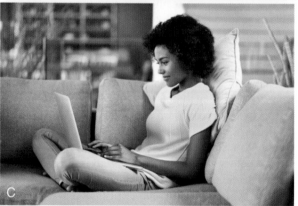

FIGURE 7-1 A, Clipboard with patient registration information form. **B,** Patient completing a patient registration form on a computer kiosk in the dental office. **C,** Patient completing a web-based registration form from home. (**A,** *Clipboard*: Copyright 2006 Devon, AllSmileMedia, Vancouver, Canada. Image from BigStockPhoto.com. *Form*: Courtesy Patterson Office Supplies, Champaign, Ill. **B,** From Hargreaves KM, Cohen S: *Cohen's pathways of the pulp*, ed 10, St. Louis, 2011, Mosby. **C,** Copyright © 2014 PeopleImages, iStock.com. All rights reserved.)

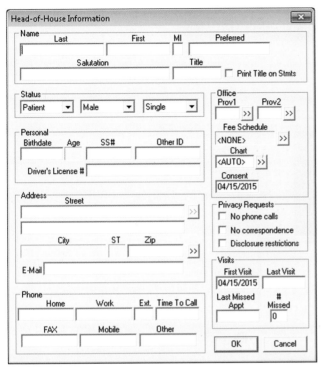

FIGURE 7-2 Head-of-House Information Window. This window shows basic information used to create a family account. The information entered on this screen pertains to the person who is financially responsible for the account (may or may not be the patient and may not be a patient of the dental practice). (Dentrix screen capture courtesy Henry Schein Practice Solutions, American Fork, Utah.)

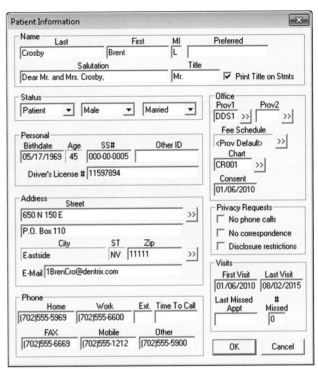

FIGURE 7-3 Patient Information Window. This window is used to enter patient information. The screen also allows the user to assign a provider, fee schedule, chart number, privacy request, and visit history. (Dentrix screen capture courtesy Henry Schein Practice Solutions, American Fork, Utah.)

Maintaining Patient Records

After an account has been established, patient information is entered (Figure 7-3). All information entered, such as address (if different from the account address), date of birth, insurance identification number, medical alert information, student status, and relationship to insurer (this information will be used to complete insurance claims), is directly related to the patient.

More than one patient can be assigned to an account (Figure 7-4). This often occurs in families whose members go to the same dentist. For example, the account number assigned to the Abbott family is ABB 100. When the computer is asked to locate account number ABB 100, it lists all members of the Abbott family who are patients. Each patient is assigned a corresponding patient number: Kim Abbott (father) ABB 101, Patricia Abbott ABB 102, and Timothy Abbott ABB 103.

Posting Transactions

The same functions are available in computerized and manual systems. After treatment has been provided, charges are posted to the patient's computer record (Figure 7-5).

The administrative dental assistant receives information from the treatment area via several different types of communications: patient routing slips, patients' clinical charts, or charge slips. The assistant uses this information during the checkout procedure.

Using a General Database

One advantage of the computerized system is that common information may be shared. Information that will be common to all accounts includes insurance carrier identification (Figure 7-6), transaction codes (Figure 7-7), and provider demographics (Figure 7-8). This information is entered only once into the system. A series of codes are assigned to the pieces of information. When it is necessary to enter information that is stored in the common database, coding is used to simplify this procedure.

Processing Insurance Claims

Insurance processing is simplified with the use of a computer. The computer system allows the user to link several different codes to complete claim forms. For example, Code on Dental Procedures and Nomenclature (CDT Code) is entered once. When it is necessary to enter information in the transaction mode, a code is entered and all pertinent information stored in the database is entered into the patient account. This code identifies the service and asks for details such as tooth number and surface. The code is linked to a fee schedule and the system selects the correct fee automatically. The provider of the service can also be linked to the code. When the corresponding code is entered, all pertinent provider demographic information is entered.

ANATOMY OF COMPUTER SCREEN ELEMENTS

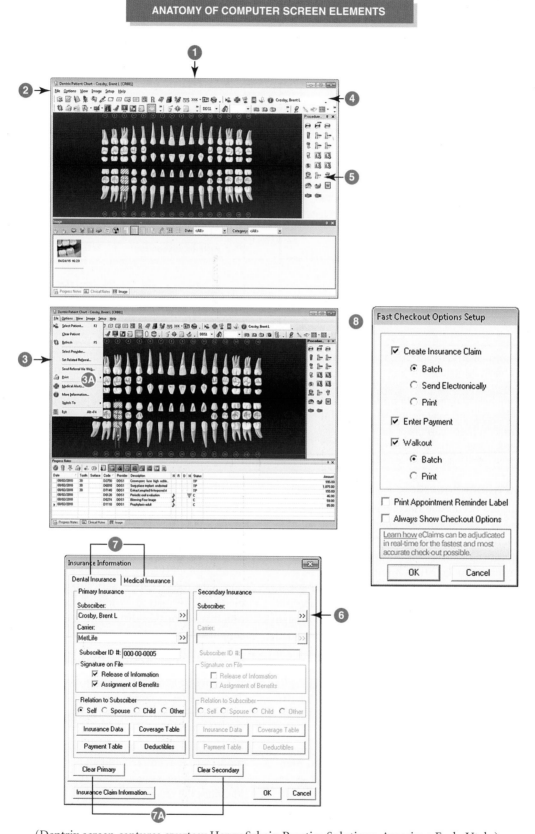

(Dentrix screen captures courtesy Henry Schein Practice Solutions, American Fork, Utah.)

1 **TITLE BAR**

The title bar identifies the software being used and the mode that is currently active.

2 **MENU BAR**

The menu bar lists the categories of options available to the user. There are two ways to reach the list of options for each category. With the mouse, place the pointer on the category title and click once on the left mouse button. Alternatively, you can use the function keys. While holding down the ALT key, press the key that matches the underlined letter of the option. Either of these operations will produce a **drop-down menu**.

3 **DROP-DOWN MENU**

A list of options available under each category on the menu bar is given in the drop-down menu. An option can be selected using the mouse or the keystroke selection method (using the key that matches the underlined letter). Options available will be in bold print. Options not available in the current mode will be gray. **3A** - A **next arrow** after the option indicates that there is a sub-menu present. To view the sub-menu, place the pointer on the function. The sub-menu will drop down.

4 **TOOL BAR**

The tool bar shows a group of icons configured as buttons that identify commonly used functions. Clicking on a button is a shortcut toward accessing these functions. Which functions are available will vary depending on the operation that is currently active. For example, if you are using a word-processing operation the buttons will be common for that operation, while the buttons for a spreadsheet operation will be different. Many programs offer an identification mode, which will allow you to identify the function of each button by placing the pointer on the button. A text box will appear to identify the function.

5 **POWER BAR**

The power bar provides quick access to selected features and reports. They normally are composed of customized icons that are unique to a particular software program. The user may have the option of activating or closing the power bar.

6 **SEARCH BUTTON**

This will give you information about the screen you are currently working in. It may identify the user who has logged on, date, time, and the current operating mode. Choose this button to open or reveal additional options.

7 **TABBED SCREENS**

Tabs are used to arrange the parts of a screen into a logical order. There may be a common area to all screens; this information will be displayed with each tab. Tabbed screens are commonly used to enter information. There will be several different fields, and you will move from field to field by using the tab key or arrows (depending on the software being used). **7A** - Buttons are also used to take the user from one screen to the next.

8 **DIALOG WINDOWS OR BOXES**

A dialog window will appear when additional input is needed, effectively asking you a question. To answer the question it will be necessary to activate the correct button. Common responses to dialog windows are yes, no, OK, and cancel.

Using information in the system, reports can be generated that will track the location and amount of the claim and will alert the administrative dental assistant when the claim has not been paid in a timely manner. The system converts all elements of an efficient manual tracking system into a highly effective computer system, providing the necessary tools for successful management of insurance claims.

Scheduling Electronically

The system allows the scheduler to be matrixed in the same way that an appointment book is matrixed. The user identifies what days of the week and what hours patients can be scheduled and customizes the schedule for each provider (dentist, assistant dentist, hygienist). Users can also program the system to schedule automatically according to procedure and can enter patient options such as time and provider (Figure 7-9).

Producing Reports

Reports can be customized to meet the needs of each office. Large dental practices with more than one provider will want the capability of generating reports unique to each provider. Reports identify production, collections, and adjustments; calculate the amount of time used to complete procedures; and track production goals. Insurance and recall tracking can be accomplished using monthly reports that identify current statuses. Reports, including accounting reports, patient reports, recall/appointment reports, provider/referring doctor reports, insurance reports, American Dental Association (ADA)/transaction/diagnosis code reports, prescription/pharmacy/laboratory reports, and practice management reports, can be customized to meet almost any need of the dental practice.

DAILY PROCEDURES WITH A COMPUTERIZED SYSTEM

One advantage of a computerized system is that it allows the administrative dental assistant and other members of the dental healthcare team to complete several functions by maximizing the computerized database, spreadsheet, and word processing functions. When these tasks are completed before the patient leaves the office, the dental practice is assured that all necessary transactions have been posted, the insurance process has been completed, and the next appointment has been scheduled. These steps improve communications with the patient by providing detailed information and help the assistant to become more organized in the completion of required tasks. Figure 7-10 provides an example of one such step in the daily office opening procedure, whereas Figure 7-11 is an example of the way an electronic system can streamline the checkout process.

The type of computer system used determines the exact order and characteristics of the start-up procedures. Each system offers different options and it is the responsibility of the administrative dental assistant to become familiar with these options. Detailed procedures are described in later chapters.

Backup System

It is necessary to have a system in place that backs up stored data. The purpose of the backup is to protect the information stored and follow established security protocols. Whether it is on an individual computer, network server, or remote server, information can be lost because of hard drive failure, power

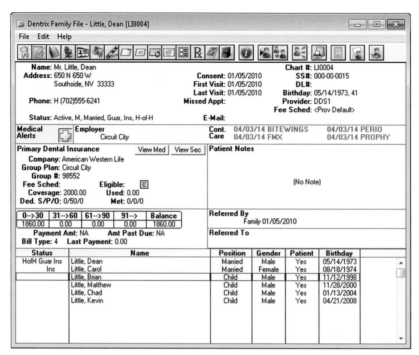

FIGURE 7-4 Family File Screen. This window identifies the head of household and all patients listed in the account. (Dentrix screen capture courtesy Henry Schein Practice Solutions, American Fork, Utah.)

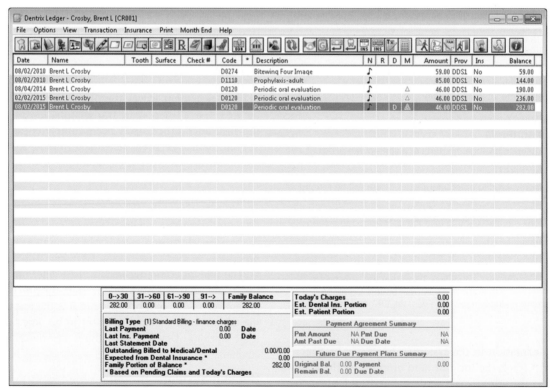

FIGURE 7-5 Ledger and History Window. This window displays individual patient history and transactions. (Dentrix screen capture courtesy Henry Schein Practice Solutions, American Fork, Utah.)

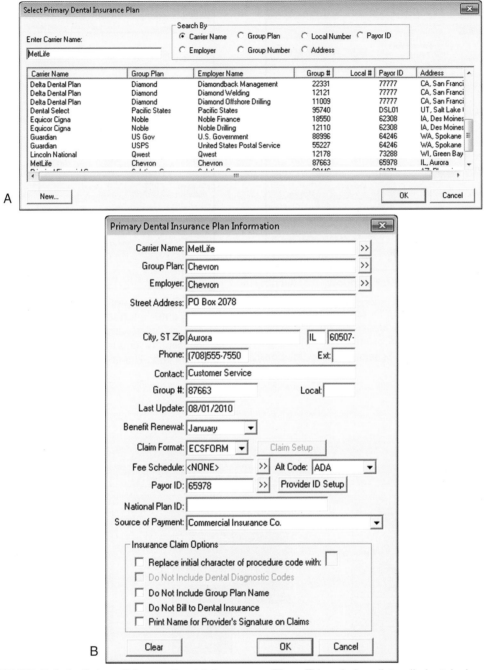

FIGURE 7-6 A, Select Primary Dental Insurance Plan. This window lists all dental plans currently stored in the software database. **B,** Dental Insurance Plan Information Window. This window is used to add a new dental plan to the software database. (Dentrix screen captures courtesy Henry Schein Practice Solutions, American Fork, Utah.)

surges, power losses, and misdirected system commands. If information is lost and there is no backup, countless hours and days are necessary to restore the lost information. In some cases, the information is never recovered. The only way to protect stored information is to back up the system consistently. Because there is such a large amount of protected data, most practices use a third party to back up their systems.

Not only can data be lost or corrupted, they are subject to outside breaches. During a security breach, unauthorized persons access vital and protected patient and practice information. If there is a security breach, there are mandated steps that need to be followed to inform patients or others that their protected information has been compromised.

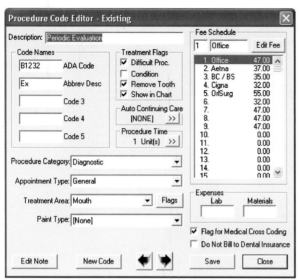

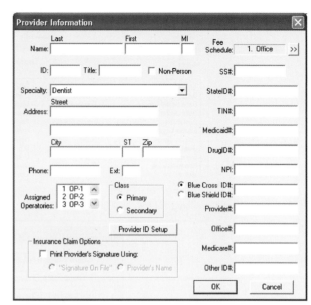

FIGURE 7-7 Procedure Code Editor Window. This window is used to add information and descriptions to a CDT code. The user is able to add information for appointment scheduling, procedure time, charting, insurance billing, fee schedules, laboratory results, and medical cross-coding. (Dentrix screen capture courtesy Henry Schein Practice Solutions, American Fork, Utah.)

FIGURE 7-8 Provider Information Window. This window is used to enter information about each provider that will be used to complete and file insurance claim forms. (Dentrix screen capture courtesy Henry Schein Practice Solutions, American Fork, Utah.)

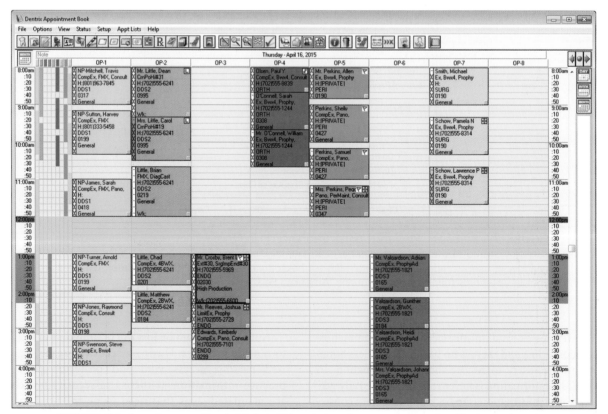

FIGURE 7-9 Appointment Book (daily). This window is an example of a filled appointment book page. The page shows dates, operatories, and color-coded providers. Each patient listed is coded to include contact information, procedure, and provider. (Dentrix screen capture courtesy Henry Schein Practice Solutions, American Fork, Utah.)

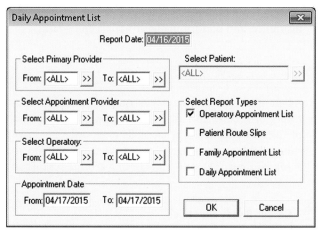

FIGURE 7-10 Daily Appointment List Window. This window is used each day during the opening procedure. From this screen, the administrative dental assistant is able to print an appointment list for each provider, a list for each operatory, and a route slip for each patient. (Dentrix screen capture courtesy Henry Schein Practice Solutions, American Fork, Utah.)

> **! REMEMBER**
>
> You never know when a computer system may fail. All members of the dental healthcare team must be prepared with a backup plan. This plan includes having an administrative dental assistant who can perform the basic skills manually (posting transactions, scheduling patients, processing insurance information, and performing basic bookkeeping tasks). These skills are important for safeguarding the practice from a loss of time and valuable information.

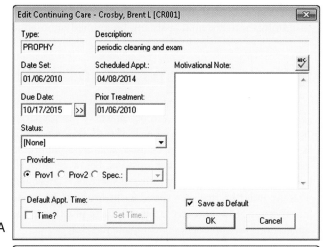

A

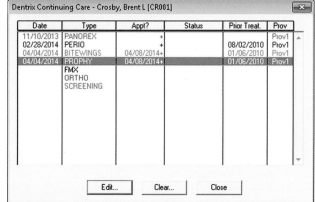

B

FIGURE 7-11 A, Edit Continuing Care Window. This window is used to identify procedures, time intervals, and providers for continuing care such as prophylaxis, radiography, periodontal care, and periodic screenings. **B,** Continuing Care Window. This window identifies which procedures the patient will require in the future. This prompts the scheduler to schedule such procedures as prophylaxis, radiographs, and screenings. (Dentrix screen captures courtesy Henry Schein Practice Solutions, American Fork, Utah.)

KEY POINTS

- Dental practice management software is available in basic and advanced software suites. Basic software suites primarily deal with the paperwork functions of the dental practice. Advanced software suites integrate business office functions with clinical functions and add greater flexibility and options. The use of an integrated system requires the cooperation of all members of the dental healthcare team and may lead to a paperless dental practice.
- Selecting a software package requires the dental healthcare team to identify its needs and express its desire to use a particular system. The team should consider different functions: general requirements, patient information, patient billing, treatment planning, insurance processing, recall and reactivation, practice management reports, electronic scheduling, database and word processing capabilities, and clinical integration.

- The role of the administrative dental assistant varies, depending on the software used. Some functions are common to all software programs. These include maintaining patient demographics, posting transactions, storing information in a general database, processing insurance claims, using an electronic scheduler, and producing reports.
- The administrative dental assistant and other members of the dental healthcare team perform daily procedures with a computerized system. These procedures rely on the computerized database and the spreadsheet and word processing functions.
- Backup procedures are vital in protecting a dental practice's information. A backup system is routinely used to protect the integrity of the computer system. The dental practice should have a plan in place that will allow the dental practice to function without the computer system

for a period of several days. This plan requires that the administrative dental assistant be trained in manually posting transactions, scheduling patients, processing insurance, and performing basic bookkeeping tasks.

■ CAREER-READY PRACTICES

Career-Ready Practices activities are designed to provide students with experiences that can be "practiced" in preparation for skills needed on the job. In each of the following exercises, a variety of approaches may be used to address the problem, rather than "right" or "wrong" answers. Below each exercise, next to the compass icon, is a listing of suggested Career-Ready Practice numbers that correspond to the listing of 12 practices in the front of the text (see p. viii-ix); these practices provide suggestions for approaches to complete the exercise.

1. Using outside information, research and compare a minimum of three dental practice management software systems. In your report, identify what you feel are basic components. Also describe some of the advanced features and explain why you would add them to the basics. Using the questions listed in this chapter on page 93, explain how these systems address these questions.

 Career-Ready Practices

    5   *Consider the environmental, social and economic impacts of decisions.*
    7   *Employ valid and reliable research strategies.*
    8   *Utilize critical thinking to make sense of problems and persevere in solving them.*

2. As an administrative dental assistant, you will be asked to perform basic and advanced computer skills to complete tasks effectively. What skills or knowledge do you think will be a challenge for you? What training do you think you need? Develop a plan to learn these skills and knowledge.

 Career-Ready Practices

    2   *Apply appropriate academic and technical skills.*
    8   *Utilize critical thinking to make sense of problems and persevere in solving them.*
   10   *Plan education and career path aligned to personal goals.*
   11   *Use technology to enhance productivity.*

3. As a new administrative dental assistant, what do you see as your biggest challenge in working with dental practice management software?

 Career-Ready Practices

    8   *Utilize critical thinking to make sense of problems and persevere in solving them.*
   11   *Use technology to enhance productivity.*

Patient Clinical Records

LEARNING OBJECTIVES

1. List the functions of patient clinical records and the key elements of record keeping. Describe the significance of each element.
2. Explain the evolution of electronic clinical records in the dental office.
3. Identify the components of a clinical record and describe the function of each component.
4. Discuss methods used in the collection of information needed to complete clinical records.
5. Discuss the function of risk management and identify situations that lead to patient dissatisfaction.

INTRODUCTION

The function of the clinical record (paper or electronic) is to provide the dental healthcare team with information. The objective of the dental healthcare team is to deliver dental treatment that takes into consideration the needs of the patient. The whole picture cannot be correctly visualized if all of the pieces are not present. The information collected during preparation of the clinical record, when complete, provides all of the necessary pieces.

The patient registration form introduces the patient to the dental practice and provides demographic and financial information that will be used to complete insurance forms and bill the patient. A comprehensive medical history alerts the dentist to drug allergies and medical conditions that may be affected by particular dental procedures. The dental history provides information about previous treatment; it also alerts the dental healthcare team to fears and apprehensions that the patient may have concerning dental treatment. The diagnostic information is used to formulate a treatment plan. Various other forms may also be used to aid the dental healthcare team.

When all of the pieces have been collected and placed together in an individual patient file folder, or an electronic file, a total picture of the patient and the patient's needs can be visualized. Once the initial information is collected and a treatment plan is developed, the next section of the clinical record documents the dental treatment. At each visit, treatment is recorded carefully and thoroughly.

In addition, the clinical record serves as a legal document. This document can be used in defense of allegations of malpractice and can provide information for forensic odontology (dental conditions used for identification). Third-party insurance carriers and managed care providers can mandate elements and organization of the clinical record.

The basic elements of all clinical records are the same, although formats and styles may vary from practice to practice. The format selected by the dentist may be determined by a specific organization, such as a professional organization, a managed care company, a corporation, an insurance company, or a practice management consultancy. The Dental Practice Act of each state may mandate required elements. Organizations may require specific forms and a predetermined format to be used by all dental offices within that particular organization. Regardless of which system is used, the key elements to success are organization, consistency, and completeness.

KEY ELEMENTS OF RECORD KEEPING

- Organization
- Consistency
- Completeness

It is the responsibility of the dental healthcare team to ensure that all aspects of the clinical record are accurate and easily accessible. In addition, the Health Insurance Portability and Accountability Act (HIPAA) Privacy Rule applies to the information contained in the patient's clinical record. The accessibility of clinical records is twofold. First, the dental healthcare team must know where the record is located at all times. Second, patients have the right to view the contents of their personal clinical records.

Each dental healthcare team member plays an important role in the collection, recording, and maintenance of clinical records. It is the responsibility of each member to ensure that the information contained within each clinical record is accurate, factual, and complete. The contents of the clinical record and all conversations with a patient are confidential and must be protected both ethically and as mandated in the HIPAA Privacy Rule (Figure 8-1).

ELECTRONIC CLINICAL RECORDS

In the past, a dental practice may have used a computer only to maintain accounting information. Now, computers are used to

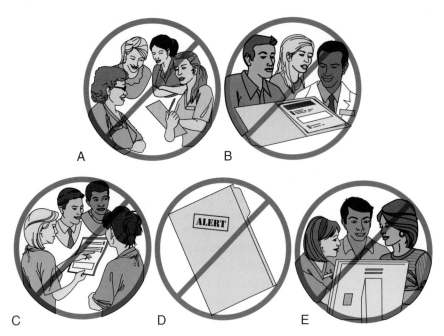

FIGURE 8-1 Safeguarding clinical records and complying with the Health Insurance Portability and Accountability Act (HIPAA) Privacy Rule. **A,** Do not ask patients questions in a place where others can hear the responses. **B,** Do not leave charts in places where others can read the content. **C,** Do not talk with staff members about patients where others can overhear the conversation. **D,** Do not place protected health information (PHI) on the outside of a clinical record. **E,** Do not have PHI displayed on a computer screen where unauthorized personnel can see it.

organize and maintain complex business and clinical records. It is no longer a luxury to have a computer system; it is a necessity. The types of records that are maintained in a computer system include patient clinical and financial information, dental examination and treatment documentation, insurance tracking, recall systems, and appointment scheduling. In addition, computers are now being used to record clinical findings, to access online services, to electronically transfer insurance information, and to communicate with patients, referring dentists, and other professional organizations.

Clinical Records

The role of computer-generated clinical records in the dental practice is limitless. The dream of a totally paperless dental practice has become a reality. Software suites have been designed to ensure the authenticity of clinical records. Digital and scanned radiographs, progress notes, periodontal charting, clinical charting, and so forth can be stored within a computer system. The advantages of a computerized clinical record include reduced storage space and less time required for shuffling papers. Charts will be permanently stored on servers (local and remote) and information can be transferred elsewhere without removal of the original document from the storage area.

The ability to easily read computer-generated progress notes takes the guesswork out of trying to interpret handwriting. Entries are stamped with the code of the person making the entry (computer signature). Computer software can be designed with safeguards that ensure that all needed information is entered before the program can be closed. This procedure helps to create documents that include all of the necessary elements of good record keeping: organization, consistency, and completeness.

Electronic Health Records

The National Health Information Infrastructure (NHII), when fully developed (scheduled for completion in 2015), will be a communications system designed to transmit patient health information (including dental). The system is designed to improve patient safety, improve the quality of healthcare, and better inform and empower healthcare consumers. Each patient's record will include a personal health record that is created and controlled by the individual or family. Healthcare providers will include information such as provider notes, clinical orders, and prescriptions. It will still be the responsibility of each provider to maintain their own patients' medical records. The confidentiality of personal health records and consumers' control over their own records is the primary component of the system. Management of the system will fall under the authority of the Department of Health and Human Services and has been defined as "an initiative set forth to improve the effectiveness, efficiency and overall quality of health and healthcare in the United States."

COMPONENTS OF THE CLINICAL RECORD

Clinical records are a crucial part of the dental practice (paper and electronic). Without accurate and well-organized clinical records, it would be impossible to determine the dental needs of each patient. The clinical record is the instrument used to communicate information on the health of the patient and the patient's dental needs, dental treatment, and financial responsibility.

Today, there are basically three ways in which clinical records are created and stored (Figure 8-2).

- Manual or paper record: The forms in this record are typically handwritten by the patient and members of the dental healthcare team and are stored in a filing cabinet.
- Electronic records (paperless): These records are digital records and are stored in a computer system. The digital forms can be a combination of forms that have been completed and signed by the patient and then scanned and uploaded into the electronic file. Forms that require signatures can also be created in a digital format and electronically signed by the patient and the dentist.

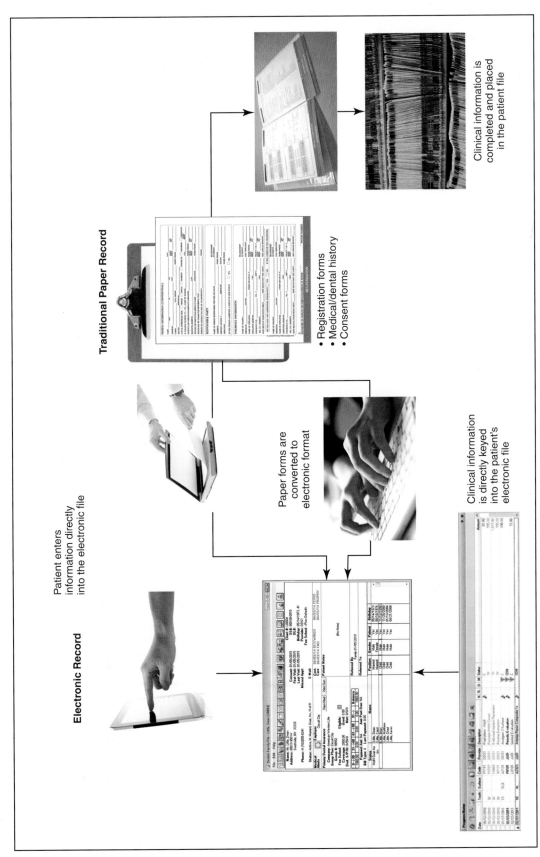

Traditional Paper Record

- Registration forms
- Medical/dental history
- Consent forms

Clinical information is completed and placed in the patient file

Electronic Record

Patient enters information directly into the electronic file

Paper forms are converted to electronic format

Clinical information is directly keyed into the patient's electronic file

FIGURE 8-2 Clinical record workflow. (*Virtual keyboard:* Copyright © 2012 blackred, iStock.com. All rights reserved. *Dentrix screen shots:* Courtesy Henry Schein Practice Solutions, American Fork, Utah. *Scanner:* Copyright © 2010 nicolas_, iStock.com. All rights reserved. *Keyboard:* Copyright © 2011 iPandastudio, iStock.com. All rights reserved. *Clipboard:* Copyright © 2010 t_kimura, iStock.com. All rights reserved. *Forms:* Courtesy Patterson Office Supplies, Champaign, Ill. *Files:* Copyright © 2006 AK2, iStock.com. All rights reserved.)

- Combination record: The information in this record is split between paper documents and electronic documents. The paper file will typically contain forms that have been completed and signed by the patient (registration forms, medical and health history, updated medical forms, consent forms, and correspondence). The electronic documents are elements of a practice management software system (examination and treatment information). The two records together are the patient's clinical record.

The order in which these forms are used and placed in the clinical record is a personal preference of the dental practice. Some forms may be consolidated to include more than one type of information. The key point is that all information must be located somewhere within the patient's clinical record. A sample electronic clinical record is provided on pp. 111–125.

✚ HIPAA

Security Standards That Apply to Electronic Clinical Records

- Administrative safeguards:
  - Identification of who will supervise compliance with Health Insurance Portability and Accountability Act (HIPAA) Security Standards
  - Staff clearance procedure that identifies which members of the staff will have access to electronic protected health information (ePHI)
  - Termination procedure
  - Security incident procedures
  - Contingency plan, including data backup plan, disaster recovery plan, and emergency mode operation plan
- Physical safeguards:
  - Protection of electronic systems, equipment, and data that contain ePHI from environmental hazards and unauthorized intrusion
  - Retention of off-site computer backups
- Technical safeguards:
  - Access control, including unique user identification (password and biometric systems)
  - Emergency access procedures
  - Audit controls

✚ HIPAA

Privacy Rules That Apply to Clinical Records

- **Access to Clinical Records:** Patients should be able to see the information in their clinical records. They may request to view the information or obtain a copy. If errors are found, they may request that they be corrected. The dental office should provide access to the records or provide a copy within 30 days of the written request. A reasonable fee can be charged for copying the records.
- **Notice of Privacy Practices:** The dental office (or any covered entity) must provide patients with a copy of the notice while explaining to patients how their personal medical information may be used and their rights under the Health Insurance Portability and Accountability Act (HIPAA; see Figures 8-5 and 8-6).
- **Limits on Use of Personal Medical and Dental Information:** Private health information (PHI) contained in the clinical

record can be shared only with other health professionals when the information is used for the care of the patient's health. PHI cannot be shared with others for purposes not related to their healthcare without written authorization from the patient.
- **Confidential Communications:** Healthcare professionals must take reasonable steps to ensure that their communications with patients are confidential. For example, when discussing PHI with a patient, do so in a private area where it cannot be overheard by others. Patients may also request that you do not contact them or leave a message at their home. The dental office must comply with such requests if they can be reasonably accommodated.

✚ HIPAA

Roles and Responsibility of the Dental Healthcare Team

- **Written Privacy Procedures:** Written privacy procedures identify which members of the staff will have access to private health information (PHI), how the information will be used, and when it may be disclosed. In addition, the policy must ensure that any business associates who may have access to the PHI will agree to follow the same procedures.
- **Employee Training and Privacy Officer:** The dental entity must provide adequate training and appoint a Privacy Officer. The plan should also state how policies will be monitored and what disciplinary actions will be taken if a policy is not followed by a staff member.
- **Public Responsibilities:** In limited circumstances, the Privacy Rule permits but does not require that covered entities continue certain existing disclosures of health information for specific public responsibilities, such as
  - Emergency circumstances
- Identification of the body of a deceased person or the need to determine the cause of death
- Research that involves limited data or that has been independently approved by an Institutional Review Board or privacy board
- Overall management of the healthcare system
- Judicial and administrative proceedings
- Limited law enforcement activities
- Activities related to national defense and security
- When no other law requires disclosures in these situations, covered entities may continue to use their professional judgment to decide whether to make such disclosures on the basis of their own policies and ethical principles.
- **Equivalent Requirements for Government:** Provisions of the Privacy Rule generally apply equally to private sector and public sector covered entities.

Text continued on page 126

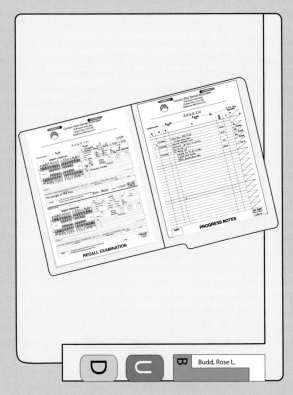

Individual Patient File

Paper: Components of the clinical record are organized and placed inside a file folder that is identified with the patient name and stored per the filing system of the office. The standard folder is 8½ × 11 inches, and a fastening system holds forms in place within the folder. Additional pockets are also included to store radiographs or other small items.

Electronic: An electronic file for each patient includes all the information contained within a traditional paper file. A single search on a patient's name pulls up all the information related to that individual, including contact and insurance information, dental images, clinical and periodontal examinations, treatment plans and progress notes, and more.

(Dentrix screen shot courtesy Henry Schein Practice Solutions, American Fork, UT.)

Dentrix Family File - Little, Dean [LI0004]

File   Edit   Help

Name: Mr. Little, Dean
Address: 650 N 650 W
Southside, NV 33333

Phone: H (702)555-6241

Status: Active, M, Married, Guar, Ins, H-of-H

Consent: 01/05/2015
First Visit: 01/05/2015
Last Visit: 01/05/2015
Missed Appt:

Chart #: LI0004
SS#: 000-00-0015
DL#:
Birthday: 05/14/1973, 41
Provider: DDS1
Fee Sched: <Prov Default>

E-Mail:

Medical Alerts

Employer
Circuit City

Cont. Care
04/03/14 BITEWINGS   04/03/14 PERIO
04/03/14 FMX   04/03/14 PROPHY

Primary Dental Insurance   View Med | View Sec
Company: American Western Life
Group Plan: Circuit City
Group #: 98552
Fee Sched: **Eligible:** E
Coverage: 2000.00   **Used:** 0.00
Ded. S/P/O: 0/50/0   **Met:** 0/0/0

Patient Notes

(No Note)

0-->30	31-->60	61-->90	91-->	Balance
1860.00	0.00	0.00	0.00	1860.00

Payment Amt: NA   **Amt Past Due:** NA
Bill Type: 4   **Last Payment:** 0.00

Referred By
Family 01/05/2010

Referred To

Status	Name	Position	Gender	Patient	Birthday
HofH Guar Ins	Little, Dean	Married	Male	Yes	05/14/1973
Ins	Little, Carol	Married	Female	Yes	08/18/1974
	Little, Brian	Child	Male	Yes	11/12/1998
	Little, Matthew	Child	Male	Yes	11/28/2000
	Little, Chad	Child	Male	Yes	01/13/2004
	Little, Kevin	Child	Male	Yes	04/21/2008

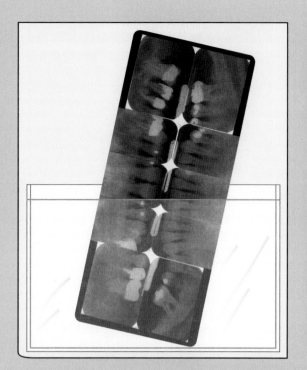

Dental Radiographs or Images

Dental radiographs or digital images are an essential element of the diagnostic process and an important part of the clinical record. They provide information about a patient's current and previous dental health and are required by insurance carriers and considered a legal document.

Paper: Original radiographs should always be stored in the dental office, generally within a pocket of the patient's file, with a copy released as needed.

Electronic: Digital images can be attached to the patient's file for easy access.

(Radiograph from Newman MG, Takei HH, Klokkevold PR et al: *Carranza's Clinical Periodontology*, ed 11, St. Louis, 2012, Saunders. Dentrix screen shot courtesy Henry Schein Practice Solutions, American Fork, UT.)

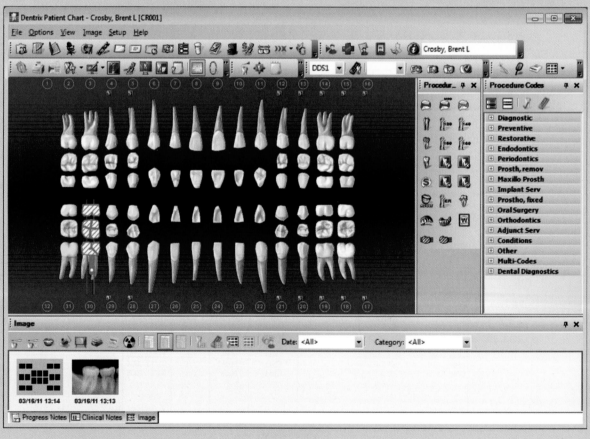

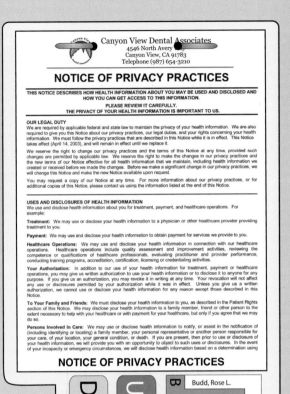

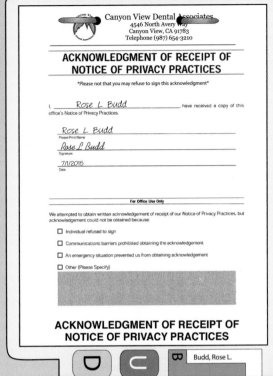

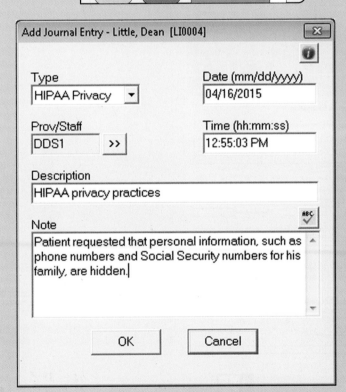

Acknowledgment of Receipt of Privacy Practices/HIPAA

All patients or representatives of patients (e.g., parents or guardians) must sign a form stating that they have received the Notice of Privacy Practices (Figure 8-5). This is required as part of the federal Health Insurance Portability and Accountability Act (HIPAA).

Paper: A formal signed acknowledgment is stored as part of the patient's record.

Electronic: The acknowledgment may be signed on hard copy and scanned into the office system or signed electronically and stored. Office staff can easily see whether this document is on file for a specific patient and will be alerted if it is required. Notations about patient preferences can also be made.

(Dentrix screen shot courtesy Henry Schein Practice Solutions, American Fork, UT.)

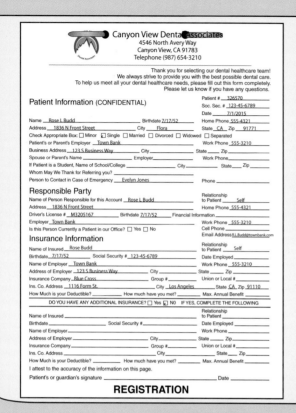

REGISTRATION

Registration Form

Registration forms provide demographic and financial information about the patient and the person or persons responsible for payment of dental fees. The form is divided into sections that help to organize the information (see Anatomy of a Registration Form).

Paper: If this form is completed by the patient, ensure that all the information is legible and complete before it is stored in the file folder.

Electronic: The information and sections of the form are the same as the paper form, and information can feed into other areas of the patient's record.

(Dentrix screen shot courtesy Henry Schein Practice Solutions, American Fork, UT.)

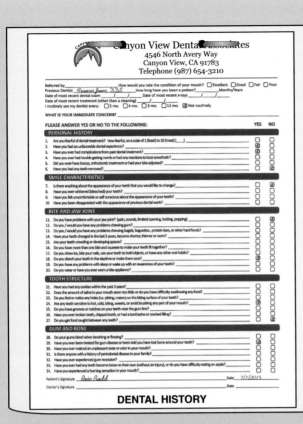

DENTAL HISTORY

Dental History Form

The dental history form provides the dental healthcare team with information about the patient's previous dental treatment and can identify patient fears and concerns. Patients are asked to provide information about the purpose of the visit, current problem(s), previous dentist(s) and radiographs, oral healthcare habits, previous orthodontic work, unpleasant dental experiences, and questions or concerns.

Paper/Electronic: The dentist interviews the patient and makes notations, and the patient and dentist sign the form. The dentist then records any adverse reactions to assist the dental healthcare team in recognizing and calming fears.

(Dentrix screen shot courtesy Henry Schein Practice Solutions, American Fork, UT.)

Dentrix Dental Practice
1220 South 630 East #100
American Fork, UT 84003

(801)763-9300

I routinely see my dentist every:
☐ 3 mo.   ☐ 4 mo.   ☐ 6 mo.   ☐ 12 mo.   ☐ Not routinely

What is your immediate concern?

Are you fearful of dental treatment? How fearful, on a scale of 1 (least) to 10 (most)

Personal History. Check all that apply:
☐ Had an unfavorable dental experience   ☐ Had complications from past dental treatment
☐ Had trouble getting numb   ☐ Had any reactions to local anesthetic
☐ Had/have braces, orthodontic treatment   ☐ Had your bite adjusted
☐ Had any teeth removed

Smile Characteristics. Check all that apply:
☐ Is there anything about the appearance of your teeth that you would like to change?
☐ Have you ever whitened (bleached) your teeth?
☐ Have you felt uncomfortable or self conscious about the appearance of your teeth?
☐ Have you been disappointed with the appearance of previous dental work?

Bite and Jaw Joint. Check all that apply:
☐ You have problems with your jaw joint
☐ You have any problems chewing
☐ Your teeth changed in the last 5 years, become shorter, thinner, or worn
☐ Your teeth crowding or developing spaces
☐ You chew ice, bite your nails, use your teeth to hold objects, or have any other oral habits
☐ You clench your teeth in the daytime or make them sore
☐ You have problems with sleep or wake up with an awareness of your teeth

page 6

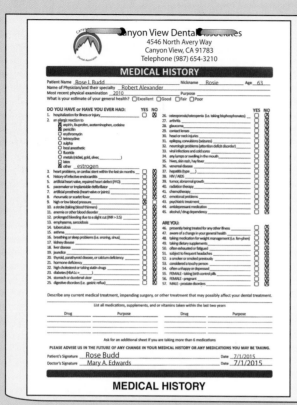

MEDICAL HISTORY

Medical History Form

A comprehensive medical history is necessary to ensure that the patient's medical needs are being met along with the dental needs. The medical history can alert the dentist to possible interactions between dental treatment and medical treatment, at which point the dentist may initiate contact with the patient's physician to ensure that any dental treatment is taking the patient's overall well-being into account.

Paper: The medical history form may use stickers, colored pens, stamps, or preprinted boxes to note any allergies or other conditions that may require special treatment. These should be done in a visual and highly consistent manner. To protect the patient's confidentiality, alerts should never be placed on the outside of the file folder where other patients may see them.

Electronic: The same sort of alerts can be placed within the patient file (see Individual Patient File screen). using colors and icons for quick and easy identification and accessible from a variety of different patient screens.

(Dentrix screen shot courtesy Henry Schein Practice Solutions, American Fork, UT.)

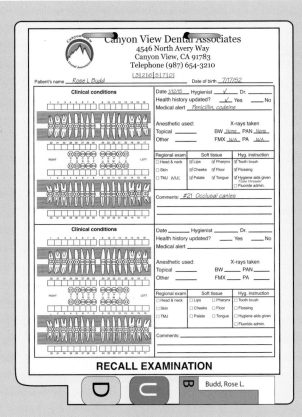

RECALL EXAMINATION

Recall Examination Form

After the initial medical history is collected, it must be updated on a regular schedule. Patients with series histories should be asked at each visit whether there has been a change in their medical status.

Paper: Some forms provide space that can be used to record changes in medical history or medications. After the update is completed, the form is signed by both the patient and dental healthcare team member.

Electronic: Changes can be noted within new appointments so that the dental healthcare team is notified of the change when the appointment is made and the information stored in the record for that day and beyond.

(Dentrix screen shot courtesy Henry Schein PracticeSolutions, American Fork, UT.)

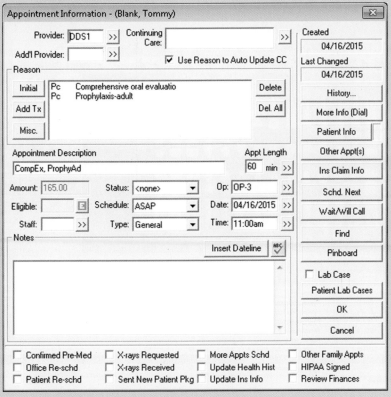

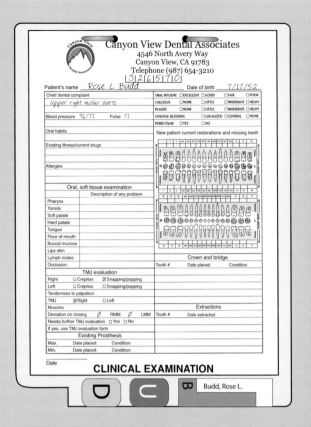

CLINICAL EXAMINATION

Canyon View Dental Associates
4546 North Avery Way
Canyon View, CA 91783
Telephone (987) 654-3210

Budd, Rose L.

Examination Form

The examination form illustrates the patient's dental condition at the time of his or her first visit to the dental practice. It is part of the permanent record and should not be altered. The form documents previous dental treatment, existing conditions, and missing teeth. In addition to oral hygiene information, the examination form lists periodontal findings and the result of soft tissue examination, plus temporomandibular joint (TMJ) and occlusion results evaluations, the patient's chief complaint, and a record of dental images and their evaluation. The information is gathered and recorded with the assistance of a dental assistant and a dental hygienist and helps the dentist develop a treatment plan.

(Dentrix screen shot courtesy Henry Schein Practice Solutions, American Fork, UT.)

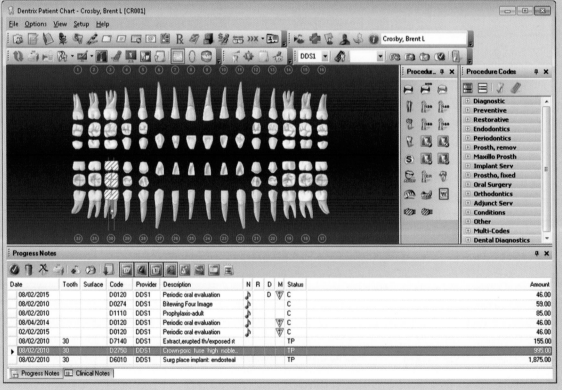

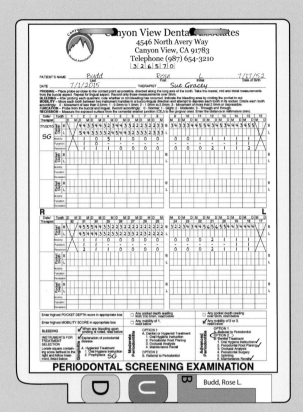

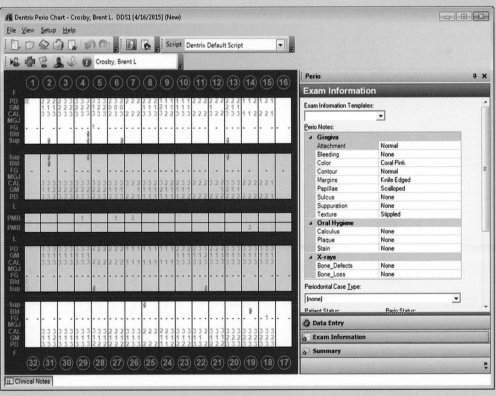

Periodontal Screening Examination

Patients who have demonstrated a need for periodontal examination may have this form completed as part of the patient file. The use of such forms varies from practice to practice.

(Dentrix screen shot courtesy Henry Schein Practice Solutions, American Fork, UT.)

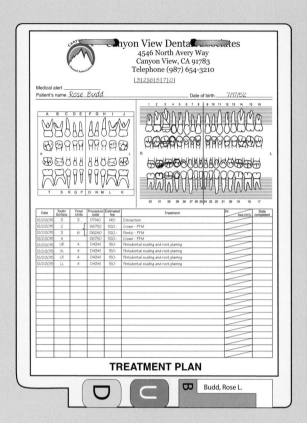

TREATMENT PLAN

Canyon View Dental Associates
4546 North Avery Way
Canyon View, CA 91783
Telephone (987) 654-3210

|3|2|6|5|7|0|

Medical alert _____
Patient's name Rose Budd   Date of birth 7/17/52

Date	Tooth/Surface	Time/Units	Procedure code	Estimated fee	Treatment	Dr.	Asst. Avg.	Date completed
12/2/2015	3	3	D7140	145.-	Extraction			
12/2/2015	2		D6750	1120.-	Crown - PFM			
12/2/2015	3	6	D6240	1120.-	Pontic - PFM			
12/2/2015	4		D6750	1120.-	Crown - PFM			
12/2/2015	UR	4	D4341	150.-	Periodontal scaling and root planing			
12/2/2015	UL	4	D4341	150.-	Periodontal scaling and root planing			
12/2/2015	LR	4	D4341	150.-	Periodontal scaling and root planing			
12/2/2015	LL	4	D4341	150.-	Periodontal scaling and root planing			

Budd, Rose L.

Treatment Plan

The treatment plan is derived from information collected in the clinical record. The dentist reviews the medical history, previous dental history, and the results of diagnostic examinations and determines the work that is needed to ensure that the best interests of the patient are protected. This form is not developed with insurance coverage or managed care contracts, and each patient is treated equally without regard to socioeconomic factors or insurance coverage. The patient is presented the full case and may then decide on alternative treatment that may meet insurance company mandates or financial needs. A treatment plan is finalized before a financial plan is prepared.

(Dentrix screen shot courtesy Henry Schein Practice Solutions, American Fork, UT.)

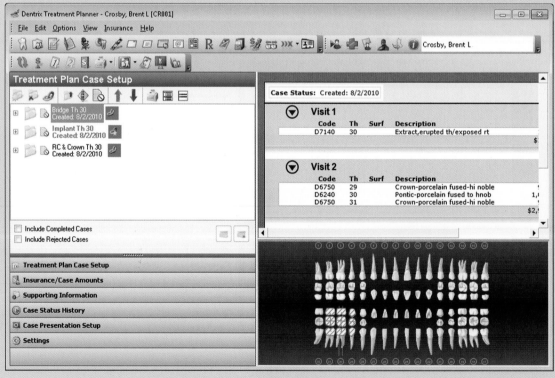

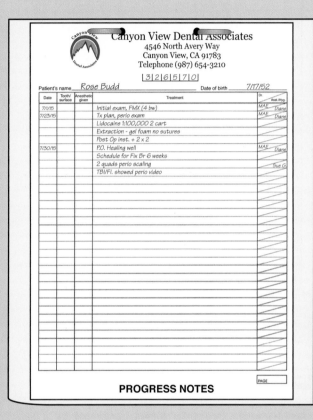

[3|2|6|5|7|0]

Patient's name __Rose Budd__   Date of birth __7/17/52__

Date	Tooth/ surface	Anesthetic given	Treatment	Dr.	Asst./Hyg.
7/1/15			Initial exam, FMX (4 bw)	MAE	Diane
7/23/15			Tx plan, perio exam	MAE	Diane
			Lidocaine 1:100,000 2 cart		
			Extraction - gel foam no sutures		
			Post Op inst. + 2 x 2		
7/30/15			P.O. Healing well	MAE	Diane
			Schedule for Fix Br 6 weeks		
			2 quads perio scaling		Sue G.
			TBI/Fl. showed perio video		

PROGRESS NOTES

PAGE

Progress Notes Form

Progress notes are used to record the course of treatment for the patient.

Paper: Each form has space for the date, tooth number, and treatment. Space should also be provided for the initials and identification number (typically license number) of the treating dentist, assistant, or dental hygienist. (These requirements vary from state to state.) Entries on the progress notes include telephone conversations, missed appointments, prescriptions, and contact with insurance carriers or other healthcare providers. Directives, prognosis, and any difficulties during treatment are also noted. All entries must be supplied in ink, preferably black, and any corrections or deletions should be marked with a single line. Progress notes will also serve as a legal document, and the information must be accurate, complete, and legible.

Electronic: The electronic notes serve the same function as the form, but some of the information indicated within the paper form may be located elsewhere within the patient's electronic file and not necessarily duplicated within this section of the file, such as the provider's initials/signature and identification number, which are stored within that provider's own file.

(Dentrix screen shot courtesy Henry Schein Practice Solutions, American Fork, UT.)

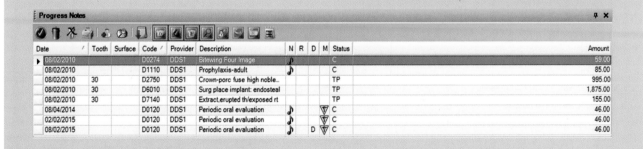

Progress Notes

Date	Tooth	Surface	Code	Provider	Description	N	R	D	M	Status	Amount
08/02/2010			D0274	DDS1	Bitewing Four Image	♪				C	59.00
08/02/2010			D1110	DDS1	Prophylaxis-adult	♪				C	85.00
08/02/2010	30		D2750	DDS1	Crown-porc fuse high noble...					TP	995.00
08/02/2010	30		D6010	DDS1	Surg place implant: endosteal					TP	1,875.00
08/02/2010	30		D7140	DDS1	Extract.erupted th/exposed rt					TP	155.00
08/04/2014			D0120	DDS1	Periodic oral evaluation	♪			▽	C	46.00
02/02/2015			D0120	DDS1	Periodic oral evaluation	♪			▽	C	46.00
08/02/2015			D0120	DDS1	Periodic oral evaluation	♪		D	▽	C	46.00

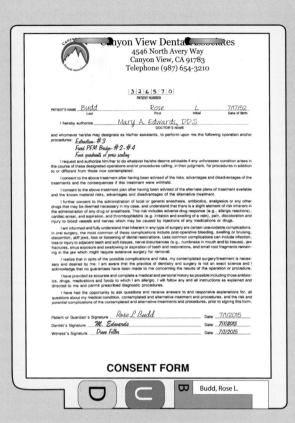

CONSENT FORM

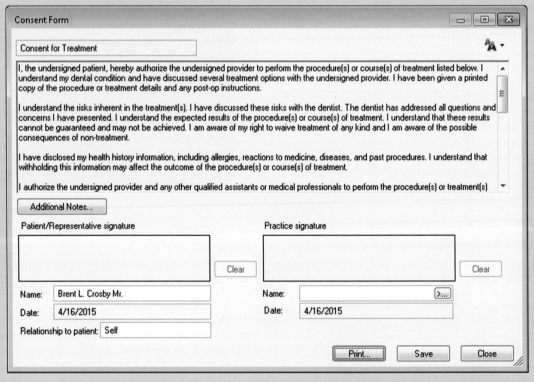

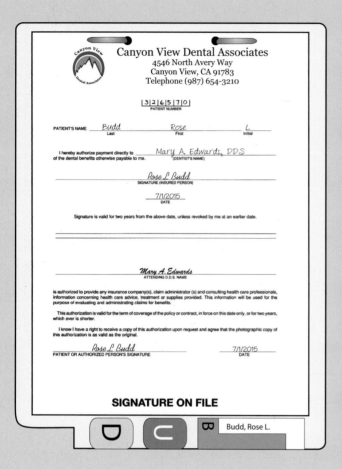

Signature on File

The purpose of the signature-on-file form is to provide a process that allows the dental practice to submit insurance forms without the patient's signature. With the use of computer-generated insurance forms and electronic submissions, it is not possible to have patients sign each form with an original signature. Therefore patients are asked to sign a form that authorizes the dentist to submit claims without the signature.

Paper: The form provides two types of authorization. The first authorizes the dentist to submit claims and request direct reimbursement. The second authorization states that the patient will release any information in his or her clinical record that will be needed by the insurance company. *Remember that all information contained in the patient's clinical record is confidential and cannot be released to anyone without the written permission of the patient.*

Electronic: In addition to the patient's authorization within the system, an electronic image of the patient's signature can also be used to attach to documents.

(Dentrix screen shot courtesy Henry Schein Practice Solutions, American Fork, UT.)

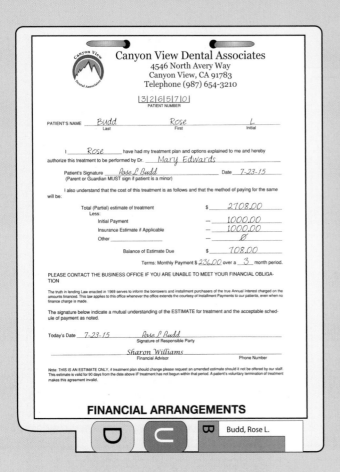

Canyon View Dental Associates
4546 North Avery Way
Canyon View, CA 91783
Telephone (987) 654-3210

[3|2|6|5|7|0]
PATIENT NUMBER

PATIENT'S NAME _Budd_   _Rose_   _L_
                  Last   First   Initial

I _Rose_ have had my treatment plan and options explained to me and hereby
authorize this treatment to be performed by Dr. _Mary Edwards_

Patient's Signature _Rose L Budd_   Date _7-23-15_
(Parent or Guardian MUST sign if patient is a minor)

I also understand that the cost of this treatment is as follows and that the method of paying for the same
will be:

Total (Partial) estimate of treatment $ _2708.00_
Less:
  Initial Payment   − _1000.00_
  Insurance Estimate if Applicable   − _1000.00_
  Other _____   − _0_

  Balance of Estimate Due $ _708.00_

Terms: Monthly Payment $ _236.00_ over a _3_ month period.

PLEASE CONTACT THE BUSINESS OFFICE IF YOU ARE UNABLE TO MEET YOUR FINANCIAL OBLIGATION

The truth in lending Law enacted in 1969 serves to inform the borrowers and installment purchasers of the true Annual Interest charged on the amounts financed. This law applies to this office whenever the office extends the courtesy of Installment Payments to our patients, even when no finance charge is made.

The signature below indicate a mutual understanding of the ESTIMATE for treatment and the acceptable schedule of payment as noted.

Today's Date _7-23-15_   _Rose L Budd_
                               Signature of Responsible Party

                     Sharon Williams
                     Financial Advisor   Phone Number

Note: THIS IS AN ESTIMATE ONLY, if treatment plan should change please request an amended estimate should it not be offered by our staff. This estimate is valid for 90 days from the date above IF treatment has not begun within that period. A patient's voluntary termination of treatment makes this agreement invalid.

FINANCIAL ARRANGEMENTS

Budd, Rose L.

Financial Arrangements Form
The use of the financial arrangements form places in writing the total estimated cost of the proposed dental treatment, when payments are expected, and the amount of each payment. It meets regulations by providing a "truth-in-lending" statement and gives instructions on what should be done if payment cannot be made. By signing the form, patients state that they understand what is going to be done, agree to the estimated fee, and accept the payment schedule.

Electronic: Practice management systems pull treatment and insurance information and easily generate printable forms.

(Dentrix screen shots courtesy Henry Schein Practice Solutions, American Fork, UT.)

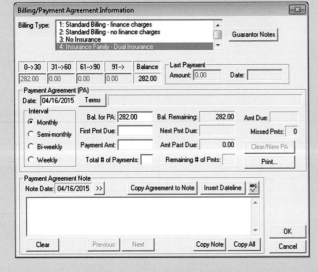

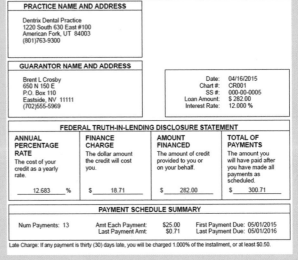

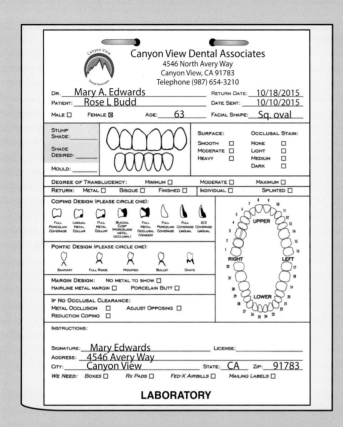

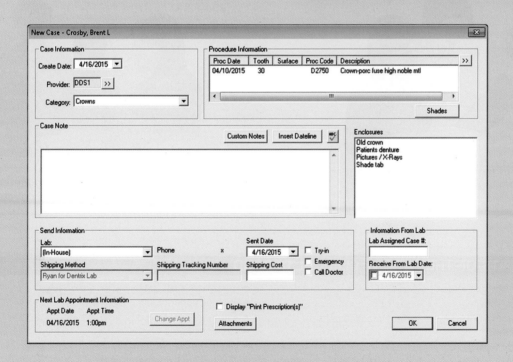

Laboratory Forms

Laboratory forms are used to communicate instructions to dental laboratory staff in the fabrication of a dental prosthesis. This form or prescription is required in most states to prevent the illegal practice of dentistry. The form contains specific information that communicates to the laboratory what needs to be done.

Paper: It is important to keep a copy of this form in the patient's chart for reference. The laboratory prescription includes the patient's name or identification number, along with date, instructions, signature, and license number of the prescribing dentist.

Electronic: As with some of the other forms, information required to be entered into the laboratory prescription may be pulled from other parts of the patient or provider files, easing the work of the dental healthcare team.

(Dentrix screen shot courtesy Henry Schein Practice Solutions, American Fork, UT.)

PROCEDURES

Steps for Collecting Information

Gathering and organizing information for clinical records can be accomplished in many different ways. Although the process and routine may vary depending on the technology used, the types of information needed remain the same.

1. **Call for first appointment.** Use a telephone information form or an electronic form to begin gathering information.
2. **Before the scheduled appointment.** If time allows, forms for registration and dental and medical histories can be sent to the patient via e-mail or a website before the first appointment. These forms can be part of a packet that also contains information about the dental practice and a welcome letter from the dentist. Electronic forms (e-forms) can be completed at the patient's leisure. The forms can be returned to the dental office electronically or printed and brought with the patient on the first visit. If forms are not completed before the appointment, the patient should be instructed to arrive 15 minutes early to complete them. To expedite form completion and prevent missing information, the patient should be informed of the types of information he or she will be required to provide, such as insurance information, types and dosages of medications being taken, and names and addresses of physicians and former dentists.
3. **Day of appointment.** When the patient arrives for the appointment, greet the patient and have all forms ready for completion (if not completed in advance). If the dental practice uses an electronic format, direct the patient to the computer kiosk or hand them an electronic tablet such as an iPad. If a manual system is used, give the patient a clipboard, a pen, and the paperwork that must be completed. Briefly explain to the patient how you would like the forms completed; this will help to answer questions in advance. If the patient is a minor, a parent or guardian must complete and sign the forms. Once the forms have been completed, they must be reviewed and checked for completeness (Figure 8-3). Another method that could be used is the interview technique. Patients are asked questions on the medical and dental history forms and answers are recorded by the assistant. If this method is used, the interview must take place in a private area (Figure 8-4).
4. **Confirmation of information.** After the forms have been completed, a member of the dental healthcare team reviews the information with the patient. Notations should be made to clarify "yes" answers and incomplete answers. During the dentist's review of the forms, he or she may ask additional medical and dental questions according to available findings.
5. **Information collected during the examination.** Additional information is recorded on the proper form by the dental assistant, as directed by the dentist. The data entered must be neat, complete, and legible. Other such records include **dental radiographs, examination forms,** and **laboratory forms.**

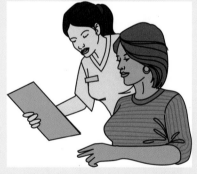

FIGURE 8-3 Administrative dental assistant and patient reviewing completed forms.

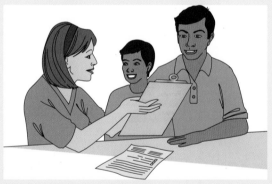

FIGURE 8-4 Patient and his father being interviewed by an administrative dental assistant in a private location.

COMPONENTS OF THE PATIENT CLINICAL RECORD

- Individual patient file folder*
- Dental radiographs*
- Acknowledgment of receipt of privacy practices notice*
- Registration form*
- Dental history form*
- Medical history form*
- Recall examination form
- Clinical examination form*
- Periodontal screening examination form

- Treatment plan form
- Problem priority list
- Progress notes form*
- Consent forms
- Signature on file form
- Financial arrangements form
- Correspondence log
- Telephone information form

* Necessary forms.

COLLECTING INFORMATION

To ensure consistency, a protocol for collection of information must be established and followed. A telephone information form, a written script, and other methods will help the administrative dental assistant to collect all information needed to compile the clinical record.

> **! REMEMBER**
>
> People outside the dental office may need to read the information contained within the clinical record. Therefore use standard abbreviations and charting terminology.

Privacy Practices Notice

Three separate communication documents must be given to a patient to describe how health information may be used and disclosed and how a patient can access his or her protected health information (PHI). The patient is first asked to read the Notice of Privacy Practices (Figure 8-5) followed by the Acknowledgment of Receipt of Notice of Privacy Practices (Figure 8-6).

Registration Forms

From a business perspective, the registration form contains information that will be used by the administrative dental assistant. The document includes demographic and insurance information needed to collect payment for dental services. It also includes key legal provisions that the patient agrees to by signing the form. There may also be separate consent forms. Study Anatomy of a Dental Registration Form to understand all of the components of this important form.

Other Diagnostic Records

Several different types of diagnostic tools may be used in the evaluation and maintenance of a patient's dental health. The most common, radiographs (x-rays), digital radiographs, and periodontal evaluations, are easily stored in the patient's clinical record. Other types of diagnostic records include intraoral photography. With an intraoral imaging system, pictures can be used to visually record the condition of the patient's teeth and surrounding tissue. The system combines an intraoral camera with a computer to record and store images. A narrative and visual report can be stored in the computer or transferred to photographs or DVD. The narrative report is included in the clinical record and a cross-referencing system is used to direct the reader to copies of the DVD, videotape, or computer record.

Diagnostic Models

Diagnostic models, or study models, are used as a tool in treatment planning. They are casts of the patient's mouth (Figure 8-7) and are not stored in the patient's clinical record; although they are part of the record, they are stored in a cabinet or box. To help locate models when needed, they should be stored alphabetically or numerically. Numeric filing works well for this purpose; the numbers are cross-referenced in the patient's clinical record and also in a master file.

CLINICAL RECORDS RISK MANAGEMENT

Risk management is a process that identifies conditions that may lead to alleged malpractice or procedures that are not in compliance with mandated regulations. Through a process of identifying and correcting possible conditions or violations, the dental healthcare team can lessen the risk of malpractice suits and deliver quality care to all patients.

Major issues that may cause the patient to question the quality of dental treatment include poor communications, poor dental healthcare team relationships, and poor record keeping. These problems can reduce the level of confidence between the patient and the dental healthcare team. During risk management evaluations, these areas should be identified and corrected before they create a need to defend in an alleged malpractice case.

A second area that can lead to legal actions or sanctions is noncompliance with statutes and regulations established by federal law, identified in the state Dental Practice Act, proscribed in professional organizations' codes of conduct, or outlined in contracts between the dental practice and third-party insurance carriers. Noncompliance can lead to fines, revocation of licenses, cancellation of contracts, and lawsuits. It is the duty of the dental healthcare team to be informed of statutes, regulations, and mandates and to follow them to the best of their ability. The American Dental Association, state dental associations, third-party insurance carriers, managed care providers, and other professional organizations have spent a great deal of time researching and developing action plans to alert the dental healthcare team to problem situations. These organizations conduct seminars and workshops to help the dental healthcare team identify problems and improve quality of care.

Maintaining Clinical Records (Manual and Electronic)

Experts in risk management have identified poor record keeping as a major justification for cases that are decided in favor of the patient. Poor records are sloppy, disorganized, and in most cases illegible. The primary reasons for keeping adequate files are to support the need for dental treatment and to justify the actions of the dentist. If the clinical record is incomplete and cannot support the need for treatment, legal cases are decided in the patient's favor. It is impossible to recount all details of each patient's treatment when you are asked questions in the future unless good records are available to which you can refer.

Canyon View Dental Associates
4546 North Avery Way
Canyon View, CA 91783
Telephone (987) 654-3210

NOTICE OF PRIVACY PRACTICES

THIS NOTICE DESCRIBES HOW HEALTH INFORMATION ABOUT YOU MAY BE USED AND DISCLOSED AND HOW YOU CAN GET ACCESS TO THIS INFORMATION.

PLEASE REVIEW IT CAREFULLY.
THE PRIVACY OF YOUR HEALTH INFORMATION IS IMPORTANT TO US.

OUR LEGAL DUTY
We are required by applicable federal and state law to maintain the privacy of your health information. We are also required to give you this Notice about our privacy practices, our legal duties, and your rights concerning your health information. We must follow the privacy practices that are described in this Notice while it is in effect. This Notice takes effect (April 14, 2003), and will remain in effect until we replace it.

We reserve the right to change our privacy practices and the terms of this Notice at any time, provided such changes are permitted by applicable law. We reserve the right to make the changes in our privacy practices and the new terms of our Notice effective for all health information that we maintain, including health information we created or received before we made the changes. Before we make a significant change in our privacy practices, we will change this Notice and make the new Notice available upon request.

You may request a copy of our Notice at any time. For more information about our privacy practices, or for additional copies of this Notice, please contact us using the information listed at the end of this Notice.

USES AND DISCLOSURES OF HEALTH INFORMATION
We use and disclose health information about you for treatment, payment, and healthcare operations. For example:

Treatment: We may use or disclose your health information to a physician or other healthcare provider providing treatment to you.

Payment: We may use and disclose your health information to obtain payment for services we provide to you.

Healthcare Operations: We may use and disclose your health information in connection with our healthcare operations. Healthcare operations include quality assessment and improvement activities, reviewing the competence or qualifications of healthcare professionals, evaluating practitioner and provider performance, conducting training programs, accreditation, certification, licensing or credentialing activities.

Your Authorization: In addition to our use of your health information for treatment, payment or healthcare operations, you may give us written authorization to use your health information or to disclose it to anyone for any purpose. If you give us an authorization, you may revoke it in writing at any time. Your revocation will not affect any use or disclosures permitted by your authorization while it was in effect. Unless you give us a written authorization, we cannot use or disclose your health information for any reason except those described in this Notice.

To Your Family and Friends: We must disclose your health information to you, as described in the Patient Rights section of this Notice. We may disclose your health information to a family member, friend or other person to the extent necessary to help with your healthcare or with payment for your healthcare, but only if you agree that we may do so.

Persons Involved In Care: We may use or disclose health information to notify, or assist in the notification of (including identifying or locating) a family member, your personal representative or another person responsible for your care, of your location, your general condition, or death. If you are present, then prior to use or disclosure of your health information, we will provide you with an opportunity to object to such uses or disclosures. In the event of your incapacity or emergency circumstances, we will disclose health information based on a determination using our professional judgment disclosing only health information that is directly relevant to the person's involvement in your healthcare. We will also use our professional judgment and our experience with common practice to make reasonable inferences of your best interest in allowing a person to pick up filled prescriptions, medical supplies, x-rays, or other similar forms of health information.

Marketing Health-Related Services: We will not use your health information for marketing communications without your written authorization.

Required by Law: We may use or disclose your health information when we are required to do so by law.

FIGURE 8-5 Notice of Privacy Practices forms are given to all patines and outlines how health information may be used and lists patients rights. The form also provides who to contact for additional information or to file a complaint.

Abuse or Neglect: We may disclose your health information to appropriate authorities if we reasonably believe that you are a possible victim of abuse, neglect, or domestic violence or the possible victim of other crimes. We may disclose your health information to the extent necessary to avert a serious threat to your health or safety or the health or safety of others.

National Security: We may disclose to military authorities the health information of Armed Forces personnel under certain circumstances. We may disclose to authorized federal officials health information required for lawful intelligence, counterintelligence, and other national security activities. We may disclose to correctional institution or law enforcement official having lawful custody of protected health information of inmate or patient under certain circumstances.

Appointment Reminders: We may use or disclose your health information to provide you with appointment reminders (such as voicemail messages, postcards, or letters).

PATIENT RIGHTS

Access: You have the right to look at or get copies of your health information, with limited exceptions. You may request that we provide copies in a format other than photocopies. We will use the format you request unless we cannot practicably do so. (You must make a request in writing to obtain access to your health information. You may obtain a form to request access by using the contact information listed at the end of this Notice. We will charge you a reasonable cost-based fee for expenses such as copies and staff time. You may also request access by sending us a letter to the address at the end of this Notice. If you request copies, we will charge you a reasonable duplication fee for staff time to locate and copy your health information, and postage if you want the copies mailed to you. If you request an alternative format, we will charge a cost-based fee for providing your health information in that format. If you prefer, we will prepare a summary or an explanation of your health information for a fee. Contact us using the information listed at the end of this Notice for a full explanation of our fee structure.)

Disclosure Accounting: You have the right to receive a list of instances in which we or our business associates disclosed your health information for purposes, other than treatment, payment, healthcare operations and certain other activities, for the last 6 years, but not before April 14, 2003. If you request this accounting more than once in a 12-month period, we may charge you a reasonable, cost-based fee for responding to these additional requests.

Restriction: You have the right to request that we place additional restrictions on our use or disclosure of your health information. We are not required to agree to these additional restrictions, but if we do, we will abide by our agreement (except in an emergency).

Alternative Communication: You have the right to request that we communicate with you about your health information by alternative means or to alternative locations. **{You must make your request in writing.}** Your request must specify the alternative means or location, and provide satisfactory explanation how payments will be handled under the alternative means or location you request.

Amendment: You have the right to request that we amend your health information. (Your request must be in writing, and it must explain why the information should be amended.) We may deny your request under certain circumstances.

Electronic Notice: If you receive this Notice on our Web site or by electronic mail (e-mail), you are entitled to receive this Notice in written form.

QUESTIONS AND COMPLAINTS

If you want more information about our privacy practices or have questions or concerns, please contact us.

If you are concerned that we may have violated your privacy rights, or you disagree with a decision we made about access to your health information or in response to a request you made to amend or restrict the use or disclosure of your health information or to have us communicate with you by alternative means or at alternative locations, you may complain to us using the contact information listed at the end of this Notice. You also may submit a written complaint to the U.S. Department of Health and Human Services. We will provide you with the address to file your complaint with the U.S. Department of Health and Human Services upon request.

We support your right to the privacy of your health information. We will not retaliate in any way if you choose to file a complaint with us or with the U.S. Department of Health and Human Services.

Contact Officer: _Canyon View Dental Associates_

Telephone: _555-0101_ Fax: _555-0202_

E-mail: _medwards@cuda.com_

Address: _4546 North Avery Way, Canyon View, CA 91783_

FIGURE 8-5, cont'd

Canyon View Dental Associates
4546 North Avery Way
Canyon View, CA 91783
Telephone (987) 654-3210

ACKNOWLEDGEMENT OF RECEIPT OF NOTICE OF PRIVACY PRACTICES

* You May Refuse to Sign This Acknowedgement*

I, _____, have received a copy of this office's Notice of Privacy Practices.

_____
Please Print Name

_____
Signature

_____
Date

_____ **For Office Use Only** _____

We attempted to obtain written acknowledgement of receipt of our Notice of Privacy Practices, but acknowledgement could not be obtained because:

☐ Individual refused to sign

☐ Communications barriers prohibited obtaining the acknowledgement

☐ An emergency situation prevented us from obtaining acknowledgement

☐ Other (Please Specify)

FIGURE 8-6 Acknowledgement of Receipt of Notice of Privacy Practices forms are provided to all patient and become part of the Clinical Record.

ANATOMY OF A DENTAL REGISTRATION FORM

Canyon View Dental Associates
4546 North Avery Way
Canyon View, CA 91783
Telephone (987) 654-3210

Thank you for selecting our dental healthcare team!
We always strive to provide you with the best possible dental care.
To help us meet all your dental healthcare needs, please fill out this form completely.
Please let us know if you have any questions.

1 Patient Information (CONFIDENTIAL)

Patient # ___326570___
Soc. Sec. # ___123-45-6789___
Date ___7/1/2015___
Home Phone _555-4321_

Name __Rose L Budd__   Birthdate _7/17/52_
Address ___1836 N Front Street___   City ___Flora___   State _CA_ Zip ___91771___
Check Appropriate Box: ☐ Minor ☒ Single ☐ Married ☐ Divorced ☐ Widowed ☐ Separated
Patient's or Parent's Employer __Town Bank__   Work Phone _555-3210_
Business Address __123 S Business Way__   City _____   State _____ Zip _____
Spouse or Parent's Name _____   Employer_____   Work Phone_____
If Patient is a Student, Name of School/College _____   City_____   State____ Zip _____
Whom May We Thank for Referring you? _____
Person to Contact in Case of Emergency __Evelyn Jones__   Phone _____

2 Responsible Party

Name of Person Responsible for this Account __Rose L Budd__   Relationship to Patient ___Self___
Address __1836 N Front Street__   Home Phone _555-4321_
Driver's License # __M3205167__   Birthdate _7/17/52_   Financial Information _____
Employer __Town Bank__   Work Phone _555-3210_
Is this Person Currently a Patient in our Office? ☐ Yes ☐ No   Cell Phone _____
Email Address _R.L.Budd@townbank.com_

3 Insurance Information

Name of Insured __Rose Budd__   Relationship to Patient ___Self___
Birthdate _7/17/52_   Social Security # _123-45-6789_   Date Employed _____
Name of Employer __Town Bank__   Work Phone _555-3210_
Address of Employer __123 S Business Way__   City _____   State _____ Zip _____
Insurance Company _Blue Cross_   Group # _____   Union or Local # _____
Ins. Co. Address __1116 Form St.__   City _Los Angeles_   State _CA_ Zip _91110_
How Much is your Deductible? _____ How much have you met? _____ Max. Annual Benefit _____

DO YOU HAVE ANY ADDITIONAL INSURANCE? ☐ Yes ☒ NO   IF YES, COMPLETE THE FOLLOWING

Name of Insured _____   Relationship to Patient _____
Birthdate_____   Social Security #_____   Date Employed _____
Name of Employer_____   Work Phone _____
Address of Employer_____   City_____   State _____ Zip_____
Insurance Company_____   Group #_____   Union or Local #_____
Ins. Co. Address _____   City_____   State____ Zip_____
How Much is your Deductible? _____ How much have you met? _____ Max. Annual Benefit _____

4 I attest to the accuracy of the information on this page.

Patient's or guardian's signature _____   Date _____

REGISTRATION

---

1 PATIENT INFORMATION SECTION

This includes demographic data that will be used in preparing financial and insurance statements.

2 RESPONSIBLE PARTY SECTION

This relates to the person or persons who are financially responsible for the payment of the dental account. This is not to be confused with insurance companies or others who will act as third party in the payment of the patient's dental fees. This concept is confusing and often misinterpreted by patients. Adult patients are responsible for their own account, and when married they are jointly responsible (in most states) along with their spouse. Minor children's accounts are the responsibility of their parents. In the case of divorced parents, the court assigns responsibility to one or both parents. Determining financial responsibility is confusing for both the dental assistant and the patient. The bottom line is that the patient or parents are responsible for payment. Insurance companies do not guarantee payment and therefore cannot be held responsible.

3 INSURANCE INFORMATION

This includes all of the information needed to complete and process dental insurance claim forms. This information is also used to determine the eligibility for and the dental insurance coverage of the patient.

4 CERTIFICATION THAT THE INFORMATION PRESENTED IS ACCURATE

This is signed by the patient or parent.

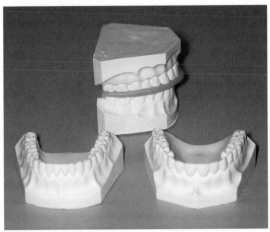

FIGURE 8-7 Diagnostic model. (From Bird DL, Robinson DS: *Modern dental assisting*, ed 11, St. Louis, 2015, Saunders.)

The administrative dental assistant plays a key role in protecting the dental practice from such lawsuits. The process begins and ends with the administrative dental assistant, as it is this staff member who collects the initial data when a patient first enters the dental practice and initiates the clinical record process. After a patient has received treatment, the clinical record is returned to the business office. It is the responsibility of the administrative dental assistant to check each chart to ensure that all necessary forms have been completed and that the entries meet mandated criteria. Through a checks-and-balances routine, the entire dental healthcare team takes part in ensuring that information is organized, complete, and legible. Regulations and mandates of record keeping vary from state to state and from organization to organization. It is therefore necessary for you to become familiar with the requirements of each state and each organization in which you work.

Procedures for Specific Tasks

Entries

All handwritten entries must be legible and entered in non-erasable ink. The entry must be signed and dated and, in some states, must include an identification number (such as a driver's license or Social Security number). If a correction is made, the error should be crossed out with a single line that is dated and initialed (Figure 8-8). When electronic records are maintained, the information must be clear, concise, and complete and the established protocol for making corrections must be followed. It is very important that the software used for patients' electronic records contain a program that tracks all entries by clearly identifying the person who entered or changed data. Abbreviations should be used consistently and a copy of definitions should be kept on file. *Rationale:* An illegible entry or the presence of whiteout can imply that something has been hidden. If abbreviations are not understood, they will confuse the reader, members of the court, or other health professionals and can lead to an incorrect interpretation.

Patient Identification

The patient's name or number should be placed on all pages of the clinical record (as illustrated in Rose Budd's clinical record) and on all radiographs, cast models, laboratory prescriptions, and correspondence. *Rationale:* If records become separated, it may be very difficult to locate the master file and vital information may become permanently lost.

Statements

Statements about patients must be truthful, factual, and objective. Guesses about how patients feel or why they did something can lead to problems if the records leave the dental practice. It is best to report only documented findings (objective findings). *Rationale:* Records can be read by patients and released to others. In a legal proceeding, they will be read by members of the court.

An example of a subjective statement is as follows:

Mary has a real attitude today.

This statement does not provide information. It is only an interpretation of an observation. Mary could have an "attitude" because of a nondental problem or this could be Mary's normal personality.

An example of an objective statement is as follows:

Mary said that she is upset because she had to wait for 20 minutes.

This statement is based on factual information given by Mary.

Progress Notes

Notations should include the diagnosis, treatment, and amount and type of anesthetic as well as the brand names of materials used. Postoperative instructions or unusual occurrences should also be noted. Spacing between entries should be consistent and limited to one or two lines (Figure 8-9).

Rationale: If spacing is inconsistent, it may appear that information was added at a later date. If it is necessary to add information, you are advised to date the entry and state that you are amending the original entry. In addition to recording treatment information, it is suggested, for good risk management, that information on correspondence, telephone conversations, missed appointment noncompliance, and prescriptions also be recorded in the progress notes.

Correspondence

Correspondence includes letters between professionals concerning the dental health of the patient, referral letters, letters between the dentist and the patient concerning dental treatment, insurance inquiries, and letters of dismissal. In addition, all correspondence received should be noted in the progress notes and a copy should be placed in the clinical record. If a correspondence log is used, information can be entered there and cross-referenced to the clinical records.

Telephone Conversations

All telephone conversations with other professionals, pharmacies, insurance carriers, and patients should be recorded and a brief description should be given stating the significance for any patient's dental care.

Missed Appointments

Documentation of missed and broken appointments establishes the intent of the dentist to complete work in a timely manner and to provide postoperative care. Missed appointments should be followed up with a letter to the patient explaining the importance of continued treatment and outlining the consequences if additional appointments are missed. Place a copy of such letters in the patient's clinical record.

Failure to Follow Instructions

Documenting postoperative or other instructions establishes that the information was given to the patient. Likewise, documenting failure of the patient to follow instructions establishes the patient's noncompliance. The consequences of noncompliance must be explained to the patient in writing; one copy is given to the patient and another copy is placed in the patient's clinical record.

Prescriptions

Records must be kept of all prescription and nonprescription drugs given to the patient. The name of the drug, quantity and dosage, and date given must be recorded in the progress notes. Other recommendations or prescriptions, such as for radiographs, laboratory tests, physical therapy, or a dental prosthesis, must be noted also and a copy of the prescription must be placed in the patient's clinical record.

> **! REMEMBER**
>
> Information left out of records is assumed, in a court of law, to have never existed.

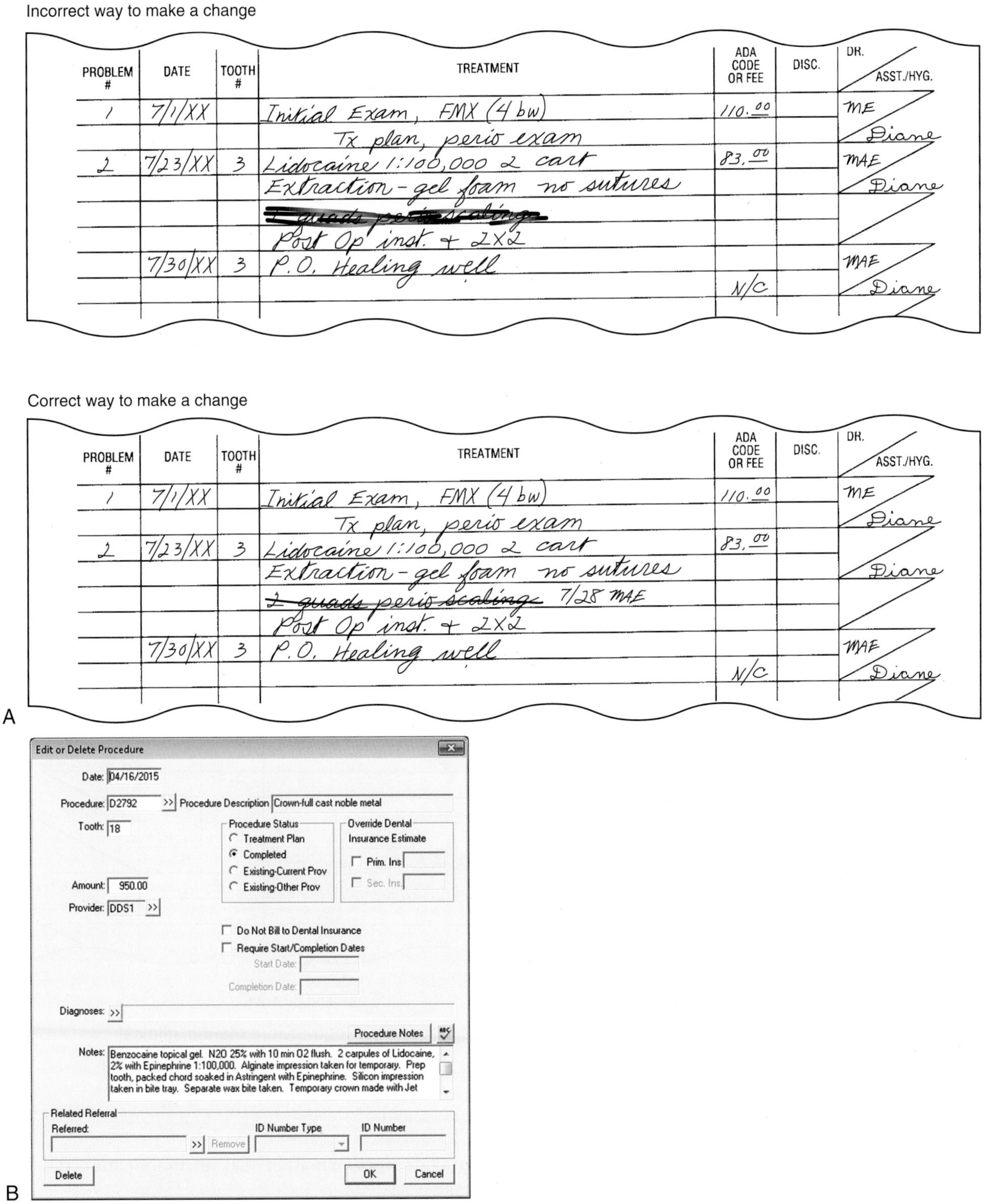

Incorrect way to make a change

PROBLEM #	DATE	TOOTH #	TREATMENT	ADA CODE OR FEE	DISC.	DR. ASST./HYG.
1	7/1/XX		Initial Exam, FMX (4 bw)	110.00		M.E.
			Tx plan, perio exam			Diane
2	7/23/XX	3	Lidocaine 1:100,000 2 cart	83.00		M.A.E.
			Extraction - gel foam no sutures			Diane
			~~2 quads perio scaling~~			
			Post Op inst. + 2X2			
	7/30/XX	3	P.O. Healing well			M.A.E.
					N/C	Diane

Correct way to make a change

PROBLEM #	DATE	TOOTH #	TREATMENT	ADA CODE OR FEE	DISC.	DR. ASST./HYG.
1	7/1/XX		Initial Exam, FMX (4 bw)	110.00		M.E.
			Tx plan, perio exam			Diane
2	7/23/XX	3	Lidocaine 1:100,000 2 cart	83.00		
			Extraction - gel foam no sutures			Diane
			~~2 quads perio scaling~~ 7/28 MAE			
			Post Op inst. + 2X2			
	7/30/XX	3	P.O. Healing well			M.A.E.
					N/C	Diane

A

B

FIGURE 8-8 A, Incorrect way to make a change and correct way to make a change in a manual clinical record. **B,** Dialogue box used to make changes to an electronic clinical record. (**B,** Dentrix screen capture courtesy Henry Schein Practice Solutions, American Fork, Utah.)

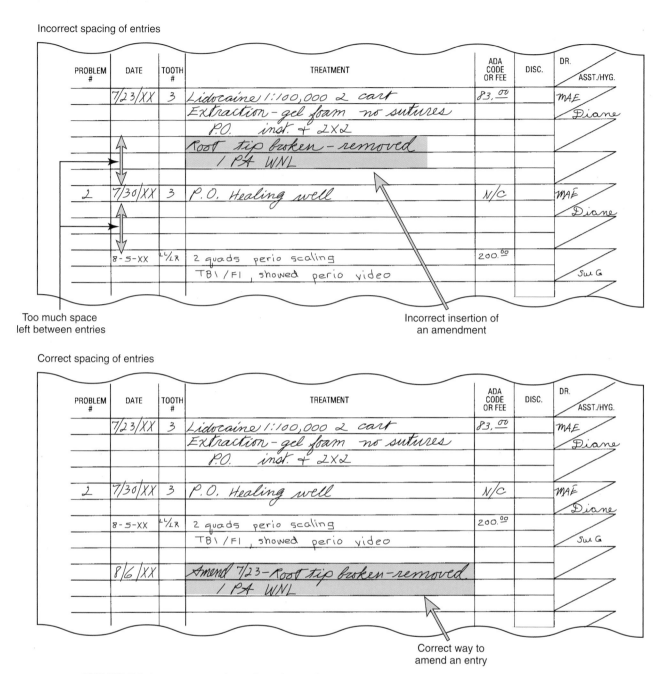

FIGURE 8-9 Incorrect spacing of entries and correct spacing of entries in a manual clinical record.

Rationale

Consider what would happen if, during an examination, a patient showed no signs of an abnormal condition and therefore no mention of the examination was added to the clinical record. An outside professional or an attorney who later reads the record may conclude that the examination did not take place. Even if no significant condition was found, a notation still needs to be made. The use of abbreviations such as **WNL** (within normal limits) and **NSF** (no significant findings) can simplify the process yet still provide documentation that an examination did in fact take place.

Other forms and documentation may be required or recommended by risk management experts. It is important to remember that all of these tools are designed to help the dental healthcare team meet the needs of the patient. By keeping good records, being organized, communicating efficiently, and establishing a partnership with patients, the dental healthcare team helps to protect the practice from alleged malpractice cases.

KEY POINTS

- The function of the clinical record is to provide the dental healthcare team with information. The registration form provides demographic and financial information needed to complete insurance forms and bill the patient. The medical history and dental history provide the dentist with information needed to diagnose the patient's condition. Treatment plans and clinical charts document necessary treatment. Progress notes document treatment that is performed. A variety of other forms help to organize and maintain a complete record for each patient.
- It is the responsibility of the administrative dental assistant to maintain organized clinical records. The administrative dental assistant collects information, organizes the clinical record, checks for completeness, and safeguards the integrity of the record.
- Risk management is a process that identifies conditions that can lead to alleged malpractice or to procedures that are not in compliance with mandated regulations. Through the process of identifying and correcting possible conditions or violations, the dental healthcare team can limit the number of alleged malpractice suits and deliver quality care to all patients. The primary reasons for keeping adequate files are to support the patient's need for dental treatment and to justify the dentist's actions.

CAREER-READY PRACTICES

Career-Ready Practices activities are designed to provide students with experiences that can be "practiced" in preparation for skills needed on the job. In each of the following exercises, a variety of approaches may be used to address the problem, rather than "right" or "wrong" answers. Below each exercise, next to the compass icon, is a listing of suggested Career-Ready Practice numbers that correspond to the listing of 12 practices in the front of the text (see p. viii-ix); these practices provide suggestions for approaches to complete the exercise.

1. Role play. Use a telephone information form as a guide and, with another student, simulate a telephone conversation according to the following scenario: A new patient calls the dental office to schedule an appointment to have a tooth checked. The tooth has been hurting for about 3 weeks.

 Career-Ready Practices
  1 *Act as a responsible and contributing citizen and employee.*
  4 *Communicate clearly, effectively, and with reason.*
  2 *Apply appropriate academic and technical skills.*

2. Mary Smith has an appointment for her first visit to the dental practice. The reception area is crowded when she arrives. Jim, the administrative dental assistant, greets Mrs. Smith.
  a. How should Jim complete the information collection process?
  b. What forms are included in the process?
  c. Form a small team and discuss situations that may arise that will require an approach that is different from the one selected by Jim. Write an action plan for each of the following situations, including statements of the problem and the solution: the patient is a minor; the patient is physically challenged; or the patient has specific medical problems.

 Career-Ready Practices
  1 *Act as a responsible and contributing citizen and employee.*
  2 *Apply appropriate academic and technical skills.*
  4 *Communicate clearly, effectively, and with reason.*
  5 *Consider the environmental, social, and economic impacts of decisions.*

3. Obtain a copy of your state's Dental Practice Act. List the mandates for clinical record keeping.

 Career-Ready Practices
  7 *Employ valid and reliable research strategies.*
  2 *Apply appropriate academic and technical skills.*
  5 *Consider the environmental, social, and economic impacts of decisions.*

4. The administrative dental assistant plays a key role in protecting the dental practice from legal actions. Describe this role and outline the duties of the administrative dental assistant that pertain to clinical records.

 Career-Ready Practices
  7 *Employ valid and reliable research strategies.*
  4 *Communicate clearly, effectively, and with reason.*
  6 *Demonstrate creativity and innovation.*

9

Information Management

LEARNING OBJECTIVES

1. List and describe the six filing methods outlined in this chapter, including demonstration of the ARMA Simplified Filing Standard Rules.
2. Compare and contrast the filing methods used for business records such as accounts payable and personnel records versus patient and insurance information.
3. List and describe types of filing equipment to store information for a paper system.
4. List and describe filing supplies, including types of file labels.
5. Prepare a new patient's clinical record for filing.
6. Prepare a business document for filing (manually and electronically).
7. Discuss how long records must be retained and the two methods of transferring records.

INTRODUCTION

The responsibilities of the administrative dental assistant in the management of information and records are multifaceted. In today's dental practice, the storage of information may involve both paper files and electronic files. Although methods of documentation may vary, the principles of a records management program will always be the same. According to the International Organization for Standardization (ISO), in *Information and Documentation—Records Management,* a general policy should involve "the creation and management of authentic, reliable and usable records, capable of supporting business function and activities for as long as they are required." The importance of collecting the correct information and preparation of a dental record were discussed in Chapter 8. This chapter discusses basic methods used in a systematic approach to the storage and retrieval of information (filing).

Once it has been created, a record (paper and electronic) should remain accessible, usable, reliable, and authentic. Systems for electronic records should also ensure that these criteria will be maintained through any type of system change for the entire period that this information will be retained, including any change in software or in the practice management system.

The purposes of following a systematic approach to information management are to simplify the retrieval process and to ensure the precise location of documents and records. In a paper environment, a storage system includes a filing system that contains metal filing cabinets and methods for organizing documents and records. In an electronic environment, the storage system includes hard drives (located on individual PCs and network servers [local or remote]) and portable devices (CDs, tapes, and portable mega storage devices).

Filing systems are used in almost all areas of daily life. Think of a supermarket. Products are divided into categories: produce, dairy, meat, frozen foods, canned goods, and so forth. Once you locate a product category, you will find that it has been subdivided into other areas. For example, when you are shopping for a can of cream of mushroom soup, you first have to locate the general area where soup is shelved. You locate the aisle by reading the overhead signs. Once in the correct aisle, you find the soup section; it will be subdivided by brands. You locate the brand of soup you are shopping for and then discover that the different types of soup are shelved alphabetically. This system helps you to find the can of cream of mushroom soup quickly and efficiently.

Filing in the dental office follows the same principles. First, you locate the file cabinet that contains the information you want to retrieve. Second, you identify the location within the cabinet that contains the subject area. Subjects may be subdivided alphabetically. This eases the retrieval process and ensures that documents are available when needed.

FILING METHODS

A filing system provides a method for placing files in a prescribed order so that they can be located and retrieved by any member of the dental healthcare team. It is the responsibility of the dental professional to safeguard the integrity and confidentiality of all documents. This cannot be guaranteed if records are misplaced or are not returned to their proper locations. It is advisable to follow one of the standardized methods for filing information. Brief descriptions of six of the basic filing systems are provided.

Alphabetic

Alphabetic filing follows strict rules. These rules have been standardized by ARMA (a not-for-profit professional organization and the authority on managing records and information) and are recognized as an American National Standard by the American National Standards Institute (ANSI). The purpose of standardization is to establish consistent methods of filing.

Standards must be applied to each and every document, patient record, or other medium that is to be stored. This is not a haphazard process; it must be followed exactly by each person who indexes, codes, and files. When these steps are followed, the integrity and safety of all records can be maintained.

All basic filing methods, with the exception of the chronological system, require alphabetic arrangement. Most of the filing within the dental practice is done alphabetically. Sometimes, a numeric filing system is used (e.g., for clinical records).

The arrangement of a name, subject, or number is referred to as indexing and constitutes a filing segment. Before a personal name, business name, or organizational name is indexed, it must be arranged in the correct order. A name, subject, or word is broken down into units. ARMA has defined a unit and filing segments as follows:

> A *filing unit* may be a number, a letter, a word, or any combination of these as stated…
> One or more filing units are a *filing segment* (i.e., the total name, subject, or number that is being used for filing purposes).

A description of what makes up each unit and the order in which units are placed follows; personal names and business or organizational names are used as examples.

- **Unit 1:** *Personal name rule:* Last name (*surname;* also known as the *family name*). *Business/organizational name rule:* First name of the business or organization (business and organizational names are filed as written).
- **Unit 2:** *Personal name rule:* First name (*given name*); can also be the initial of the first name. *Business/organizational name rule:* Second name as written.
- **Unit 3:** *Personal name rule:* Middle name or initial. *Business/organizational name rule:* Third name as written.
- **Unit 4:** *Personal name rule:* Titles, appendages, and degrees (e.g., Prince, Sr., DDS). *Business/organizational name rule:* Fourth name as written.

NAME AS WRITTEN	NAME AS FILED			
	Unit 1	**Unit 2**	**Unit 3**	**Unit 4**
Robert A. Weingart, DDS (Personal name rule)	Weingart	Robert	A.	DDS
Robert A. Weingart, DDS (Business name rule)	Robert	A.	Weingart	DDS

Chart Label (Personal Name)

Weingart, Robert A., DDS (comma is placed between the last name and the first)

File Label (Business Name)

Robert A. Weingart, DDS

The following are examples based on the ARMA **Simplified Filing Standard Rules for Personal Names.**

Names with prefixes. When a surname has a prefix, such as De, La, Mac, Mc, O', or Van, the prefix is indexed and filed as one unit with the surname. Business and organizational names follow the same rules as personal names.

Personal and professional titles and suffixes. Titles and suffixes are not used as a filing unit except when they are needed to distinguish between two or more identical names. When used, titles and suffixes are placed in the last filing unit and are filed as written. (Punctuation is ignored.) Specific filing guidelines specify that suffixes are filed in numeric sequence when needed for identification.

When college degrees are used, they are placed in the last unit and are used for indexing only, to distinguish between two identical names.

Hyphenated names. Hyphenated surnames are treated as one unit.

NAME AS WRITTEN	NAME AS FILED			
	Unit 1	**Unit 2**	**Unit 3**	**Unit 4**
Allen	Allen			
A. C. Allen	Allen	A.	C.	
A. C. Allendale	Allendale	A.	C.	
Alice Allendale	Allendale	Alice		
Charles Allendale	Allendale	Charles		
Charlotte Allendale	Allendale	Charlotte		

NAME AS WRITTEN	NAME AS FILED			
	Unit 1	Unit 2	Unit 3	Unit 4
Mark De Anza	De Anza	Mark		
Josie De La Cruz	De La Cruz	Josie		
James M. El Camino	El Camino	James	M.	

NAME AS WRITTEN	NAME AS FILED			
	Unit 1	Unit 2	Unit 3	Unit 4
James Hall	Hall	James		
James C. Hall	Hall	James	C.	
James C. Hall, Sr.	Hall	James	C.	Sr.
James C. Hall, Jr.	Hall	James	C.	Jr.
James C. Hall, III [third]	Hall	James	C.	III [third]
James C. Hall, V [fifth]	Hall	James	C.	V [fifth]

NAME AS WRITTEN	NAME AS FILED			
	Unit 1	Unit 2	Unit 3	Unit 4
Judith L. Green	Green	Judith	L.	
Judith L. Green, DDS	Green	Judith	L.	DDS
Judith L. Green, DMD	Green	Judith	L.	DMD
Julia J. Green	Green	Julia	J.	
Julia J. Green, Ed.D	Green	Julia	J.	Ed.D

NAME AS WRITTEN	NAME AS FILED			
	Unit 1	Unit 2	Unit 3	Unit 4
Lynn Marie Jones	Jones	Lynn	Marie	
Mary Ann Jones-Scott	Jones-Scott	Mary	Ann	
Mary Kelly	Kelly	Mary		
Sandra Kelly-Jones	Kelly-Jones	Sandra		

NAME AS WRITTEN	NAME AS FILED			
	Unit 1	Unit 2	Unit 3	Unit 4
Duchess of York	Duchess (of)	York		
Father O'Malley	Father	O'Malley		
Madame Curie	Madame	Curie		
Pastor Ralph	Pastor	Ralph		
Sister Mary Frances	Sister	Mary	Frances	

Royal and religious titles. When royal and religious titles are followed by a single name, they are filed as written.

Rarely are titles such as Mr., Mrs., Ms., and Miss or military titles used in indexing, unless they are required to distinguish between two identical names. When they are used, these are indexed in the last unit and are alphabetized in the abbreviated form.

When filing records with properly indexed names, one should follow these basic rules:

- The first *letter* that is different in *any unit* determines the alphabetic order.
- Single names are filed before the same name followed by an initial or name.
- Initials are filed before the spelled-out name.
- Abbreviations are filed as if they were spelled out. Example: St. becomes Saint, 3rd becomes Third.
- Nicknames are treated as first (given) names.
- Business and organizational names are filed as written; the business letterhead should be used as a guide.

Numeric

Numeric filing is used for very large numbers of records. In this system, records are filed according to the number assigned. A key component to this system is cross-referencing. Cross-referencing is a method that identifies what other name (or number) a record may be filed under. In numeric filing, an alphabetic listing of all records is used to match names with numbers. Most practice management computer software programs use a numeric system. When a new patient name is entered into the system, the computer assigns the patient a number. The computer can locate patient records by entering a number or an alphabetic configuration (name).

In the numeric system, the order in which the number falls determines its place in the filing system. This is much like counting: 100, 101, 102. Groups of numbers may be assigned to letters of the alphabet that correspond with surnames (last names)—for example, 100 to 999 may be assigned to surnames beginning with *A;* 1000 to 1999 may be assigned to surnames beginning with *B;* and so forth. File guides are used in the filing cabinet to identify specific numeric sections.

A computer system works well with this method because it can assign numbers and provide cross-referencing.

Geographic

Geographic filing categorizes records according to a geographic location, such as city, zip code, area code, state, or country. Each document is coded and filed according to the selected geographic locator.

Subject

The purpose of subject filing is that it allows the retrieval of information according to subject. In this system, files are arranged alphabetically by subject and then within each subject by subgroup (e.g., company name). This system works well for business records (Figure 9-1).

Chronological

Chronological filing allows one to locate documents according to date, month, or year (Figure 9-2). Files are first sorted alphabetically by subject and then within each subject by chronology.

Electronic

In today's business environment, the majority of records and documents will be created, stored, and transmitted electronically. The primary advantage of using electronic file types, including documents, e-mail, databases, and websites, is the ease and efficiency with which information can be accessed and shared. With the added advantages of electronic media come the same issues and problems one encounters in a paper-based system. In order for the information to be accessed easily, it has to be easy to find. It is just as easy to lose an electronic document as it is to lose a paper document. A key difference is that in an electronic environment you can use advanced computer searches to locate files, but you still need to know how to filter and sort information. Therefore the same principles and practices used in a paper system need to be applied in an electronic system. You will still need to be consistent in the way your folders are organized and how you file information. In an electronic filing system, a folder is where you place subfolders and files. Files are individual items such as a Word document, picture, database, or e-mail attachment.

Questions to Ask

1. *Where will the electronic folders be kept?* Electronic folders can be stored in different ways, from single users to multiple users. If the folder is located on an individual computer, access is limited to that computer. If you want the folder to be available to users at other computers in the dental office or in a remote location, the folder needs to be placed on a network. Placing folders on networks may require different security levels depending on the nature of the information and whether it needs to be protected. Sometimes access is password protected and documents may be locked so that information cannot be changed.

2. *How will the folders and files be organized and classified?* The folders need to be organized in a systematic way that is consistent with other filing systems established by each dental office, provided that they are effective and efficient. Most operating systems will allow you to organize folders and files in a file hierarchy similar to the way you would store paper documents. If you have a paper filing system that uses a subject or functional records classification for business functions, your electronic business folders need to be classified and organized in the same manner. Different categories of folders may have different classifications and coding. For example, business folders are organized by function; correspondence is organized by individual and filed alphabetically; account numbers are used to file individual patient account information.

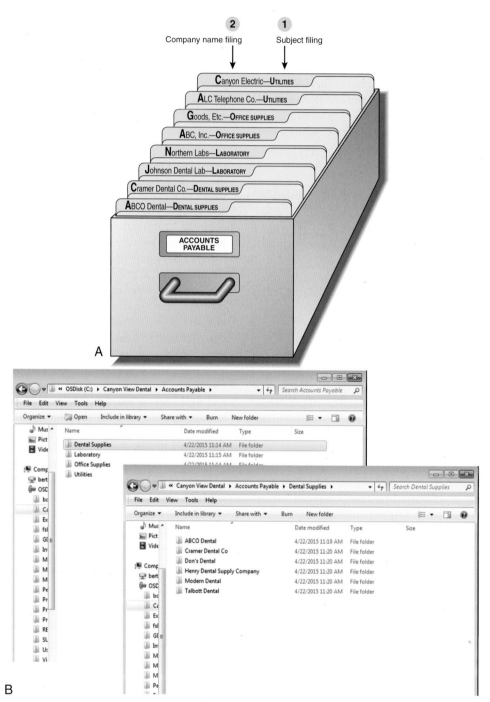

FIGURE 9-1 Subject filing. **A,** Traditional subject filing: accounts payable, with general headings and subheadings. **B,** Computerized subject filing: accounts payable, with general headings and subheadings.

3. *How will folders, subfolders, and files be named?* If the system is going to be useful, the naming of the folders, subfolders, and files must be consistent and have meaning. It is helpful to develop a common naming protocol for the dental office so that all of the folders and files follow the same format. This is extremely helpful when there are many different people working with the same folders. There is a limit to how much information can be included when naming electronic folders and files, which varies with the software being used. As long as files are being saved to the appropriate folders, the folder structure can be used to provide further information. When naming an individual file, stick to the details of that specific file and allow the folders it is placed in to provide context. For example, the folder is named *Dental Supplies*, the subfolder is the name of the vendor, and the files placed in the

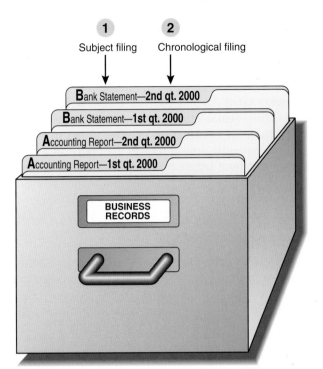

FIGURE 9-2 Chronological filing: financial reports, with *1*, general headings (subject filing) and *2*, subheadings (chronological filing).

vendor file are named by year and month. Because computers can sort folders and files alphabetically or numerically, be consistent in how you start folder and file names. The computer can sort by date, number, name, or symbol and you will be able to set the sorting parameters.

TYPES OF INFORMATION

Information that is stored in either a paper or an electronic system can be divided into two broad categories: business and patient information. Within each of these two categories, subjects are divided into more specific topics.

Business Records

Business records consist of all documents that pertain to the operation of the dental practice. Business records are divided into several different topics and a variety of methods exist for their retrieval and storage.

Accounts Payable

Accounts payable records, tracks, and stores information about the money the practice pays to others for services and supplies (see Chapter 16). Records are divided and categorized by subject and then by vendor, according to the filing system selected. For example, an office may divide accounts according to general headings, such as dental supplies, laboratory, office supplies, and utilities. Once major headings have been developed, it is necessary to subdivide by vendor (see Figure 9-1).

Accounts Receivable

Accounts receivable records and tracks money that is owed to the dental practice (see Chapter 17). Accounts receivable records are stored in a different location or file from accounts payable. When a computerized system is used, these records are stored within the computer under the heading of "Patient Accounts." If a peg board or manual system is used, ledger cards are filed alphabetically in a small metal file box (see Chapter 14).

Bank Statements and Financial Reports

Bank statements and financial reports are financial records that are filed according to subject and then subdivided chronologically (see Figure 9-2).

Personnel Records

Personnel records relate to matters that pertain to the employees of the dental practice. These records include payroll records, which document financial information about each employee. The records are filed by subject (payroll) and then subdivided alphabetically by employee name. Each employee file is subdivided chronologically (by payroll period).

Confidential personnel records contain information about the employee's work record. These files contain employment contracts, performance reviews, and documentation of noncompliance. They must be secured and cannot be made available to nonauthorized people.

Tax Records

Tax records are filed by subject and then subdivided into types of reports or records. These records usually cover a specified period of time and therefore are subfiled chronologically. Tax reports include payroll, business, and corporate tax reports.

Business Reports

Business reports include profit and loss statements, practice production, and other specified reports that categorize a subject area. Reports are filed by subject and then subdivided chronologically.

Insurance Records

Insurance records include contracts with third-party carriers (insurance companies) and insurance policies that cover areas of the dental practice. These contracts and policies are filed according to subject.

Professional Correspondence

Professional correspondence includes correspondence between individuals and professional organizations. Files are organized by subject (e.g., Dental Specialty) and then divided into specific subject areas (e.g., Endodontics). Specific subjects are then subdivided according to individual or organization (Figure 9-3).

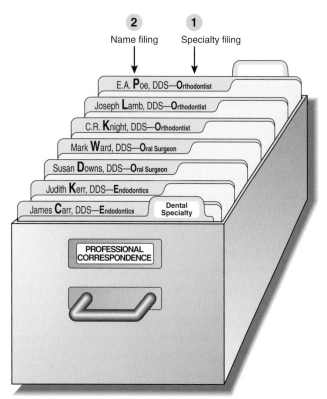

FIGURE 9-3 Professional correspondence filing: organized by subject, subdivided into specific areas, and then subdivided by individual or organization.

Patient and Insurance Information

Patient Information

Patient information is stored within the clinical record (see Chapter 8). Information contained within the record deals strictly with treatment of the patient. The record does not include financial accounts or insurance forms. Clinical records are filed alphabetically or numerically in a variety of different storage cabinets.

Insurance Records

Insurance records are stored separately from patients' clinical records. Insurance forms are filed in a manner that is specified by each dental practice (see Chapter 15). Forms can be filed by insurance company and then subdivided by patient. Chronological filing categorizes the forms according to the date on which the work was completed or the date on which the claim was filed. Once a claim has been paid, it is pulled from the original file and refiled in the Paid Claims file.

> ### WHAT WOULD YOU DO?
>
> Your dental office has decided that it is going "green" and will convert its current paper filing system for business records to an electronic filing system. How will you design the new electronic filing system?

FILING EQUIPMENT FOR A PAPER SYSTEM

Storage of information is achieved by putting documents in the correct file folder and placing the folder into the filing unit. The purposes of the filing unit are to store documents safely and to provide a system for easy retrieval. Most dental offices use more than one type of system. Business information may be stored in vertical files while patients' clinical records are placed in a lateral filing unit. Patient ledger cards are stored in small metal boxes and recall cards may be filed in an index box. Sizes and configurations of filing cabinets vary according to the needs of the dental practice.

Vertical Files

Vertical files are cabinets that consist of one to five drawers that are arranged one on top of another. When these cabinets are used for storage of business records, a frame can be inserted into each drawer to accommodate hanging files. Hanging files can be labeled and then individual files can be organized within each hanging file (see Figure 9-1).

Lateral Files

Lateral files, or open files, are very popular with dental professionals. They can take the form of modular units or built-in shelving systems. They take up less floor space and blend with the current trend in office design (Figure 9-4). File folders used in this system have side tabs.

Card Files

Card files, or Rolodex files, are designed for quick reference of telephone numbers and addresses and can be used in a recall system. Their small size allows them to be set on a desk or countertop.

FILING SUPPLIES

Once a filing method and appropriate filing equipment have been selected, supplies are needed to complete the system.

File Folders

File folders come in a variety of formats. They are usually made of heavy stock paper, which adds durability. File folders are used to store documents, patient record forms, and business reports.

Vertical File Folders

Vertical file folders are used with vertical filing systems and have tabs located at the top of the file (see Figure 9-2). Labels are placed on the tab to identify the contents of the folder. The location of the tab varies from folder to folder; this provides a means of looking at more than one tab at a time. Folders that have a series of three tabs—far left, center, and far right—are referred to as ⅓ cut. Folders with a series of five tabs are referred to as ⅕ cut.

Organization of the filing cabinet can involve a hanging file system. This system uses a frame from which files hang.

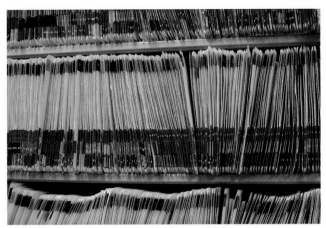

FIGURE 9-4 Lateral filing system. (Copyright © 2006 AK2, iStock.com.)

Hanging files can hold several file folders, can provide tabs for indexing, and can be moved easily to accommodate rearranging of files. Hanging files work well in systems in which files must hold more than one file folder.

Lateral File Folders

Lateral file folders are used for clinical records and come in a variety of formats and designs. Tabs are located on the sides of the folders. Indexed labels and color-coded labels are placed on the tabs (Figure 9-5). Each folder consists of one or two fasteners designed to keep patient record forms in place (see Chapter 8). Each also has one or two pockets in which radiographs and loose papers can be kept. Some file folders have dividers that help to organize forms within the clinical record.

Guides

Guides are used to divide filing systems into small sections. The guide is typically made of heavy stock paper and may be laminated for durability. In the alphabetic system, each letter of the alphabet has a guide. When files are large, additional guides or dividers can be used to subdivide the sections. Smaller sections have less chance of being misfiled.

Out-Guides

Out-guides are used to fill the space occupied by a file that has been removed from the system. The out-guide can simply denote that a record has been removed or it may contain information stating the location of the record, who removed it, and when it will be returned. The primary purpose of the out-guide is to signify that a record has been removed from the system (see Figure 9-5).

File Labels

The style and location of file labels are based on the filing system and must be used consistently. You must be careful to select the correct label for the file folder and to index it according to the selected method. Labels can be typed or computer generated.

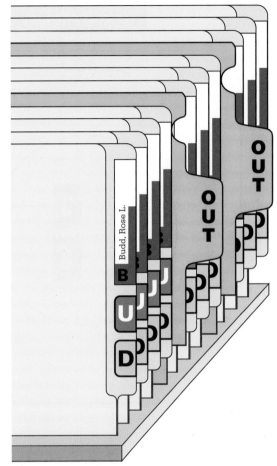

FIGURE 9-5 Lateral file with out-guides showing where records have been removed.

Color Coding

The purpose of color coding in a filing system is to provide visual identification. Charts are marked with color tabs. If the charts are filed properly, a uniform pattern will be visible. When a chart is filed incorrectly, the colored pattern will be broken, alerting you to the error. Typically, a color coding system uses a different color for the first 13 letters of the alphabet and then repeats the color with a mark, such as a wide band, for the second half of the alphabet. Systems may use one to three colors per file. Color coding can be used in vertical and lateral systems but it is more effective when used within a lateral filing system.

Aging Labels

The use of aging labels allows for quick and easy visual identification of when a patient was last seen in the dental practice. This type of identification allows the transfer of charts from active to inactive files. A label is put on a new patient's chart to indicate the year the patient was first seen. The next year that the patient is seen, a new label is placed over the old. At designated intervals, charts are removed from the active files and placed in the inactive files. Time lapse varies from practice to practice.

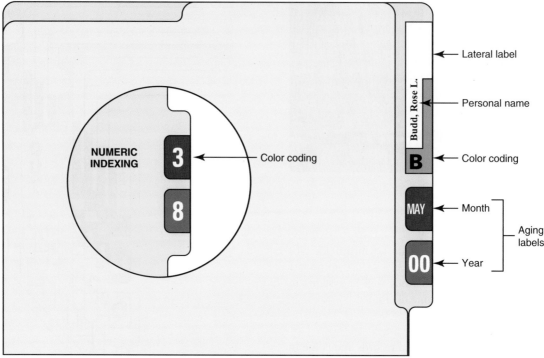

ANATOMY OF AN INDEXED FILE FOLDER

NUMERIC INDEXING

3

8

Color coding

Lateral label

Budd, Rose L.

Personal name

B

Color coding

MAY

Month

00

Year

Aging labels

Aging labels can also be used to track patient treatments. When a treatment is completed, the chart is flagged with the appropriately colored label. If a patient does not complete a treatment, the chart can be easily identified and the proper steps can be taken to reschedule the patient. By adding a month label, the chart can be flagged for recall. The use of colored labels can also distinguish the primary dentist and the type of insurance. The most important element of a successful coding system is that it be kept simple. Every member of the dental healthcare team should be able to use the system.

PREPARING THE PAPER CLINICAL RECORD

When a patient visits the office for the first time, the administrative dental assistant, in addition to collecting the correct data each time a patient visits the office, is responsible for placing all forms in a file folder and correctly labeling the folder. See Chapter 8 for information on preparing an electronic patient record.

General Guidelines

1. Check each form for the necessary information.
2. Make sure each form within the clinical record can be identified by the patient's name or account number. This provides a way of identifying forms if they should become separated from the folder.
3. Fasten forms in the correct order.

Preparing the Label

1. Determine the indexing method to be used (i.e., alphabetic or numeric).
2. Type the name or number on a label. (Become familiar with the different rules of indexing. It is very important to follow the same rules and to be concise in their application.)
3. Place the label on the file folder.

Coding the File Folder

1. Place corresponding color tabs according to the guidelines of the selected color coding system.
2. Place other coding labels according to preset guidelines (e.g., aging, year, month).

Cross-Referencing (Numeric Indexing)

Record the patient's name and chart number on your cross-reference list.

A computer system can aid in the preparation of file folders by printing labels according to the guidelines of the indexing system, assigning account numbers, and creating cross-referencing lists.

PREPARING BUSINESS DOCUMENTS FOR FILING

Business documents are prepared for filing using the steps outlined in Box 9-1. When an electronic filing system is used, the majority of the documents and records will already be in electronic format. You will classify name and place electronic files in the correct folder, eliminating the steps for preparing paper documents described in the following section.

PREPARING PAPER DOCUMENTS FOR FILING

Inspecting

Inspecting involves checking the document and making sure that it is ready to file. You will need to develop a method by which you can indicate that the document is ready to be placed in the filing system. This may include the initials of the dentist or other team member who has been working with the document, a simple checkmark, or a stamp.

Indexing

Once the document has been released for filing, the next step is to determine where the document should be filed and what method of indexing is required. A file folder will have to be prepared for a document that is to be filed for the first time (see Figures 9-1 and 9-2).

Coding

If you are using a subject method of filing, you may want to write the subject in the upper right corner of the document. If the subject appears in the heading of the document, you can simply underline or highlight it. Subheadings can also be identified and coded.

Filing Procedures

Filing is more than putting away documents. You must follow the steps below to ensure that files are *concise, consistent,* and *convenient.*

- The first step is to be *concise* when preparing clinical records for filing. This includes labeling the clinical record according to the indexing rules for the selected method of filing.
- The second step is to be *consistent* in placing the record in the filing system. This is done by following the simplified rules for filing that are established and outlined for each dental practice. If everyone follows the same rules in filing documents, documents will be returned consistently to the same place each time.
- The third step is to store files in *convenient* locations so that they can be accessed easily. When files are indexed concisely and are consistently placed in the correct order

in a convenient place, documents are easy to find and are safeguarded against loss or damage.

Sorting

After records and documents have been indexed and coded, they are sorted. During the sorting phase of the process, records and documents are separated into categories according to the filing method and the location of the files. This is a systematic step that will save time during filing. Records and documents are separated and placed in the same order in which they will be filed.

Sorting speeds up the filing process because you will not have to move back and forth from one end of the filing system to the other, opening and closing file drawers. Instead, you will work in order from one end of the system to the other, saving time and steps. Many accessories, such as a basket with file guides, can aid you in the sorting process. The key is to select a method that works well for you.

Putting Records and Documents in Their Final Place

The final step in the filing process is putting away records. Most people dread this process because they find it time consuming, boring, and unfulfilling. If you approach this part of filing with a positive attitude and are well organized, you will move quickly through the task.

How to Safeguard Records

As previously stated, clinical, business, and tax records are important elements of the dental practice. If they are lost, damaged, or poorly maintained, they can serve no useful purpose. It is your responsibility to safeguard each and every document and to maintain the integrity of the contents.

✚ **HIPAA**

HIPAA Privacy Rule

The Health Insurance Portability and Accountability Act (HIPAA) Privacy Rule covers the protection of all protected health information (PHI) in paper form and the HIPAA Security Rule applies to all electronic protected health information (ePHI).

Know where records are at all times. Records should never be removed from the office. Copies of records can be made when the information is needed for work outside the office.

Records should be returned to the file cabinet at the end of each day. The chance of losing or destroying them is reduced when records are kept in the file cabinet. Vertical files offer some protection from fire and water damage if files are tightly compressed and drawers are locked. Lateral files stored in cabinets provide the best protection; drawers should be closed and locked. Ledger cards and other file cards that are usually set out during the day should be placed in a file drawer at night for storage and protection.

A computerized system should be backed up on a regular basis and the backup files stored off site. It is costly, time consuming, and almost impossible to recapture information that is lost in a computer system.

 HIPAA

Security Rule

Ensure the integrity and confidentiality of electronic protected health information (ePHI).

Protect against any reasonable anticipated threats or hazards to the security or integrity of the ePHI.

Protect against unauthorized uses or disclosures of the ePHI.

Retention and Transfer of Records

The quantity of records in storage can become large and cumbersome. A policy must be established for the systematic removal of records. Most records must be retained for a particular length of time; however, inactive records do not have to be stored in active files. Active files should be located to provide easy access for business office staff. When files become inactive, they should be moved to a less convenient area, such as the bottom filing drawers or a cabinet located away from the business office.

Retention

Which records must be retained and for how long vary from state to state, according to the type of record. Retention of patient records also depends on the extent of treatment, whether radiographs have been taken, and regulations established by third-party insurance carriers. It is advisable to keep records of patients who have received extensive dental treatment and to retain full mouth radiographic surveys indefinitely because of their significance in forensic dentistry.

Federal regulations and state statutes of limitations determine the retention of business records. Each state establishes periods during which records can be used in legal proceedings; this is referred to as the *statute of limitations*. After the statute of limitations expires, records can no longer be used in legal matters. Records that fall into this category are contracts, open accounts, and accident reports.

The federal government has assembled a set of regulations that determine the length of time that records that deal with federal issues must be kept. These records include payroll reports, tax reports, receipts and bank statements, and other documentation used in the preparation of reports.

It is the responsibility of the administrative dental assistant to become familiar with regulations and statutes that govern the place of employment. Before you destroy any files, you should seek the advice of an accountant or an attorney. You should destroy records and files only under the direct order of your employer. Once files have been released for destruction, care should be taken to destroy them appropriately. Services are available that destroy records or you can do so by yourself. A cross-reference list should be kept to denote the types of documents being destroyed, the time period that the documents represented, and the method used for destruction. It is essential that records be destroyed appropriately, so that they can never be used for fraud.

Transfer Methods

A filing system works best when the storage area is accessible and the files are not overcrowded. Therefore this space should be used only for active files. So that there is space for active files, a routine must be developed for the systematic removal of inactive files. Two types of transfer methods have been developed for the systematic removal of inactive files.

The perpetual method uses a system that identifies files and records that have been inactive for a predetermined length of time or that are no longer required for quick reference. As soon as a file or record reaches this interval, it is removed from the active filing system and placed in the inactive filing system. For example, if you are using aging labels, you will be able to visually identify records that are ready to be removed from the active filing system. You have predetermined that all charts will be placed in the inactive file if a patient has not been seen in the practice for a period of 3 years. Monthly, you quickly scan the files and pull all charts of patients who have not been seen for the past 3 years. This method will ensure that you do not overcrowd your filing space. Computer systems can also generate monthly reports that list all records that should be removed from the active file.

The periodic method works well for business records. At a determined time, usually the end of the year, all files are transferred to the inactive file and the same types of files in the inactive file are transferred to storage boxes. For example, all financial reports, payroll records, and other monthly reports are transferred to the inactive file to make room for the new year's reports and records. The previous year's reports are removed from the inactive file and boxed for storage. Boxes that go into storage can be marked with the year in which they can be legally destroyed. When new boxes go into storage, old boxes marked for destruction can be removed and destroyed. Once again, a well-organized cross-referencing system is needed to track boxes and their contents.

Active and inactive files must be kept in the dental practice for easy access. The chance that records will need to be accessed drops significantly with the passing of each year but they still must be retained. Storage of countless boxes of files becomes expensive and serves no useful purpose unless they are properly cross-referenced. A solution to this problem is imaging.

This process places images of the contents of files and records on storage disks, microfilm, or magnetic tape. Scanners and other imaging equipment transfer images via computer to storage disks. Microfilming takes pictures of documents and reduces the size of the image, resulting in the ability to store several hundred documents on a reel of film. Disks, tapes, and reels, which have the capability to hold thousands of records, take up a fraction of the space that is required to store the original records. When an imaging system is used, it also cross-references the contents, which makes it possible to search documents quickly and easily, even 30 years later. Storage of original documents and radiographs may or may not be necessary, depending on the type of document. Each dental practice must establish a protocol that describes its policies on document storage.

KEY POINTS

- The purposes of developing a systematic approach to filing are to simplify the retrieval process and to ensure the precise locations of documents, in both a paper and electronic system. Guaranteeing integrity and safeguarding all documents are primarily the responsibilities of the administrative dental assistant.
- Within the dental practice, more than one type of filing system may be used. The filing system will be determined by the type of information that must be filed. Information can be divided into two broad categories: (1) business documents and patient-related documents and (2) clinical records and patient insurance forms. The six basic filing methods are as follows:
  - Alphabetic
  - Geographic
  - Numeric
  - Subject
  - Chronological
  - Electronic
- Personal names and business or organizational names are indexed according to ARMA Simplified Filing Standard Rules. The arrangement of a name, subject, or number is referred to as indexing. Names are broken down into units; a group of units is a segment. When filing documents with properly indexed names, follow these basic rules:
  - The first letter that is different in any unit determines the alphabetic order.
  - Single names are filed before the same name followed by an initial or name.
  - Initials are filed before the name spelled out.
  - Abbreviations are filed as if they were spelled out.
  - Nicknames are treated as first names.
  - Business and organizational names are filed as written.
- Effective storage of information is achieved by matching the type of document with the correct file folder (electronic or paper) and placing it within the filing unit. Documents can be stored electronically in folders and subfolders or in vertical files, which have one to five drawers. Vertical files require the use of file folders with tabs located at the top. Lateral file units make up a shelving system that uses side tab folders. The lateral unit is popular for the storage of clinical records because several different coding methods can be applied.
- Documents must be stored for a specified length of time, depending on the type of document and the legal requirements. A policy must be developed that systematically identifies documents that should be moved from active to inactive files.

CAREER-READY PRACTICES

Career-Ready Practices activities are designed to provide students with experiences that can be "practiced" in preparation for skills needed on the job. In each of the following exercises, a variety of approaches may be used to address the problem, rather than "right" or "wrong" answers. Below each exercise, next to the compass icon, is a listing of suggested Career-Ready Practice numbers that correspond to the listing of 12 practices in the front of the text (see p. viii-ix); these practices provide suggestions for approaches to complete the exercise.

1. Apply what you have learned in this chapter to create an electronic and paper filing system for the following business documents. Describe how you would arrange the documents and identify the method you would use for each system. In the electronic format, create folders and subfolders and place the files in the corresponding folders. For the paper system, write file labels and arrange them in the correct sequence for the chosen method.
   - Monthly bank statements from ABC National Bank (January to December 2016)
   - Quarterly bank statements from RBB for the same period (January to December 2016)
   - Monthly business reports: practice production reports, practice collection reports, hygiene production reports, associate dentist's production reports, and primary dentist's production reports

 Career-Ready Practices
   2 *Apply appropriate academic and technical skills.*
   6 *Demonstrate creativity and innovation.*
   11 *Use technology to enhance productivity.*

2. Correctly index the following names and write them as you would on a filing label. Arrange the indexed names in alphabetic order.
   - W.P. Hazelton
   - Victor J. Carlucci, Jr.
   - Sung Kim
   - Robert James McCarty
   - R. Davison
   - Mary Anne Lucchesi
   - Mark Sandwell
   - Liz Famillian
   - James Lloyd

- Damian Carmona
- Brook M. Calloway
- Ben DeFrank

 Career-Ready Practices

2 *Apply appropriate academic and technical skills.*

3. Using the names listed above, develop a numbering system.
   - Assign each patient a different six-digit number.
   - Index the numbers (each number is a different unit).

- Create a cross-reference list.
- Place the numbers in sequence.

 Career-Ready Practices

2 *Apply appropriate academic and technical skills.*
6 *Demonstrate creativity and innovation.*
8 *Utilize critical thinking to make sense of problems and persevere in solving them.*

10

Dental Patient Scheduling

LEARNING OBJECTIVES

1. Describe the mechanics of scheduling, including the criteria required for matrixing an electronic scheduler or manual appointment book.
2. Discuss the art of scheduling and how to maximize scheduling efficiency, including the different methods used to identify when specific procedures should be scheduled.
3. Explain the seven different scenarios of appointment scheduling and formulate an action plan to solve the problems.
4. Describe the four ways that patients may schedule an appointment, including the use of traditional and alternative types of appointment cards and reminders.
5. Explain how use of a call list and daily schedule sheets can save time in the dental office.
6. List the steps to be followed in performing the daily routine associated with the appointment schedule.

INTRODUCTION

Developing and implementing an organized, functional schedule for a dental practice requires time, experience, and the cooperation of the entire dental healthcare team. The process of scheduling appointments involves more than entering names in a book or keying into a computer. Scheduling is a complex process that has two main elements. The first is the mechanics of scheduling, which includes selecting the appointment book (manual or electronic), outlining or matrixing, and entering information.

The second is the "art" of scheduling. The first step in the art of scheduling is to work with the dental healthcare team and answer a few questions. These questions, such as how much time is required to complete a procedure (i.e., total time from patient to patient), help to identify when the dental healthcare team is the most productive. The second step is to develop a process for monitoring and adjusting the schedule to meet the goals set by the dental healthcare team.

Scheduling can be done by anyone but effective scheduling is a skill that must be developed. Traditionally, scheduling was assigned to a single individual with little input from other members of the staff. In today's integrated dental practice, the use of electronic schedulers allows scheduling to be performed from any computer terminal. Although several members of the dental healthcare team may perform scheduling, the ultimate responsibility for reviewing and maintaining an efficient schedule typically will be assigned to the administrative dental assistant.

MECHANICS OF SCHEDULING

Selecting the Appointment Book (Manual and Electronic)

The appointment book in today's dental practices can be either manual or electronic and is a tool that, when used efficiently, helps to organize the daily schedule of the dental practice. The book identifies who will be performing which tasks, on what date, and at what time. The book outlines which treatment rooms are available and at what times. It identifies who will be seen, the treatment that will be performed, and the amount of time required to complete the treatment.

✚ HIPAA

Privacy Rule: Protect the Confidentiality of Patient Treatment

Appointment books contain protected health information (PHI) and must be kept out of sight. Ensure that patients cannot see an open appointment book or computer screen when you are scheduling appointments.

The electronic scheduler or computerized system incorporates many of the same features as those in the manual appointment book. During the system setup, a series of questions will be asked that are designed to customize the scheduler to the individual practice, including the number of practitioners or treatment rooms, time blocks for specific procedures, operating hours of the dental practice, days of the week, and production goals (Figure 10-1). Once the

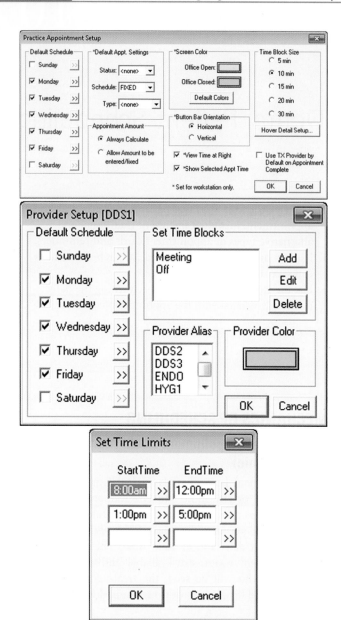

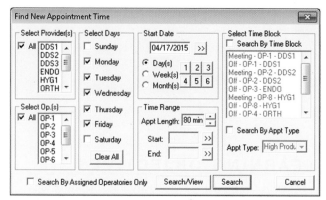

FIGURE 10-2 Once the practice information is set up, the program can be run manually or can automatically choose the day and time for the next appointment. (Dentrix screen capture courtesy Henry Schein Practice Solutions, American Fork, Utah.)

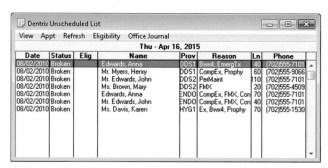

FIGURE 10-3 The system automatically searches the patient database for unscheduled recalls, saving time. (Dentrix screen capture courtesy Henry Schein Practice Solutions, American Fork, Utah.)

FIGURE 10-1 A, The electronic scheduler allows the administrative dental assistant to set up practice days. **B,** During the setup process, hours of business for each of the providers can also be set. (Dentrix screen captures courtesy Henry Schein Practice Solutions, American Fork, Utah.)

system is programmed, it may operate in a number of modes, such as manual selection, in which the assistant selects the appointment day and time, and automatic mode, in which the assistant enters the procedures and the computer selects the day and time for the appointment (Figure 10-2). In addition, the electronic scheduler will track missed appointments, provide up-to-date call lists at the push of a key, and search the database for incomplete treatment plans and unscheduled recalls (Figure 10-3). The primary difference between the manual appointment book and the electronic scheduler is the method in which data are entered and the ability, with the electronic scheduler, to perform a variety of specialized tasks efficiently.

Manual appointment books come in several different styles. The most common style is the week at a glance. When the book is open, this style allows the assistant to view the full week, Monday through Saturday. When fully opened, books range in size from 9 × 22⅞ inches to as large as 11 × 35¼ inches. When selecting a style, you must consider the number of practitioners you are scheduling for and the amount of desk space that is available for the opened book. In a large practice with several practitioners, it may be necessary to have an individual book for each practitioner.

! REMEMBER

Appointment books are considered legal documents and can be a valuable tool in the defense of alleged malpractice; therefore they must be kept in storage for the prescribed length of time.

Common Features of an Appointment Book

Both the electronic scheduler and the manual appointment book have the same key components in the organization of the daily office schedule. Visually the pages are very similar. The pages are divided into columns; identify who will be seen, at what time, the work to be done, and whom the patient will see. The primary difference is in the way the information is entered into the electronic system or written in the manual appointment book.

Columns

Pages of the appointment book are divided into **columns** (Figure 10-4). The function of the column is to organize the schedule and identify who is performing the treatment, who the patient is, why the patient is being seen, and what will be done. Columns can be assigned to an individual practitioner or treatment room or can be used to record additional information about the patient. The number and size of the columns in an appointment book depend on the style selected by the dental practice—for example, Canyon View Dental Associates employs two dentists, Dr. Edwards and Dr. Bradley, and two dental hygienists, Vivian and Diane. These employees work at different times. Because more than two practitioners are never in the office at one time, the practice can use a two-column appointment book. If the practice expands its hours or wants to include more information in the appointment book, a new appointment book style with additional columns would be needed.

Another way to schedule is to assign each treatment room a column in the appointment book. This means that the number of columns would equal the number of treatment rooms. (This form of scheduling requires advanced techniques and should not be attempted without a full understanding of the principles.)

Units or Time Blocks

Each column is divided into time segments. Each segment represents a unit (**units/time blocks** are either 10- or 15-minute intervals).

There are *four units per hour* when scheduling 15-minute intervals (see Anatomy of an Appointment Book Page and Figure 10-4) and *six units per hour* when scheduling 10-minute intervals (see Anatomy of an Electronic Appointment Book). The dental healthcare team will usually refer to the number of units needed for a procedure instead of the amount of time. For example, three units may be requested for a procedure. If a 15-minute unit is being used, a 45-minute block of time is needed to complete the procedure (30 minutes if using a 10-minute unit). Consistency is very important; everyone needs to speak the same language.

> ### ◢ FOOD FOR THOUGHT
> The dentist has just told you that he needs four units to complete a procedure. Is that 1 hour or 40 minutes?

Additional Appointment Book Features

Color is used in both systems to identify different practitioners, treatment rooms, and the type of treatment. The color of the manual appointment book can be used to distinguish one book from another at a quick glance. These same features are incorporated into the electronic scheduler as a quick way to visualize who is scheduled, what room is in use, or if there is an opening in the schedule. Once you are familiar with the color-coding it becomes very easy to quickly find specific information at a glance.

Bookmarks, colored tabs, and other accessories are easy ways to divide the appointment book according to day, month, or week. For example, a **month tab** makes it easy to turn to a given month. This is especially handy when you are scheduling a few months in advance. **Bookmarks** are used to identify the current week so it can be turned to quickly.

The manual appointment book can be ordered with or without dates. **Predated appointment book pages** are convenient and are used when schedules stay consistent. **Undated appointment book pages** are used when flexibility is needed. For example, flexibility is needed when a practitioner works only a few days a week at a given location. With undated pages, the administrative dental assistant can customize the design of the appointment book. Loose-leaf appointment books accommodate undated pages well because they can be added easily.

Codes can be customized to fit the needs of any dental practice but they are useful only if each member of the dental healthcare team understands them. Be careful not to use too many codes or other information that may clutter the entry and make it very difficult to read.

> ### ❗ REMEMBER
> When using both electronic and manual systems, identify the patient and the procedure and indicate the time the patient will be in the dental treatment room. When listing additional information, carefully use the space provided to ensure that the entry remains legible and easy to read.

THE ART OF SCHEDULING

The art of scheduling is important when the rules are established and maintained. The key to the art of scheduling is to determine when the dental healthcare team is the most productive and how, through effective scheduling, the goals and

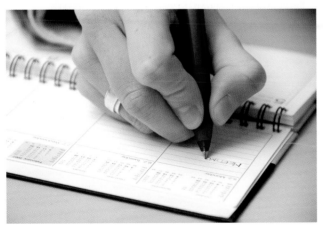

FIGURE 10-4 A manual appointment book is set up in columns with blocked time periods throughout the day. (Copyright © 2007 SilviaJansen, iStock.com. All rights reserved.)

ANATOMY OF AN ELECTRONIC APPOINTMENT BOOK

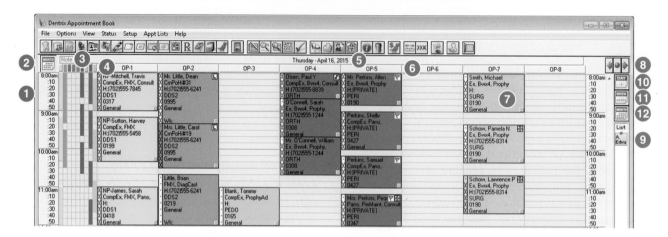

1. The Time Bars on the left and right sides of the Appointment Book separate hour intervals into selected time block size.

2. Click the Calendar button to open a monthly Calendar. From the Calendar dialog, you can view production goals, scheduled production, and actual production, making it easy to quickly evaluate your progress in meeting production objectives. In addition, you can click a date square to quickly move to the selected date in the Appointment Book.

3. Click the Note button to enter a note applicable for that day. The Note button turns yellow when a note is entered, indicating to staff members that a note has been entered for that day. There is also an option to print the Appointment Book Day Note when printing the Appointment Book View.

4. A unique color can be used for each treatment provider in your office. These colors will be used to flag each appointment, so you can tell which provider the patient is seeing. Similarly, on the left side of the Appointment Book is a color column for each provider. A colored block in that column indicates that the provider is scheduled to be working on a patient during the blocked time.

5. The Date Bar displays the date being viewed.

6. A column is displayed for each operatory added to the system. Operatories are displayed in numerical, then alphabetical, order by Operatory ID.

7. Each time an appointment is scheduled, a colored block appears in the appropriate operatory column for the amount of time scheduled. This new appointment will be the color assigned to the provider in the Provider Setup. Depending on the length of the appointment, up to nine lines of customizable information may be displayed, including Name, Appointment Reason, Home Phone, Work Phone, Provider, Production Amount, Appointment Type, Staff, Chart Number, Preferred Name, Name/ Preferred Name, Referred By, and Social Security Number. In addition, a red cross on the appointment block indicates that the patient has a Medical Alert. Similarly, a blue musical note indicates that the patient has a note attached to the displayed appointment.

8. The Navigation buttons are used to move from day to day in the Appointment Book. Click the left arrow button to move back one day. Click the right arrow to move forward one day. Click the circle button to return to the current day.

9. The Appointment Book pin board can be used to temporarily store appointment information until a new appointment time can be found. An appointment can be quickly moved to a different day by dragging the appointment to the pin board, switching to another date, and then dragging the appointment to a new time. A scheduled appointment can be moved to any place on the schedule by clicking and dragging the appointment to a new time, a new operatory, or a new day (using the pin board).

10. Opening the Appointment Book in the day view allows you to see detailed information pertaining to an individual day and its scheduled appointments. Appointments can be scheduled by double clicking an available time.

11. The week view option allows you to see a week's worth of appointments. In the week view, the Appointment Book window displays large columns for each day of your work week. Each day column is further divided into operatory columns that show provider color blocks, indicating already scheduled appointments, making it easy to see free scheduling opportunities. To schedule an appointment, doubleclick an available time.

12. Click the **Month** button to display an entire month's worth of appointment times for each provider. On the left side of the Appointment Book, each provider is listed by ID for each workday in the month. On the top of the Appointment Book, the time of day is shown. To view the appointments on a particular day, click the desired date to move to that date in the day view.

ANATOMY OF AN APPOINTMENT BOOK PAGE

Mon. 3/20

Time	Dr. Edwards	Vivian (hyg)
8 00	Jacob Henry	
15		Judy Carr
30	Cr. prep #24	
45		
9 00		Jon Ford
15		
30	Martha Sterling	
45		Jason Ward
10 00	Br. prep 12-14	Michael Ward
15		
30		
45		Jeniffer Vail
11 00		
15		
30		
45		
12 00		
15		
30		
45		
1 00	Kathy Bader	Jim Butler
15	F. Imp	
30		
45		
2 00	Christopher Darling	Carol Aguilar
15	Comp 8-9	
30	Sealants	
45		
3 00	Dawn Savage	Kathy Campbell
15	Ag #14	
30	Julie Singer - ok	
45	Mark Dryer - ok	Pat Perez
4 00		
15		
30		Frank Williams
45		
5 00		
15		
30	Rio Vista Dist. Inservice	
45	No school	
6 00		

Tues. 3/21

Time	Dr. Edwards	Vivian (hyg)
8 00	Louise Brook	
15		Carrie James
30	f.imp	
45		
9 00	Dorothy Starr	Al Parker
15		
30	Comp, 8 & 9	
45	Francisco Lopez	Maria Gonzales
10 00	Cr. Prep 30	
15		
30		Jody Tan
45	Maria Gonzales	
11 00		
15	Amal. 14 & 18	Sarah Martin
30		
45		
12 00		
15		
30		
45		
1 00	Lloyd Barber	Mark Kemp
15	Try-in	
30	Jim Becker	
45	Ext	Sue Le
2 00	(tp 1:45 pre-med)	
15		
30	Mary Thomas	Anita Vasquez
45	Amal 3 & 4	
3 00	Comp 7	
15		Larry Smith
30		
45		
4 00		Rob Hills
15		
30		
45		
5 00		
15		
30		
45		
6 00		
15		
30	ADAA meeting	
45	Canyon View Civic Center	
7 00	Dr. Wagner, Patient	
15	Management	
30		
45		

Wed. 3/22

Time	Dr. Edwards	Dr. Bradley
8 00	Kyra Robb	comp
15		
30		sealants
45		
9 00	Phil Kidd	
15		Crns
30		
45		
10 00		
15	Jeff Painter	
30		
45	Br prep	
11 00		Max Golden
15		Adj
30		Sadie Collins
45		Comp
12 00		
15		Ann Buffam
30		Comp
45	Lions Club	mar L/R
1 00		
15		
30	Kathy Bader	
45	Bite L	
2 00	Seth Thomas	
15		
30	Ags	
45		
3 00	Laura Allen	Comp
15	Comp	
30		
45		
4 00		Sandra Michaels
15		Cr prep
30		
45		
5 00		
15		
30		Randy McNally
45		
6 00	Dental Study Group	RCT
15	Society Office	BU
30		
45		
7 00		Will Dodge
15		Ag
30		
45		

Appointment Book Matrix

Once the style of the appointment book is selected, the next step in the organization of the appointment book is to custom configure the pages. This is referred to as the **appointment book matrix**. The purpose of the matrix is to configure or outline the pages. Electronic schedulers are matrixed during the initial computer set-up function. The program will customize the appointment book following the specifications of the dental practice.

Steps in matrixing an appointment book

1. Assign each practitioner a column for the day and clearly identify. If you are scheduling by treatment room, identify the treatment room assigned to each column.

2. Mark the columns so it can be easily determined by anyone looking at the appointment book what time the first procedure begins, when lunch or dinner will be scheduled, and when the last procedure ends.

3. During the course of the day it may be necessary to schedule emergency patients. The appointment book can be matrixed to identify a specific block of time each day in anticipation of an emergency. Dovetailing is another method used for short appointments and emergencies. For example, the dentist will need to wait 10 to 20 minutes after giving anesthetic before proceeding with the procedure, allowing time to check another patient.

4. With careful planning and attention to detail, the appointment book can be matrixed to identify when and where specific procedures should be scheduled. Colored highlighters, small colored sticky notes or colored book tabs (sticky notes and book tabs can be reused) will help identify blocks of time and procedures to be scheduled. When using a computerized scheduler, this type of function can be programmed into the system.

5. Identify when the local schools are on break or have days off. This is useful because teachers and children will be available for appointments without missing school.

6. Information other than patient appointments can be placed in the appointment book, which will help organize the function of the office. Items included are: professional meetings for the dentist and auxiliary, such as dental society meetings, dental assistant and dental hygienist society meetings; study clubs and continuing

Continued

education courses; vacations; and important deadline dates, such as quarterly taxes, payroll deposits, or other dates important to the dental office.

7 When making entries in the appointment book, care should be taken to write legibly and in pencil. Entries include the patient's name (both the first and last name), the amount of time needed for the procedure (indicated by an arrow), and a code for the procedure. It may also be advisable to include a telephone number for confirmation (especially for a new patient), a code to indicate if lab work is needed for the procedure, and if the lab work has returned from the lab. It may be necessary to indicate if the patient requires premedication, or any other information that is vital to the case.

Some common codes are:

C – appointment needs confirmation
C̸ – confirmed
cr – crown
ag – amalgam
comp – composite
ext – extraction
prophy – prophylaxis
RP – root planing
rc – root canal (rct)
fl – fluoride treatment
p.o. – post operative appointment
br – bridge
prep – preparation (crown, bridge, inlay, or onlay)
ins – insertion (placement of crown, bridge, inlay, or onlay)
tp – told patient
L – lab work
Ⓛ – lab work returned from the lab

philosophy of the dental practice can be met. This is not a simple one-step procedure. It takes time and the cooperation of all members of the team. The process is ongoing, allowing for adjustments when needed to meet the goals of the dental practice.

Productivity

Productivity in dentistry is a complex concept. There are two types of **productivity.** The first is determined by the amount of dental treatment that is completed and the second is determined by the amount of money collected. The amount of treatment that is provided can be increased by efficient scheduling and the amount of money collected can be increased by effective collection methods. Maintaining efficiency in both areas is a function of the administrative dental assistant. In this chapter, ways to increase productivity through efficient scheduling are discussed. (See Chapter 14 for a discussion of collection productivity.)

The answers to four key questions will help you to maximize scheduling efficiency:

1. *At what time of day does the dental healthcare team work smarter and faster?* This can be determined by selecting the time of day that the dentist performs best. Some dentists are "morning people." They wake up early and are eager to start work. Because this type of person is most productive in the early morning, difficult and challenging work should be scheduled then. The dentist will be able to remain focused on the task and will complete the procedure without becoming overly stressed or fatigued. As the day passes and the dentist's ability to remain focused decreases, the type of procedure scheduled should be changed. This is an appropriate time for shorter appointments and less challenging work. For the dentist who wakes up later and is less focused in the mornings (also known as the "I don't do mornings" person), schedule the easier tasks first. Increase the difficulty of the procedure according to the dentist's internal clock to enhance productivity and reduce stress. Synchronization of work

schedules with team members' internal work clocks will help to increase productivity and meet the needs of patients.

2. *How much time is needed to complete a procedure?* This question is not easy to answer. Theoretically, the same procedure should consistently take the same amount of time. All patients are different, however, and what takes three units of time for one patient may take four units for another. To determine procedure times, you must average the times over several different patients. Once the average procedure time is determined, a list can be made to identify the amounts of time to allot for specific treatments. This process requires constant monitoring and adjusting. In addition to the amount of time it takes to complete the procedure, the amount of time it takes to properly clean and ready the room for the next patient must be considered. This time varies by procedure (the minimum is 10 minutes). More complex procedures require longer clean-up times to ensure that proper infection control protocol is followed.

3. *Which procedures may require the assistance of an extended function dental assistant?* Depending on the duties dental assistants are allowed to perform (these are outlined in the Dental Practice Act of each state), the assistance of an extended function dental assistant may be needed. When extended function dental assistants are used, the amounts of time they will spend with patients must be considered when procedures in which they will assist are scheduled. For example, for a procedure that requires four units of chair time, the dentist may spend three units with the patient and the assistant may spend one unit. The dentist is then available for one unit with another patient. (This unit would be a good time for procedures such as examinations, postoperative check-ups, and appointment adjustments.)

4. *Who will do the scheduling?* In both systems, the scheduling process requires the cooperation of the entire dental healthcare team through constant monitoring and adjustment of

procedural times. The initial entering of information in the appointment book can be assigned to one or two persons. It will be their responsibility to set up and matrix the appointment book and to schedule as efficiently as possible according to the guidelines developed by the dental healthcare team. The advantage of an electronic scheduler is that more than one person can schedule appointments and still maintain an effective system.

Scenarios for Scheduling

Scheduling would be easy if every patient and every procedure could be treated in exactly the same way, but this is not the case. Dental healthcare teams are continually faced with complex problems that require well-established guidelines that are also flexible. The scheduler must maintain control of the appointment book and must be creative in meeting the needs of both the dental healthcare team and the patient. At times, it is very difficult to accommodate everyone.

Scenario One: The Emergency Patient

Dorothy Star calls the office and informs you that she has a "pounding toothache" and has to see the dentist today.

With the help of a telephone information form, questions can be asked to determine where the pain is located, how long the pain has been present, if there is swelling, and whether there are other symptoms that will help to determine if the patient must be seen "today." If the appointment book has been matrixed to allow for emergency patients, the patient can be informed of the appointment time. It is advisable to tell emergency patients that the dentist can see them for the immediate problem and relieve the discomfort. If more extensive work is needed, another appointment must be made.

If emergency time has not been worked into the daily schedule, a time will need to be selected. Find a scheduled procedure that will allow the dentist to leave this patient momentarily to attend to the emergency patient without interfering with the amount of time scheduled for the first patient (this type of scheduling requires experience).

> ### ! REMEMBER
>
> "Dentists shall be obliged to make reasonable arrangements for the emergency care of their patients of record. Dentists shall be obligated when consulted in an emergency by patients not of record to make reasonable arrangements for emergency care. If treatment is provided, the dentist, upon completion of treatment, is obligated to return the patient to his or her regular dentist unless the patient expressly reveals a different preference."—American Dental Association: *Principles of ethics and code of professional conduct*, January 2010, Chicago, Ill.

Sometimes patients cannot come in during a period when you can work them in. If these patients can wait, they can be scheduled for another day. However, the dental healthcare team may need to be flexible and schedule the patient at a different time, such as during someone's lunch hour or at the

end of the day. This type of scheduling should be avoided and done only after all other options have been explored. (Caution: Other patients should not be inconvenienced because of the poor planning or lack of flexibility of another patient. You may help one patient but lose others in the process.)

> ## SCHEDULING OPTIONS FOR EMERGENCY APPOINTMENTS
>
> Matrix the appointment book with cushion times, one in the morning and the other in the afternoon, that can be used for emergency appointments or to help readjust the schedule on a busy day.
>
> Check the schedule for a time when the dentist can momentarily leave a patient, for example:
> - When waiting for anesthesia
> - When the extended function dental assistant is completing a procedure
> - When there is a patient who is scheduled for multiple procedures and his or her appointment could be shortened without causing inconvenience
>
> Make sure a treatment room is available for radiographs and treatment.
>
> Check the schedule of other dentists in the practice.

Scenario Two: The "Afternoon Only" Patient

Francisco Lopez must have extensive dental work performed and he is concerned about the amount of time he will lose from work. Mr. Lopez is a production manager and is in charge of the production line from 8:00 AM to 12 NOON. He expresses an interest in scheduling his appointments in the afternoon.

A treatment plan must be prepared for each patient and the steps in the treatment must be prioritized. When scheduling appointments, the assistant can clearly identify from the priority list the order in which treatment steps must be performed and can determine the types of procedures that have to be scheduled.

The assistant can explain to the patient that the more extensive work, the crown and bridge, must be scheduled in the morning because this is when the dentist performs more extensive procedures. The less extensive work can be scheduled in the afternoon. By explaining the scheduling process to the patient and showing a willingness to divide the work so that part of it can be completed in the afternoon, the assistant demonstrates concern for the patient while maintaining control of the appointment book.

Scenario Three: The Chronically Late Patient

Julie Singer is a very busy professional woman. If you schedule her for a 2:00 PM appointment, she will rush into the office at 2:08.

Several factors enter into scheduling chronically late patients. First, the patient who is late even by as short a time as 8 minutes can and will affect the schedule. Second, patients who rush have racing pulses. Their higher-than-normal blood pressures may cause other problems if they are given local anesthetic before their vital signs return to normal.

The one thing you can do with patients who you know will be late is to schedule them 15 minutes early for their appointment. Inform the patient who is scheduled to see the dentist at 2:00 PM that the appointment is at 1:45. This will allow time for the patient to arrive late and rest before he or she is seen by the dentist.

> ### ! REMEMBER
>
> This technique can backfire if patients discover you are scheduling them early. The entire dental healthcare team must know when you have done this in case a patient should call and ask the time of the appointment. Place a notation in the appointment book that clearly identifies the time the patient was told (e.g., "tp 1:45" to indicate "told patient 1:45").

When patients are always late for their appointments, dental healthcare team members should ask themselves why. In some cases, the dental office is the cause for late arrivals. Patients who consistently must wait to be seen by the dentist may develop the attitude that it does not make any difference if they arrive late; after all, they always wait for the dentist. It is very important to set the example. If we expect our patients to be on time, then we must be on time for them. Occasions will arise when it is impossible to see a patient within 10 minutes of arrival. When this occurs, the patient should be informed of the delay and given an approximate time at which the dentist will be available. It may be necessary to give the patient the option of rescheduling the appointment.

Scenario Four: The Canceled Appointment

Al Parker often cancels his appointments at the last minute because he cannot leave work.

When patients cancel appointments often, look beyond the reasons they give. Fear is frequently the reason that appointments are canceled. When this occurs, steps can be taken to relieve the fear through an established patient management protocol. These steps should be outlined by the dentist and may include premedication to relieve anxiety. Other reasons for cancellation include inability to pay for the visit, a lack of understanding of the importance of keeping appointments, and a lack of understanding of the consequences that may occur when prescribed dental treatments are not received. Once the reasons for constant cancellations have been determined, steps can be taken to help patients keep their appointments.

> ### ! REMEMBER
>
> For legal reasons, document all missed, broken, and rescheduled appointments.

Scenario Five: The Student Who Cannot Miss School

Kyra Robb is a student and her mother wants her scheduled for appointments after 3:00 PM.

Most patients, if given a choice, would schedule their appointments when it is the most convenient for them. Peak appointment times usually occur in the later afternoon, early evening, and holidays when the dental office is open. Controlling these time slots is difficult.

> ### ! REMEMBER
>
> The dental assistant must maintain control of the appointment book while meeting the needs of patients. Peak time slots should be given only to those who cannot possibly come at any other time. If the appointment book has been matrixed, it is essential that the types of procedures scheduled in particular time slots are the types for which the slots are designed. Again, when patients understand the reasons why they need to be scheduled at less than ideal times (because it is in their best interest), they are usually willing to compromise.

> ### TREND IN OFFICE HOURS
>
> Historically, dental practices have scheduled patients between the hours of 8:00 AM and 5:00 PM. In today's society, many patients are unwilling to change their schedules to meet the needs of dental practices. In addition, the number of dental practices is increasing. The need to attract and keep patients has resulted in the establishment of extended hours. It is not uncommon to find dental practices that are open in the evenings and on weekends to meet the needs of dental patients.

> ### ↗ WHAT WOULD YOU DO?
>
> The dentist has asked you to research and report back to him on the latest trends in scheduling patients, especially when the office is closed.

Scenario Six: The Patient Who Arrives on the Wrong Day

Jeff Painter arrives for his appointment. When you check the schedule, you discover that he is due on Wednesday at 10:00 AM, not on Tuesday.

It is always a delicate situation when a patient arrives on the wrong day or at the wrong time; this must be treated with tact and diplomacy (no matter who is at fault). First, inform unexpected patients that you have them on the schedule at a different time and ask if they have their appointment card with them. (It is crucial to give all patients an appointment card.) Check the appointment card and determine who is at fault. If it is the patient, politely point out the error and offer your condolences. If it is a short procedure that you can work into the schedule without inconveniencing other patients, offer to do so. If the error was made by a member of the dental healthcare team, offer your condolences and try to work the patient into the schedule. (Flexibility in the schedule may be needed at this time.)

Scenario Seven: Unscheduled Appointments

Mrs. Sarah Martin is an older patient with a lot of free time. She will drop by the dental office wishing to see the dentist for a "quick appointment" to adjust her partial. It is very difficult to say no to Mrs. Martin.

Patients who drop in and request service can create a very difficult situation. If they have a true emergency and cannot wait until another time, they will have to be accommodated. It works best if you agree to have the dentist see them, tell them when the dentist will be available for an emergency situation, and explain that they will have to wait until that time.

Patients who can very easily be seen on a different day must be informed that it is not office policy to see drop-in patients for nonemergency appointments because it takes time away from the patients who are scheduled and that it is the dentist's philosophy to give all patients full attention during treatment. This is a very delicate situation and must be explained to the patient without causing an angry reaction.

In addition to unscheduled patients, unscheduled procedures can cause problems. For example, a patient who is scheduled for a recall appointment is discovered to need a couple of simple restorations. Instead of having the patient return on another day, the dentist may wish to squeeze the patient's procedures into the schedule. This technique works only if the dentist has enough time to properly attend to the patient. This practice generally does more harm than good. The only person who appreciates this addition to the schedule is the patient. The dental healthcare team will be stressed by the added procedures and other patients will be inconvenienced by having to wait.

During the day, the dentist's schedule can be interrupted for a variety of reasons—for example, by telephone calls, visits from sales representatives, and friends who "just stop by." All of these situations, if not controlled, add stress to the day for the dental healthcare team and for patients. When interruptions get out of control, the situation must be addressed. Identify the problem and work out a solution.

Other Patients Who Require Flexibility

Children. Schedule short appointments for children in the morning. Once children are comfortable and trust the dental healthcare team, the length of the appointment can be increased. Cranky children are not easy for the dentist to treat; try to schedule them when they are at their best.

Patients who need extra time. Many patients may require extra time when scheduling. Special needs patients and patients with disabilities may require additional time and specific times of the day to accommodate their needs. Some patients question everything the dentist does and thus the dentist will need additional time to answer all of their questions. Some patients cannot sit still, some constantly complain, some are fearful and need extra reassurance, and some will not stop talking (even when their mouths are full of dental materials).

Results of Poor Scheduling

Problem	Results
Patients have to wait longer than 10 minutes before they are seen by the dentist.	• Patients will arrive late because they always have to wait for the dentist. • Patients are offended when the dentist does not consider their time valuable. • Patients feel the stress of the dental healthcare team. • Patients will look for another dentist who will respect their time and is less stressed.
There is not enough time to complete the scheduled treatment.	• Patients begin to question the quality of the work the dentist is performing. • Patients have to make more trips to the dentist than needed because their treatment was not scheduled efficiently. • Care is not taken to provide quality work. • Members of the dental healthcare team become stressed and overworked. • Patients will look for another dentist who will provide quality care. • Members of the dental healthcare team will look for another employer who will respect their time and develop a true team spirit in the delivery of dental care.

> **! REMEMBER**
>
> Effective scheduling is a powerful practice builder. Patients want service. When the schedule serves the needs of only a few, the system of scheduling must be reevaluated and adjusted.

MAKING APPOINTMENTS

Appointments can be made in one of four ways: (1) The patient calls or is called for an appointment. (2) The patient is present in the dental office and needs follow-up work in the near future. (3) The patient schedules an appointment through a web-based program from his or her computer or mobile device. (4) The patient preschedules an appointment at the conclusion of a recall appointment. Each of these situations requires a slightly different approach.

1. *Patient calls for an appointment.* With the use of the telephone information form (manual or electronic), the assistant can quickly identify the nature of the patient's call and ask the necessary questions in a logical manner to determine what type of appointment should be scheduled and to record the necessary information for follow-up. Once the appointment has been made and recorded

in the appointment book or electronic scheduler, the assistant should repeat the information and the time of the appointment: "Mrs. Thomas, I have scheduled you for an appointment on Tuesday, July 3rd, at 2:30 PM. You are scheduled with Dr. Edwards. At that time, she will be replacing your old restorations and you can plan on spending about one and one-half hours with us. Are there any other questions I can answer for you? Thank you for calling and we will see you on July 3rd." It is important to record all relevant information on the telephone information form, enter the name and procedure in the appointment book or electronic scheduler, and repeat the information back to the patient before the call is ended. It is easy to become distracted by another phone call or patient and it is very embarrassing to have a patient show up for an appointment that was not entered in the appointment book.

2. *Patient schedules follow-up appointment.* The patient has completed treatment for the day and is checking out at the front desk. The assistant records all necessary information in the appointment book or electronic scheduler, completes the appointment card, and hands it to the patient. As the assistant then repeats the information (date, day of the week, time, and procedure), the patient reads the appointment card and confirms that the information is correct.

3. *Patient schedules an appointment through a web-based program from his or her computer or mobile device.* Secure websites are making it possible for patients to schedule or request an appointment at any time from the convenience of their computers. Much like other online scheduling, patients will log in to their account, select a day on which they would like to be seen, and check to see if that time is available. The secure information is transferred to the dental office and the appointment is scheduled and confirmed. This is extremely helpful for scheduling routine check-ups and initial appointments (Figure 10-5) but does not work for all appointment types.

4. *Patient preschedules a routine check-up appointment at the conclusion of a recall appointment.* When patients schedule an appointment 4 to 6 months in advance of the date, you handle it in the same way as the previous situations. You schedule the appointment, inform the patient, give him or her an appointment card, and verify that the information on the card is correct (Figure 10-6). In addition, you explain the recall procedure and tell the patient that he or she will receive a card in the mail or an e-mail a few weeks before the appointment. You may want to remind the

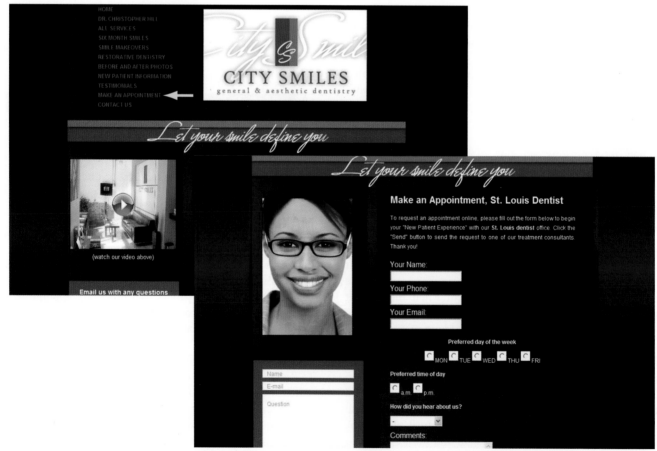

FIGURE 10-5 Many dental offices now have websites that allow patients to request an appointment time online. (Courtesy Dr. Christopher Hill, St. Louis, Mo.)

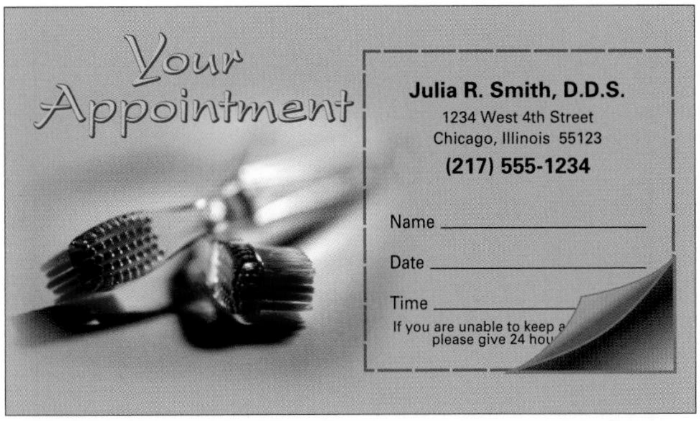

FIGURE 10-6 A sample appointment card provides the patient with the date and time of the next appointment. This particular version is produced as a sticker and can be affixed to a calendar. (Courtesy Patterson Office Supplies, Champaign, Ill.)

patient of the importance of keeping the appointment and notifying the dental office if there is a need to change it. This type of an appointment must be confirmed.

> **! REMEMBER**
>
> Scheduling recall appointments in advance requires careful monitoring and special consideration. Caution: Do not fill the schedule to capacity 6 months out; you will not be able to accommodate new patients or reschedule appointments in a timely manner.

Appointment cards are written reminders to patients of their next appointments. The design and style of the card vary widely from practice to practice. The card is usually the size of a business card and is printed on medium-weight paper. Information that should be included on the card is shown in Figure 10-7.

In addition to the traditional appointment card, many innovative ideas have been developed to help patients remember their appointments. Appointment cards may have a sticky

HAS AN APPOINTMENT ON

☐ MON.   ☐ TUES.   ☐ WED.   ☐ THUR.   ☐ FRI.   ☐ SAT.

A.M.
DATE _____ AT _____ P.M.

PARK AVENUE PROFESSIONAL GROUP
GENERAL DENTISTRY

2000 MILL STREET   Telephone
NEENAH, WISCONSIN 54957   (123) 555-2000
IF UNABLE TO KEEP APPOINTMENT KINDLY GIVE 24 HOURS NOTICE.

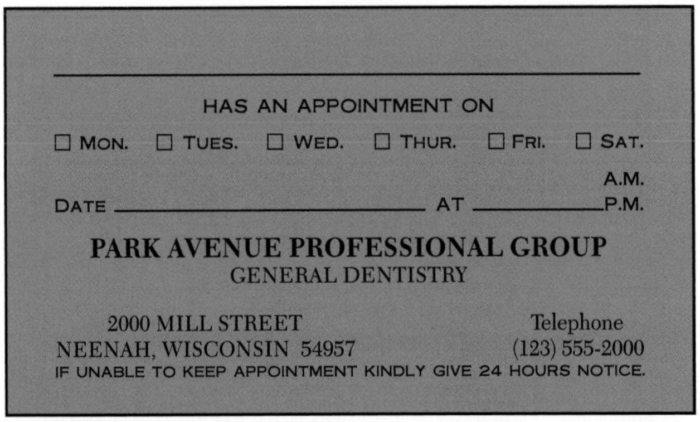

FIGURE 10-7 A sample back of the appointment card provides detailed information about the patient's next appointment. (Courtesy Patterson Office Supplies, Champaign, Ill.)

patch on the back so that patients can place them on a calendar. Refrigerator magnets are another popular form of appointment card. A card can also be sent to the patient's e-mail address or to his or her mobile devices. Short Message Service (SMS) is a type of text messaging that can be used to inform patients of their appointment. The appointment card comes in many colors and styles and can be delivered in a variety of methods but the purpose is still the same: to remind patients of the day, date, and time of their appointments.

TIME-SAVING FUNCTIONS

Previously, tracking patients who missed appointments, had unscheduled dental treatment, were waiting for insurance authorization, or who wanted to come at a different time than scheduled required manual flagging. The administrative dental assistant would work very hard to maintain current and comprehensive lists. With the adoption of practice management software, many of these lists can be generated quickly and accurately because the information has been tagged in the patient database (see Figure 10-3). No matter what system is incorporated, the goal is still the same: efficient and effective appointment scheduling. You may have several different lists of patients who need follow-up care but they will only be scheduled for an appointment if they are contacted.

Develop Call Lists

A **call list** is a tool used by the administrative dental assistant to help identify patients who are in need of a dental appointment. The purpose of the call list is to be able to quickly identify these patients and schedule them for an appointment (Figure 10-8). Typically the list is used to fill holes in the daily schedule. This may be because of a last-minute change or cancellation or when there are time blocks still open a few days ahead of time. For example, patients who are scheduled in the future but who would like to come in sooner can be flagged and then placed on the call list. You can also track patients who have called and canceled an appointment but who have not scheduled another appointment. Patients who have uncompleted treatment plans can be identified easily and contacted for an appointment. You can even track patients who are waiting for insurance authorization.

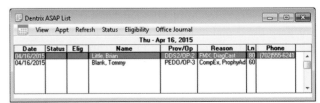

FIGURE 10-8 A call list in the electronic schedule quickly identifies the names of patients in the database who are in need of an appointment. (Dentrix screen capture courtesy Henry Schein Practice Solutions, American Fork, Utah.)

Maintain Daily Schedule Sheets

Daily schedule sheets contain information transferred from the appointment book or electronic scheduler and are used in treatment rooms, doctors' private offices, laboratories, and other work areas. These sheets contain patients' names, scheduled procedures, and amounts of time needed. Any other reminders for the day may be included (Figure 10-9). If changes or additions to the schedule are made during the day, the assistant simply revises each schedule sheet.

✚ HIPAA

Privacy Rule: Protect the Confidentiality of Patient Treatment

Schedule sheets contain protected health information (PHI) and must be kept out of sight.

Establish a Daily Routine

Develop a routine in accordance with the guidelines established by the dental healthcare team. Certain tasks should be completed every day.

1. Pull patients' clinical records and review procedures that are going to be completed on the following day. In a chartless practice, you can review from the computer monitor or print a summary of the treatment with special notes.
2. Check patients' charts (manual or electronic) for any information that may not have been included on the schedule, such as need for premedication, payments due, or updated insurance and medical information.
3. Confirm the return of laboratory work.
4. Confirm or remind patients of their upcoming appointments.
5. Use the call list to fill any openings in the day's schedule.
6. Type the daily schedule (or print it from the computer).
7. Give patients' clinical records to the dental assisting staff to review before they see the patients.
8. Spend 5 to 10 minutes with the dental healthcare team and review the daily schedule. Review vital information about procedures and patients to help provide quality care and relieve stress factors before patients begin to arrive. If this cannot be done first thing in the morning because of staggered schedules, plan a time to meet the day before, when the entire dental healthcare team is together.
9. Update schedules throughout the day as changes occur.
10. Keep the dental healthcare team and patients informed of any changes that will affect their schedules.

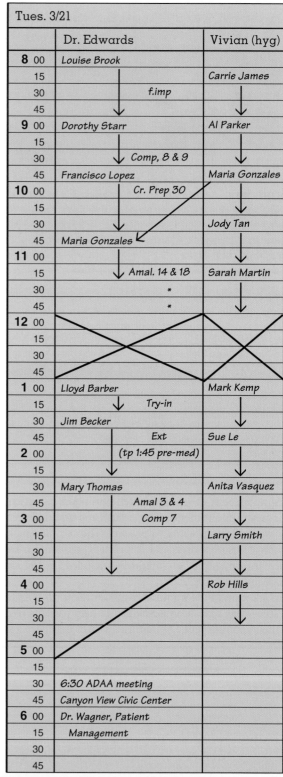

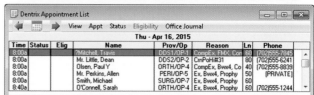

FIGURE 10-9 A manual (**A**) and computer-generated (**B**) daily schedule. (**B**, Dentrix screen capture courtesy Henry Schein Practice Solutions, American Fork, Utah.)

KEY POINTS

- The development and implementation of an organized, functional schedule for a dental practice requires time, experience, and the cooperation of the entire dental healthcare team. There are two components to scheduling: the "mechanics of scheduling" and the "art of scheduling."
- The mechanics of scheduling involves selecting the appointment book or electronic scheduler that is best tailored to the daily schedule of the dental practice and then matrixing it properly. The book identifies who will perform which tasks, on what date, and at what time. The book outlines which treatment rooms are available and at what times. It identifies patients who will be seen and what treatment will be performed, including the amount of time required to complete the treatment. The appointment book is divided into days and each day is divided into time segments. Time segments are referred to as *units* or *time blocks*. Either four units per hour (15-minute intervals) or six units per hour (10-minute intervals) are used when scheduling patients.
- The art of scheduling includes establishing the rules for scheduling. The objective of this process is to determine when the dental healthcare team is the most productive and how, through effective scheduling, the dental healthcare team can meet the financial goals of the dental practice.
- Effective scheduling takes into consideration the best time of day to perform procedures and how to meet the needs of patients while maintaining control of the appointment book.

CAREER-READY PRACTICES

Career-Ready Practices activities are designed to provide students with experiences that can be "practiced" in preparation for skills needed on the job. In each of the following exercises, a variety of approaches may be used to address the problem, rather than "right" or "wrong" answers. Below each exercise, next to the compass icon, is a listing of suggested Career-Ready Practice numbers that correspond to the listing of 12 practices in the front of the text (see p. viii-ix); these practices provide suggestions for approaches to complete the exercise.

1. Consider the following scenario: You have just started working for Canyon View Dental Associates. The dental practice employs two dentists, Dr. Edwards and Dr. Bradley, as well as two dental hygienists, Vivian and Diane. Dr. Edwards works 2 days per week and Dr. Bradley works 3 days per week. Dr. Edwards works from 8 AM to 5 PM (2 days per week). Dr. Bradley works from 11 AM to 7 PM (2 days per week) and on Saturdays from 8 AM to 2 PM. The hygienists also work 2 days per week. Diane works 1 day with Dr. Edwards and Vivian works 1 day with Dr. Bradley. Both dentists take 1 hour for lunch unless they are attending luncheon meetings.

- Identify what further information is needed to matrix an appointment book. With the information given in the scenario and the information you add, matrix a week in an appointment book for Canyon View Dental Associates. Use the workbook or your instructor will provide appointment sheets.
- Schedule the following patients (see the table below) during 1 week in your matrixed appointment book. The number of patients listed will not fill the week. You may wish to add additional patients to the schedule and identify which dentist and hygienist each patient will see. For further practice, add emergency patients, study clubs, staff meetings, luncheon meetings, and other appointments that will need special consideration in the schedule.

 Career-Ready Practices

8 *Utilize critical thinking to make sense of problems and persevere in solving them.*

11 *Use technology to enhance productivity.*

2 *Apply appropriate academic and technical skills.*

Patient	Treatment	Units of Time	Tooth No.	Special Instructions	Telephone No.
Carol Aguilar	Recall	3		Hygienist	503-555-3376
Christopher Darling	Composite sealants	4	8 & 9 max and mand	After school	503-555-3256
Dawn Savage	AMAL	2	14		503-555-9987
Dorothy Starr	Comp	3	7, 8, & 9	Premedication	503-555-0087
Francisco Lopez	Cr prep	3	18		503-555-0980
Frank Williams	Recall	3		Hygienist	503-555-3382
Jacob Henry	Cr prep	6	24	Premedication	503-555-3245
Jason Ward	Recall/Fl tx	2		Schedule with brother	503-555-7533
Jennifer Vail	NP	3		Early AM	503-555-6743
Jim Beckner	Extraction	4	14, 15, & 16	Schedule 15 min early	503-555-3356
Jim Butler	Recall	3		Hygienist	503-555-9923

Continued

Patient	Treatment	Units of Time	Tooth No.	Special Instructions	Telephone No.
Jon Ford	Recall	3		Hygienist	503-555-4428
Judy Carr	Recall	3		Hygienist	503-555-8833
Julie Singer	Check/po	½		Patient late	503-555-7774
Kathy Bader	Final imp	4	FUD	PM	503-555-8763
Kathy Campbell	Recall	3		Hygienist	503-555-2245
Lloyd Barber	Try-in	2	FUD		503-555-6634
Louise Brooke	Final imp	4	PUD	Before noon	503-555-2953
Maria Gonzales	Prophy	3		Hygienist	503-555-7245
Maria Gonzales	Amalgam	4	2, 3	Following hygiene appt	503-555-7245
Mark Dyer	Check/adj	½		Late afternoon	503-555-1123
Martha Sterling	Bridge prep	8	12–14		503-555-6578
Michael Ward	Recall/Fl tx	2		Schedule with brother	503-555-7533
Pat Perez	Recall	3		Hygienist	503-555-4720
Mary Thomas	Amalgam composite	6	12, 14, 24, 25	Fearful of injections	503-555-5572
Carrie James	Prophy	3		Hygienist	503-555-8965

11

Recall Systems

LEARNING OBJECTIVES

1. Define recall system and explain the benefits of a continuing care (recall) program for patients and the financial health of a dental practice, including the elements that are necessary for an effective recall system.

2. List the different classifications of recalls.
3. Identify the methods for recalling patients and explain the barriers and solutions for each method.

INTRODUCTION

A **recall system** is an organized method of scheduling patients for examinations, prophylaxis, or other dental treatments. The success of a recall system is dependent on several factors: (1) Patients must be willing to return to the dental practice for follow-up care and examinations. (2) The dental practice must follow the procedure consistently to schedule patients at the prescribed time. (3) The dental practice must have an efficient method for tracking and contacting patients who fail to return at the scheduled time.

The function of a dental **recall appointment** system is to automate the scheduling of a patient for preventive dental treatment or for reevaluation of other dental conditions. A routine recall appointment, for the purpose of an examination and prophylaxis (cleaning), is scheduled every 6 months. The prescribed length of time between appointments may vary from patient to patient. The dentist and dental hygienist determine the appropriate length of time between appointments on the basis of the dental needs of each patient.

Patients must understand the importance of the recall appointment before they are compelled to follow the advice of the dentist. Patients who seek dental treatment only when they are in pain are not likely to follow through with a recall appointment. The dental healthcare team has an obligation to all patients to educate them about the benefits of good oral health. Once patients understand and accept the benefits of good oral health, they are more likely to return for regular check-ups and prophylaxis.

The role of a dental healthcare team is to provide comprehensive, professional treatments through a system of dental examinations, preventive care measures, restorative treatments, and education. By educating patients about the benefits of home dental care and the benefits of establishing good dental health habits, the dental healthcare team forms a partnership with patients. When a team approach is used, the patient, as a team member, is more likely to accept his or her role in the prevention of dental disease, which includes regular examinations and prophylaxis.

Conditions that lead to a successful recall system do not just happen. Organization and commitment from the patient and the dental healthcare team are required if they are to occur.

The benefits of a recall system for the patient include the following:
- By maintaining good oral health, the patient will be free from dental disease, pain, and discomfort.
- Once optimal oral health has been achieved, the patient's cost of dental care is minimal.
- Insurance carriers encourage preventive dentistry. Most insurance policies provide 100% coverage for preventive procedures (radiographs, prophylaxis, and examinations).
- Some insurance carriers offer the incentive of providing higher percentages of coverage in increments for dental treatment to reward patients when they undergo examinations and prophylaxis on a regular basis (70% the first year, 80% the second year, and 100% after 4 years).
- The amount of time a patient must spend at the dental office is reduced when dental disease is detected and treated early, which prevents the need for more extensive treatment.

The benefits of a recall system for the dental practice include the following:
- It forms a partnership between the patient and the dental healthcare team (the patient is a person and not just a "mouth").
- It increases referrals from patients because they feel comfortable and satisfied with the quality of the dental care they are receiving (accomplished through patient education).
- It ensures a steady flow of patients through regularly scheduled appointments.
- It results in a partnership with other dental professionals because the total care of the patient is shared. Patients who are referred to a dental specialist for treatment are then referred back to the general dentist when that treatment is completed. When treatment continues for longer than a few months, the patient is referred back to the general dentist for a regular recall appointment.

163

CLASSIFICATION OF RECALLS

The average recall appointment includes an examination, radiographs (at prescribed intervals), and prophylaxis. For children, the appointment may also include a fluoride treatment.

During recall appointments, the dentist reexamines patients and evaluates their dental health. If dental disease is detected, it can be treated while it affects only a small area, which saves the patient time and money. Dental flossing and toothbrushing techniques should be discussed to optimize patients' home care.

In addition to the routine recall appointment, patients may be scheduled for follow-up of previous dental treatments or for monitoring of a dental condition. Treatments that may require follow-up appointments include the following:

- Endodontic treatments
- Dental implants
- Crowns and bridges
- Partial and full dentures
- Surgical procedures
- Orthodontic evaluations

Additionally, patients who have been referred to specialists for treatment should subsequently be seen by the general dentist for regular check-ups.

METHODS FOR RECALLING PATIENTS

Once patients have been educated about and motivated to participate in preventive dentistry, the next step in the recall system is to formulate a process that ensures that each patient has the opportunity to return to the dental practice at the prescribed time. Several different types of systems can be used to identify when a patient should be seen, the type of appointment needed, and whether the patient followed through with the appointment. Manual and computerized systems have been developed for these purposes and vary widely from practice to practice.

> **! REMEMBER**
>
> The best system is the one that works.

General Information Needed for a Recall System

- Type of recall
- Month in which the patient is due for an appointment
- Who the appointment should be scheduled with: the dentist or the hygienist
- The amount of time needed for the appointment and what treatment will be performed
- What method of recall each patient prefers: prescheduled appointment, reminder by mail, or reminder by telephone call

Prescheduled Recall System

One of the most effective recall methods is to have a patient schedule his or her next appointment before he or she leaves the office, after his or her current recall appointment is finished. This method (the **prescheduled recall system**) is highly successful because patients have personally participated in the

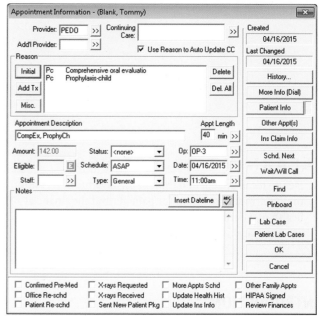

FIGURE 11-1 The Appointment Information window allows the administrative dental assistant to record all necessary data about a patient's next appointment. Having patients preschedule their appointments before leaving the office is a highly successful practice. (Dentrix screen capture courtesy Henry Schein Practice Solutions, American Fork, Utah.)

scheduling of their own appointment (Figure 11-1). Although schedules change and some appointments must be rescheduled, they are very seldom broken.

> **! REMEMBER**
>
> Once patients have failed to make or to keep a recall appointment, they are sometimes too embarrassed to call and reschedule a new appointment.

Barrier to the Success of Prescheduled Recall

Barrier	Solution
The hygiene schedule is booked 6 months in advance and it is difficult to work in other patients.	Do not fill any one schedule completely. Designate appointment times that are not to be filled until 1 to 2 weeks before the date. Rationale: This leaves space to schedule patients who are new to the practice. Patients do not like to wait for appointments and may seek another dentist if they cannot get an appointment in a reasonable length of time (2 weeks is the average). Keep a call list. If you get an opening sooner, you can call the patient and fill the opening.

> **! REMEMBER**
>
> When talking to patients, never tell them you have a cancellation. This only raises questions: "Why was the appointment canceled? Was something wrong?" Tell patients that you have an opening in the schedule or that you have rearranged the schedule.

PROCEDURES

Steps in Prescheduling the Recall Appointment

Manual System

1. Have the patient self-address a recall postcard.
2. Mutually schedule the next appointment before the patient leaves the office.
3. Enter the date and time on the recall postcard (Figure 11-2).
4. Place the recall postcard in a monthly filing system. File the card according to the month the patient is due back for the appointment. (The month, date, and time of the appointment should also be recorded in the clinical chart.)
5. Mail cards to the patients 2 to 4 weeks before their appointment. Patients who must reschedule their appointment will call the office and a new appointment can be scheduled.

Automated System

1. Tag the patient's computer file for recall (referred to as *continuing care* in the Dentrix system).
2. The practice management system will prompt recall information during the patient checkout process and schedule the recall appointment before the patient leaves the office.
3. The information is stored in the system database.
4. The practice management system has been programmed to follow a set of conditions used to identify the recall patient and when and how to send the reminder (electronically via e-mail [Figure 11-3] or text message or by generating a notice that can be mailed). The information can be viewed in the patient file.
5. Mail cards for patients who have requested this form of appointment notification. Most practice management systems will prompt you when the cards need to be printed and sent.

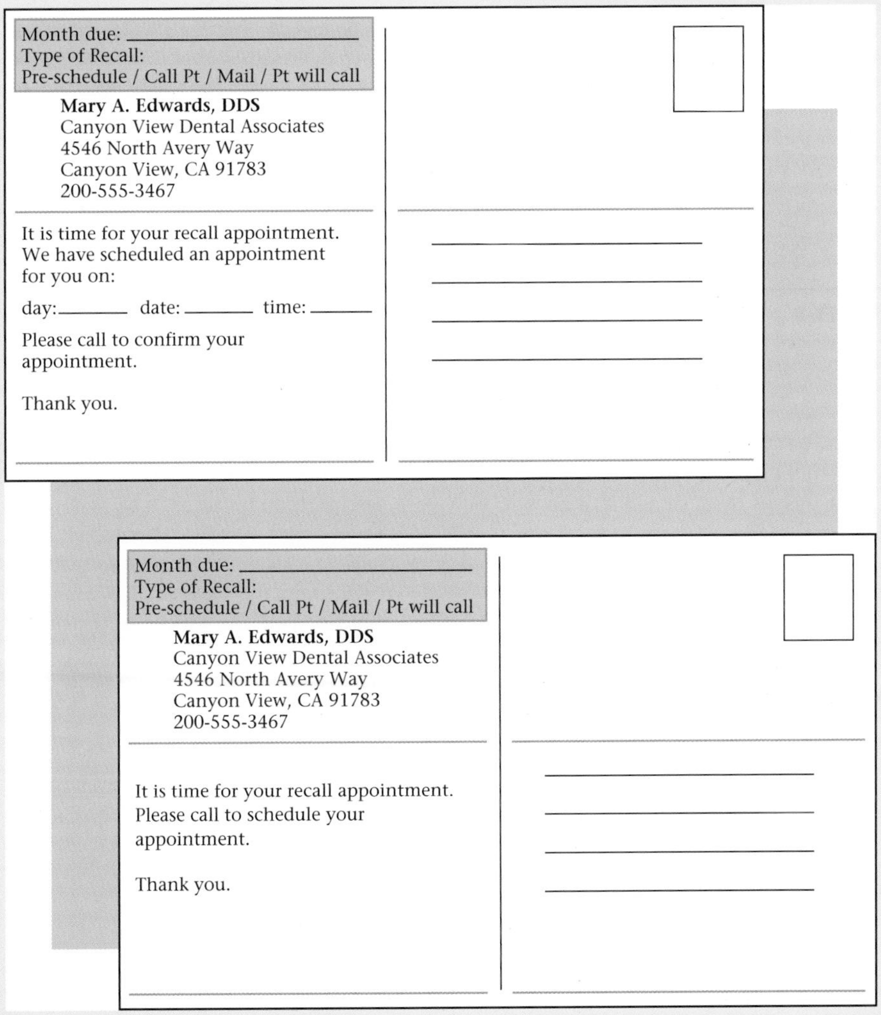

Month due: _____
Type of Recall:
Pre-schedule / Call Pt / Mail / Pt will call

Mary A. Edwards, DDS
Canyon View Dental Associates
4546 North Avery Way
Canyon View, CA 91783
200-555-3467

It is time for your recall appointment. We have scheduled an appointment for you on:

day: _____ date: _____ time: _____

Please call to confirm your appointment.

Thank you.

Month due: _____
Type of Recall:
Pre-schedule / Call Pt / Mail / Pt will call

Mary A. Edwards, DDS
Canyon View Dental Associates
4546 North Avery Way
Canyon View, CA 91783
200-555-3467

It is time for your recall appointment. Please call to schedule your appointment.

Thank you.

FIGURE 11-2 Two types of messages are used on recall cards. Selection depends on whether a specific date and time has already been scheduled.

Continued

PROCEDURES—cont'd

Steps in Prescheduling the Recall Appointment

From: Canyon View Dental Associates
To: RLBudd@townbank.com
Date: Mon, July 18, 2016 3:44:05 PM
Cc:
Subject: New dental appointment for Rose - Please reply!

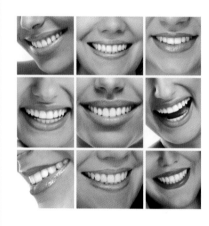

Put this on your calendar, please

Dear Rose,

We have reserved the following appointment especially for you - please add it to your calendar.

Date: Wednesday August 31, 2016
Time: 4:00 PM

Please click on a response below so we'll know you received this e-mail, or call our office at 987-654-3210 if you need to arrange a better time.

- ■ *It's on my calendar, but please remind me again a few days before the appointment.*
- ■ *Yes, I'll be there. I don't need another e-mail or phone call.*
- ■ *I have a question or concern about this appointment - please contact me.*

Thank you!

Canyon View Dental Associates
4546 North Avery Way
Canyon View, California
Telephone (987) 654-3210

FIGURE 11-3 Appointment reminders can be sent via e-mail for patient convenience. (Composite photo copyright © 2013 LuckyBusiness, iStock.com. All rights reserved.)

Manual System

6. Enter pertinent information on the tracking form.
7. Call a patient 2 days before his or her appointment to confirm the date and time. This lessens the chance that a patient will miss an appointment.

Automated System

6. The practice management system automatically tracks recall patients. You will be able to print a list of patients who are due for recall (typically at preset intervals such as weekly, biweekly, or monthly). The list will identify the patient (including contact information), the service to be performed, the provider, and when his or her appointment is scheduled. The list can also identify patients who are overdue for their appointments.
7. Call a patient 2 days before his or her appointment to confirm the date and time. Patient appointments can also be confirmed electronically via e-mail and text message (Figure 11-4).

From: Canyon View Dental Associates
To: RLBudd@townbank.com
Date: Fri, August 12, 2016 7:01:08 AM
Cc:
Subject: Confirming Rose's dental appointment - Please reply!

Confirming your appointment with us

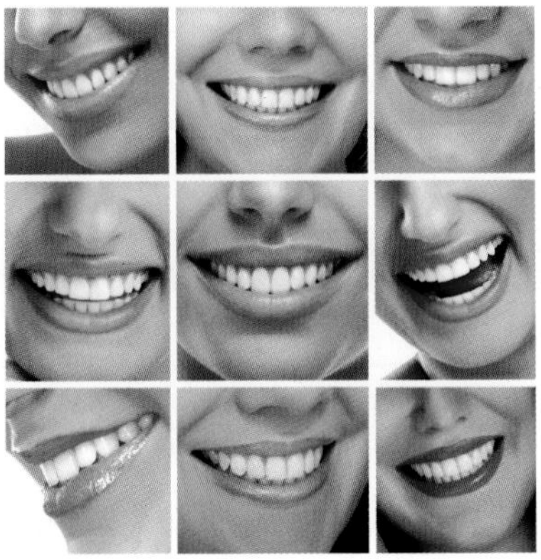

Dear Rose,

We have reserved time for your professional cleaning, examination, and oral cancer screening on **Wednesday August 31, 2016 at 4:00 PM. Please click on a response below so we'll know you received this e-mail**, or call our office at 987-654-3210. We look forward to seeing you!

- *It's on my calendar, but please remind me again a few days before the appointment.*
- *Yes, I'll be there. I don't need another e-mail or phone call.*
- *I have a question or concern about this appointment - please contact me.*

Thank you!

Canyon View Dental Associates
4546 North Avery Way
Canyon View, California
Telephone (987) 654-3210

FIGURE 11-4 Appointment confirmations may be sent via text message to ensure that they reach busy patients; patients may have the time to text a confirmation when they would not have enough time to make a phone call to confirm the appointment. (Composite photo copyright © 2013 LuckyBusiness, iStock.com. All rights reserved.)

Telephone Recall System

The **telephone recall system** requires that an assistant call each patient before the month in which he or she is due for recall to schedule the appointment. This system provides immediate feedback about the needs of the patient.

Barriers to the Success of Telephone Recall

Barrier	Solution
Patients are difficult to reach at home.	In today's society, it is difficult to reach patients at home. Often both spouses work. The best time to call is in the early evening but then you may interrupt the dinner hour. With this type of recall system, it is best to know your patients' preferences. You may need to ask their permission to call them at work or in the early evening.
The recall system is time consuming.	Select a time to make phone calls when you have someone to answer the telephone and schedule patient appointments for you. Alternatively, schedule an evening when you can make calls. Evenings are usually less hectic and you can accomplish a great deal in a short time. You will find patients at home and be free of interruptions.
Only one person should make the calls.	Telephone scheduling is usually more successful if only one or two assistants are in charge of the calls. Although this may seem burdensome for one person, it does have an advantage. Patients are more comfortable when they are familiar with the assistant who is making the call. Over time, assistants get to know the needs and schedules of their patients and this is comforting to patients. It eventually saves time in scheduling patients.

Barrier

Assistants can become frustrated after making several back-to-back calls. (They can begin to sound like a computerized message.)

Solution

Remember that this is not a telemarketing job. When you become frustrated, your patients detect it. It is best to pace yourself and not spend hours at a time on the telephone. If you develop a negative attitude while making the calls, go back to them when you feel more positive.

✚ HIPAA

Privacy Rule: Confidential Communications

Patients can request limitations to communications, including place and type of telephone calls and messages.

Mail Recall System

A **mail recall system** requires the mailing of recall cards to patients to remind them that they are due in the dental office for an appointment (see Figure 11-2, *bottom*).

PROCEDURES

Steps in Using the Telephone Recall System

1. Select a time when you can make telephone calls with very few interruptions. (Remember to smile when you are talking to your patients on the phone. Smiles, as well as poor attitudes, travel over phone lines.)
2. Contact the patient and schedule an appointment.
3. Confirm the information you have, such as insurance coverage, and remind the patient to bring any necessary forms.
4. Follow up with a confirmation recall card.
5. Record the new information in the tracking system.

PROCEDURES

Steps in a Mail Recall System

1. Select recall cards that catch the eye of the receiver (Figure 11-5). Several companies print a wide selection of recall and other promotional cards.
2. Have patients self-address cards at the time of their appointment. If a computerized method is used, enter the date into the system and the computer will generate recall cards at the appropriate time.
3. Place the card in a card file according to the month in which the patient is due for recall.
4. Mail the card before the month in which the patient is due for recall.
5. Enter the information in a tracking system.

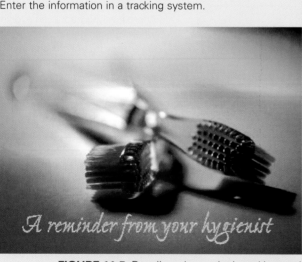

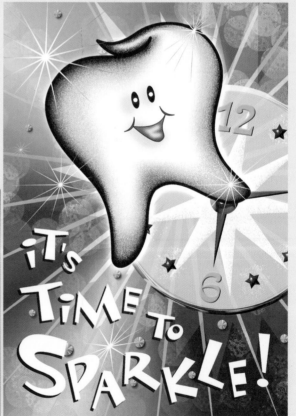

FIGURE 11-5 Recall cards are designed in a variety of styles and colors. They should be selected to catch the patient's eye. (Courtesy Patterson Office Supplies, Champaign, Ill.)

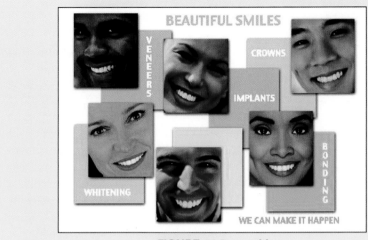

FIGURE 11-5, cont'd

TIPS FOR MAINTAINING A SUCCESSFUL RECALL SYSTEM

- Form a partnership with the patient. (Education = Motivation = Acceptance)
- Use the type of recall that works best for the individual patient.
- Follow through with a tracking system (manual or computerized).
- Always remain flexible.
- Coordinate recalls with insurance coverage. If an insurance carrier will pay for a prophylaxis only every 6 months, do not schedule the patient for one in 5 months unless the dentist recommends that the patient be seen more often for dental health reasons and only after the patient understands that the insurance company may not pay for the visit. *Always inform the patient.*
- Never lose contact with patients. They will not call you until they are in pain.
- Develop a system that can be used by all members of the dental healthcare team. Remember, the administrative dental assistant is the organizer of the system but it takes a team effort to make it work smoothly (Figure 11-6).

Automated Recall Systems

Many dental practices are using computers to schedule and track recall patients. The **automated recall system** uses a database to identify and track recall patients. The system combines all of the components of an effective recall system into one seamless function that can save the dental practice time and money.

Barrier to the Success of Mail Recall

Barrier   **Solution**

Patients do not call.   This system relies on patients' taking the initiative to call the dental office to schedule an appointment. When patients are given sole responsibility, it is highly unlikely that they will call for the appointment. If you use this system, you will need to have a very good tracking system in place and follow through often to ensure that patients are scheduling their appointments

FLOW CHART FOR A MANUAL RECALL SYSTEM

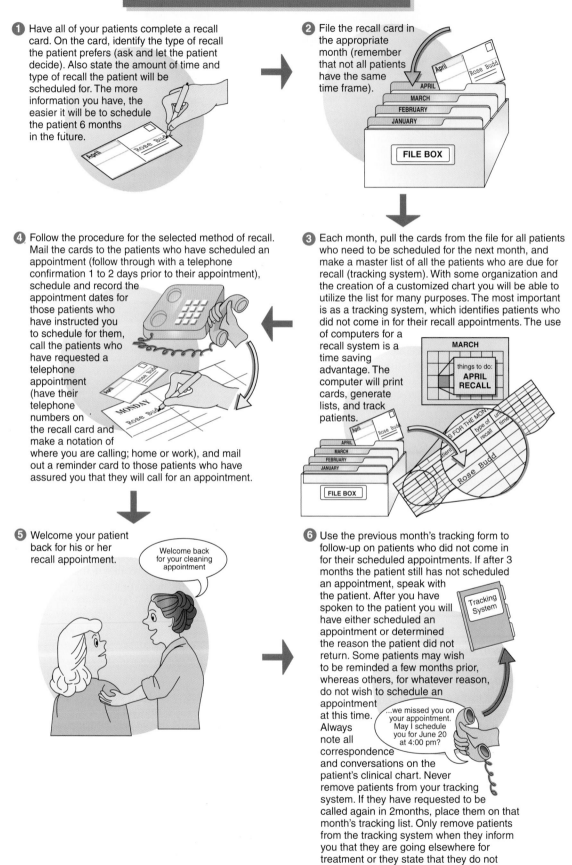

① Have all of your patients complete a recall card. On the card, identify the type of recall the patient prefers (ask and let the patient decide). Also state the amount of time and type of recall the patient will be scheduled for. The more information you have, the easier it will be to schedule the patient 6 months in the future.

② File the recall card in the appropriate month (remember that not all patients have the same time frame).

③ Each month, pull the cards from the file for all patients who need to be scheduled for the next month, and make a master list of all the patients who are due for recall (tracking system). With some organization and the creation of a customized chart you will be able to utilize the list for many purposes. The most important is as a tracking system, which identifies patients who did not come in for their recall appointments. The use of computers for a recall system is a time saving advantage. The computer will print cards, generate lists, and track patients.

④ Follow the procedure for the selected method of recall. Mail the cards to the patients who have scheduled an appointment (follow through with a telephone confirmation 1 to 2 days prior to their appointment), schedule and record the appointment dates for those patients who have instructed you to schedule for them, call the patients who have requested a telephone appointment (have their telephone numbers on the recall card and make a notation of where you are calling; home or work), and mail out a reminder card to those patients who have assured you that they will call for an appointment.

⑤ Welcome your patient back for his or her recall appointment.

Welcome back for your cleaning appointment

⑥ Use the previous month's tracking form to follow-up on patients who did not come in for their scheduled appointments. If after 3 months the patient still has not scheduled an appointment, speak with the patient. After you have spoken to the patient you will have either scheduled an appointment or determined the reason the patient did not return. Some patients may wish to be reminded a few months prior, whereas others, for whatever reason, do not wish to schedule an appointment at this time. Always note all correspondence and conversations on the patient's clinical chart. Never remove patients from your tracking system. If they have requested to be called again in 2months, place them on that month's tracking list. Only remove patients from the tracking system when they inform you that they are going elsewhere for treatment or they state that they do not want you to call.

...we missed you on your appointment. May I schedule you for June 20 at 4:00 pm?

FIGURE 11-6 Flow chart for a manual recall system.

ANATOMY OF A RECALL TRACKING SYSTEM

The ultimate purpose of the tracking system is to ensure that all patients who are in the recall system return for their recall appointments. It is easy for any member of the dental healthcare team to pick up the book and contact the overdue recall patients. Any member should be able to identify who has completed the recall and who has not. A system, manual or computerized, is set up that identifies the type of second notice, third notice, and so on until the patient is seen or removed from the system. When the system is used to its fullest extent, the status of the patient is always known and the patient is not lost.

				① Monthly Recall Tracking Form										
RECALLS FOR THE MONTH OF APRIL, 20XX														
Patient	type of recall	unit time	x-rays	telephone #	prescheduled appointment	call patient	pt will call	recall completed	other work	appt Dr./Hyg.	1st notice	2nd notice	3rd notice	
②	③	④	⑤	⑥	⑦	⑧	⑨	⑩	⑪	⑫	⑬	⑭	⑭
Rose Budd	prophy	3	no	555-1233(H)	4/4/99			4/4/XX	bridge	hyg	####			
Bill Frank	endo	1	yes	555-4987(W)		x		4/22/XX	crown	doctor	####			
Jose Gomez	prophy	3	bw/2	555-6794(VM)			x	4/18/XX		hyg	####			
Sam Jones	prophy	3	FMX	555-0908(W)			x			hyg	####			

① MONTH

Identify the month and year the patient is due for recall.

② PATIENTS' NAMES

Patients' names are listed in alphabetical order. Adding an account number will help to locate the patient in the computer file, or the numerical number of the patient if the dental practice utilizes a numerical filing system.

③ TYPE OF RECALL

Identifies the category of recall needed.

④ UNIT TIME

States the amount of time that will be needed to complete the appointment.

⑤ X-RAYS (radiographs)

Indication of whether x-rays are needed and what type.

⑥ TELEPHONE NUMBER

The telephone number of the patient. Indicate if the telephone is home, work, voice mail, or message center.

⑦ PRESCHEDULED

Type of recall method. The appointment was made at the patient's last recall appointment. In a modified version of this system, the patient selects a general day of the week and time for the next appointment. When the recall cards are processed for a given month the assistant schedules the appointment. The patient is notified by mail and has the opportunity to keep the selected time or call the office to reschedule.

⑧ CALL PATIENT

Type of recall method. The patient has indicated that he or she wants to be called a few weeks prior to the recall to schedule an appointment.

⑨ PATIENT WILL CALL

Type of recall method. The patient has stated that he or she will call for an appointment after receiving a reminder in the mail.

⑩ RECALL COMPLETED

The date the patient is seen in the office for the recall. This is the most important element of the system. If this portion is not completed it will be impossible to determine if the patient has returned as scheduled. Time must then be taken to check the clinical record or the computer system.

⑪ OTHER WORK

Identify if there is any other treatment that needs to be scheduled at the time of the recall. It is also a good tracking tool for clinical treatment. Patients may delay treatment for a variety of reasons.

⑫ APPOINTMENT WITH

Identify which dental professional needs to see the patient.

⑬ 1ST NOTICE

Record the date that the first recall card was sent or telephone call was made.

⑭ 2ND NOTICE, 3RD NOTICE

The dates that follow-up contacts were made with the patient regarding the recall appointment. A system is designed by the dental practice to notify patients (via post-card, letter, or personal telephone call) that they need to schedule an appointment. For example, a 2nd notice is mailed if they have not returned to the dental practice within 3 months of their original recall month. At 6 months, a third attempt is made. This can be a combination of a reminder card or letter followed by a telephone call. At this point, patients on a 6-month recall have not had their teeth cleaned or examined for 1 year.

(Dentrix screen capture courtesy Henry Schein Practice Solutions, American Fork, Utah.)

KEY POINTS

- A recall system is necessary to ensure that patients return to the dental practice at scheduled intervals for preventive treatment and examinations. The recall appointment benefits patients by helping them to maintain good oral health, thus reducing their cost of dental treatment over the long term. It benefits the dental practice by promoting partnerships with patients, increasing referrals, and ensuring a steady flow of patients.
- Types of recall systems include the following:
  - Prescheduled
  - Telephone
  - Mail
  - Automated
- Tips for maintaining a successful recall system include the following:
  - Customize the recall method for individual patients.
  - Follow through with a tracking system.
  - Remain flexible.
  - Coordinate recalls with insurance coverage.
  - Never lose contact with a patient.
- Computerized recall systems combine the elements of a manual system and are programmed to perform steps automatically.

CAREER-READY PRACTICES

Career-Ready Practices activities are designed to provide students with experiences that can be "practiced" in preparation for skills needed on the job. In each of the following exercises, a variety of approaches may be used to address the problem, rather than "right" or "wrong" answers. Below each exercise, next to the compass icon, is a listing of suggested Career-Ready Practice numbers that correspond to the listing of 12 practices in the front of the text (see p. viii-ix); these practices provide suggestions for approaches to complete the exercise.

1. A successful recall program depends on several factors, one of which is the ability to educate patients on the benefits of preventive dental care. Describe the strategies you would use to explain the benefits to a reluctant dental patient.

 Career-Ready Practices
  1 *Act as a responsible and contributing citizen and employee.*
  3 *Attend to personal health and financial well-being.*
  5 *Consider the environmental, social and economic impacts of decisions.*

2. In a small group, share your ideas and strategies and create a presentation for a group, such as school-aged students at a community health fair, or for an individual patient that explains the benefits of preventive dental care.

 Career-Ready Practices
  8 *Utilize critical thinking to make sense of problems and persevere in solving them.*
  6 *Demonstrate creativity and innovation.*
  4 *Communicate clearly, effectively, and with reason.*

3. What do you think are the important steps that need to be followed to have a successful recall system?

 Career-Ready Practices
  9 *Model integrity, ethical leadership, and effective management.*
  8 *Utilize critical thinking to make sense of problems and persevere in solving them.*
  5 *Consider the environmental, social, and economic impacts of decisions.*

12

Inventory Management

LEARNING OBJECTIVES

1. Explain how to establish a successful inventory management system, including:
   - List the information needed to order supplies and products and discuss how this information will be used.
   - Define rate of use and lead time.
   - Describe the role of an inventory manager.
   - Analyze the elements of a good inventory management system and describe how elements relate to the organization and overall effectiveness of a dental practice.
2. Identify the types of supplies, products, and equipment that are commonly purchased for a dental practice.
3. Discuss the selection and ordering process of supplies, products, and equipment, including:
   - Compare the advantages and disadvantages of catalog ordering and supply house services and explain when it is appropriate to use the two services.
   - List the information that should be considered before an order is placed for supplies and products.
   - Explain how shipments should be received and proper storage techniques.
4. Explain the role of the Occupational Safety and Health Administration (OSHA). Describe the various sections of an effective hazard communication program and discuss what information is important to an inventory manager.

INTRODUCTION

Ordering and managing supplies in a dental practice requires organization, communication, and the cooperation of the entire dental healthcare team. Inventory control is not limited to supplies in the clinical area. Those in the laboratory and business office must also be managed. Because the financial health of the dental practice depends on controlling costs, it is necessary to establish and maintain an inventory management system (IMS) that is cost effective, efficient, and easy to manage. Having the proper supplies on hand at all times is necessary in order to offer patients the best possible care.

ESTABLISHING AN INVENTORY MANAGEMENT SYSTEM

An effective IMS, manual or automated, will provide similar outcomes. In a small dental practice it may not be necessary to use a fully automated web-based system to manage the practice's inventory effectively. On the other hand, a large multispecialty practice will require an advanced system to track and control inventory. To establish most types of systems, the dental practice will be required to spend some time setting up the system. After the dental practice researches and determines the type of system and the functions that will be used, the next step is to inventory the current supplies and discard items that are obsolete and products that have expired.

To effectively manage and monitor inventory, you need to know what you have, when you will need to reorder, where

ESTABLISHING AN INVENTORY MANAGEMENT SYSTEM (IMS)

- Research and select the type of IMS that fits the needs of the dental practice
- Inventory current supplies
  - Discard (or recycle) obsolete and expired products
- Create a database (list) of inventory items
  - Name of product (generic)
  - Brand name
  - Supplier (vendor)
  - Contact information
- Establish maximum and minimum levels to create a baseline for reordering
- Export the database into the new IMS

KEY FUNCTIONS OF AN INVENTORY MANAGEMENT SYSTEM

- Track inventory supply purchases and usage
- Use data communication technology to transfer information such as barcoding
- Efficiently track items by usage and expiration date
- Use data communication to place orders, track shipments, and pay accounts
- Interface with practice management software to generate multiple reports (financial and operational)
- Interface with vendor catalogs and point-of-sale options
- Provide information required for Occupational Safety and Health Administration (OSHA) hazard communications compliance
- Store data on individual computers, network servers, or web-based Cloud hosting

inventory is stored, and when it will expire. This function begins when the information is entered into a database (electronic or manual). The database can be as simple as a handwritten index card or an Excel spreadsheet or as complex as a customized database in an inventory management software program. The average IMS uses a database that identifies the product, tracks the minimum and maximum supply levels, and alerts you when it is time to reorder. The data are entered into a database via a form of data communication technology (barcodes and radio-frequency [RF] tags) or recorded directly by the administrative dental assistant. The system may produce a weekly list of supplies to be ordered or reports that alert you when supplies fall below the minimum supply level or are about to expire. Some programs link your account directly to the vendor and automatically place an order when a product reaches the minimum level

Data Communication Technology

An IMS uses a system of data communications that is able to transfer data quickly across both small and large distances. For this communication to work, a system must be in place that transfers the information from point A to point B. One type of data communication is the barcode. A barcode is an optical machine-readable image of symbols and shapes that represents data relating to the object to which it is attached. Barcode technology is widely used to communicate information, from supermarket checkout to ensuring that your luggage arrives at the correct destination. In healthcare, barcodes are used to identify patients, track medications, and control inventory. Barcodes are read by a line of sight produced by a handheld scanner or by passing the item over a fixed scanner (Figure 12-1).

In an IMS, barcoding is used to simplify and automate the tracking of supplies and products by transferring the information from point A (the item) to point B (the IMS database). Most supplies will arrive precoded; if they are not

precoded, it will be the administrative dental assistant's responsibility to create a code. Once the item is coded, it is scanned before it is placed in storage and again when it is used. When the item is scanned, the attached data are transmitted to the IMS database and inventory data are updated (Figure 12-2). Handheld scanners are mobile and can be easily placed in areas where items are stored. The key advantages to using barcodes are that it is a fast and efficient system and can be used by any member of the dental healthcare team.

Another type of data communication technology is radio-frequency identification (RFID). This technology uses radio waves to identify or track objects. Typically, a small chip (RF tag) stores data that can be scanned by a reader in any direction. The RF tag is reusable and the data can be refreshed. This technology is often used in a fully automated system that uses secure centralized locations for supplies. Items with RF tags are automatically scanned as the items leave the storage area.

Once the information is stored in the database, the IMS can be programmed to do a wide array of tasks. The information can be used to track the use of products down to the individual patient encounter, providing data that can be analyzed to determine actual procedure costs.

The IMS also has the ability to use data communication to connect directly to suppliers and vendors via a web-based system. When an item reaches a reorder point, the data are communicated and the item is reordered automatically. The same system can be used to place orders directly, check the status of an order, track backorders, and pay the account.

The information in the IMS database can also be exported to practice management systems to generate a number of reports that can be used to analyze inventory cost, patient usage, and overall effectiveness of the IMS. Business managers use the information to help control the cost of supplies and add to the financial health of the dental practice. When items are overstocked, become obsolete, or

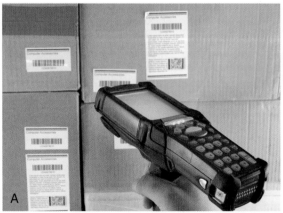
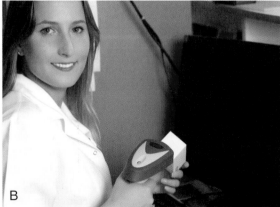

FIGURE 12-1 A, A barcode system can be used to scan every piece of inventory. **B,** The information is then stored in a computer database for easy management. (**A,** Copyright © 2011 ermingut, iStock.com. All rights reserved. **B,** Copyright © 2010 energyy, iStock.com.)

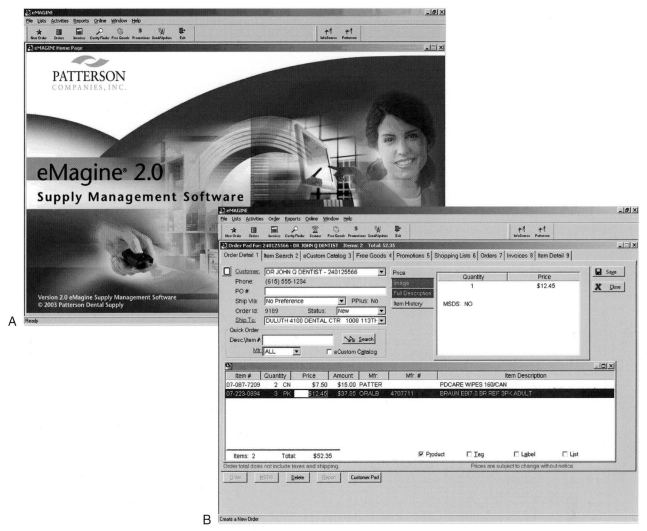

FIGURE 12-2 A, An electronic inventory management system (IMS) is designed to store and track lists of products within the dental office. **B,** Products that the office uses regularly can be searched, stored in a user account, and quickly reordered online. (Screen views of eMagine ordering system courtesy Patterson Dental, St. Paul, Minn.)

expire, they add unnecessary and avoidable expenses to the dental practice.

The computer software required and the way in which data are accessed will depend on many factors and the level of information required. The software program may be housed on an individual computer, which would require that all functions originate from that computer. The application software can also be located on a local network, which would allow the program to be accessed from any computer that is on the network and interfaces directly with other practice management programs. A web-based IMS is accessed virtually from anywhere using a variety of devices (computers, smartphones, and tablets); this is also true when the data are housed in a Cloud. Refer to Figure 12-3 for a visual example of the steps taken when using an IMS.

Manual Inventory Management Systems

When the practice does not have a computer or has a limited computer program, manual systems can be used. A manual system is effective but in most cases is far more time consuming than a good software program.

A simple card index system can be used to track the use of supplies and products (Figure 12-4). An index card is formatted to include all vital information needed to track and reorder the correct supplies and products. A simple Excel spreadsheet can also be designed to include the same vital information recorded on the index card. When a spreadsheet is used, it is easy to sort information and track usage and expiration dates. Because the data are limited and the functionality of a computerized system is not available, it will be necessary to manually compute reorder points and determine what needs to be ordered.

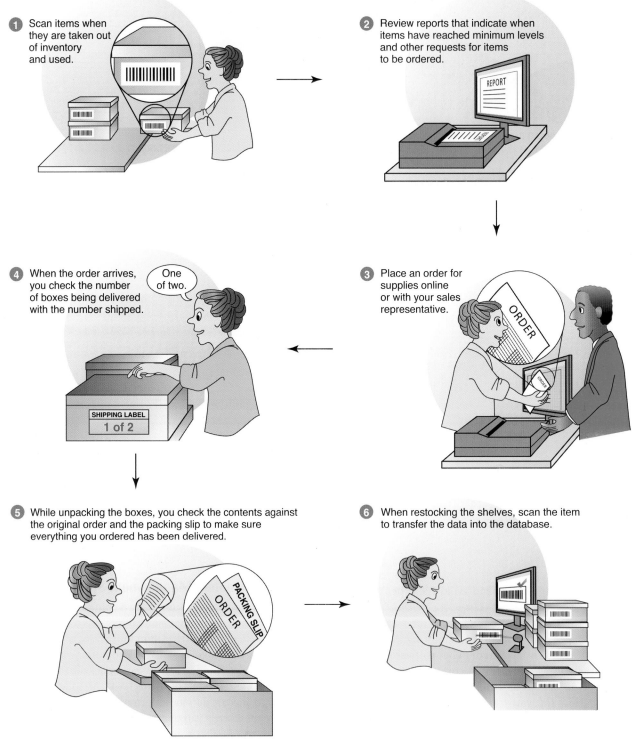

FIGURE 12-3 Steps to be followed when using an inventory management system (IMS).

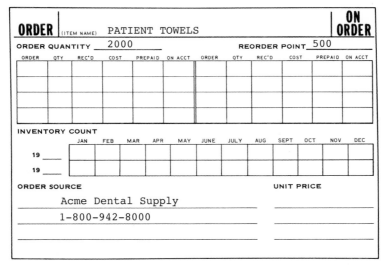

FIGURE 12-4 A sample inventory control card for a manual inventory system.

PROCEDURES

Steps in Determining When to Reorder

1. Determine how much of the product is used and how quickly it is used (**rate of use**). Some supplies arrive in quantities that will last at least 1 week and other supplies will last much longer, depending on how frequently they are used. The dental healthcare team can help to determine how rapidly supplies and products are used.
2. Determine how long it will take for supplies to arrive at the office once the order has been placed (**lead time**). Depending on the product and the supplies, this time will vary. It is a good management skill to establish a list of your vendors and record their average delivery times. Remember to add a few extra days as a margin of safety.

Selecting an Inventory Manager

PERSONAL CHARACTERISTICS OF AN INVENTORY MANAGER

- Is organized
- Has time to carry out duties
- Is able to communicate with others
- Is a team player
- Is a good shopper

DUTIES OF AN INVENTORY MANAGER

- Develops and maintains an accurate inventory system
- Seeks input from other members of the dental healthcare team
- Monitors inventory
- Maintains an accurate and current database (manual or electronic)
- Processes orders
- Receives orders and verifies invoices
- Organizes and maintains storage areas
- Tracks backorders

ELEMENTS OF A GOOD INVENTORY MANAGEMENT SYSTEM

- A qualified inventory manager is in charge.
- Supplies and products that are used in the dental practice can be identified quickly via a computer system, organized list, or card index.
- Products are stored according to the manufacturer's and Occupational Safety and Health Administration's (OSHA's) requirements (cool dry place, refrigerated, away from heat).
- Supplies are located for easy access by all members of the dental healthcare team (a master list identifies the location of each product or cabinets and shelves are clearly labeled).
- Reorder points are clearly identified in a database or with labeled tags, cards, or tape.
- A protocol has been clearly defined for notifying the inventory manager when a product or supply should be ordered.
- A process is in place for identifying which products need to be ordered, have been ordered, or are on backorder (tracking system).

It is easy to turn over all responsibility to one member of the dental healthcare team and simply say "handle it," but this method is not always a good dental business strategy. There is much more to a well-organized and efficient system. It is acceptable to have one person in charge but he or she must be given direction, guidance, and cooperation from other members of the dental healthcare team. Each member of the team has the duty and responsibility to help maintain the IMS. This includes selecting products and following the established protocol for the management of inventory.

Inventory Management System Protocol

Several points must be considered when an IMS protocol is developed. It may be the primary duty of one person to maintain the system but cooperation from the entire dental healthcare team is required to develop the protocol.

Steps in Developing an Inventory Management System Protocol

1. Identify products and supplies that are needed.
2. Select the vendor or vendors to be contacted.
3. Develop ordering guidelines.
4. Establish a receiving protocol.
5. Organize the storage area.
6. Check for compliance with Occupational Safety and Health Administration (OSHA) regulations.

TYPES OF SUPPLIES, PRODUCTS, AND EQUIPMENT

Consumable Supplies and Products

Consumable supplies and products are those items that are used and must be replenished (Figure 12-5). In the clinical area, such items as x-ray film, anesthetics, dental materials, and infection control products are used or consumed (not eaten). When the product is gone, it has to be replaced with fresh material. In addition, disposable supplies are used only once. These products include needles, saliva ejectors, and suction tips. Usually, for health and safety reasons, these supplies are not reused. A supply that comes in direct contact with a patient can be reused only if it can be sterilized (which involves complete destruction of all living organisms—not to be confused with disinfecting, which is only partial destruction of organisms).

Supplies for the business office include paper, envelopes, insurance forms, business cards, patient billing statements, business checks, clinical records forms, and charts. Impression material, gypsum products, and wax are among the supplies needed in the dental laboratory.

Nonconsumable Products

Nonconsumable (expendable) products are supplies and products that can be reused for a specific length of time before they must be replaced (Figure 12-6). Instruments, handpieces, and small equipment fall into this category. These items can be used for a year or two before they must be replaced because of wear and tear.

Major Equipment

Major equipment includes equipment that can be used for longer than 1 to 2 years (Figure 12-7). This equipment, such as dental chairs, radiology units, computers, office equipment, and laboratory equipment, can be depreciated on the business's tax returns.

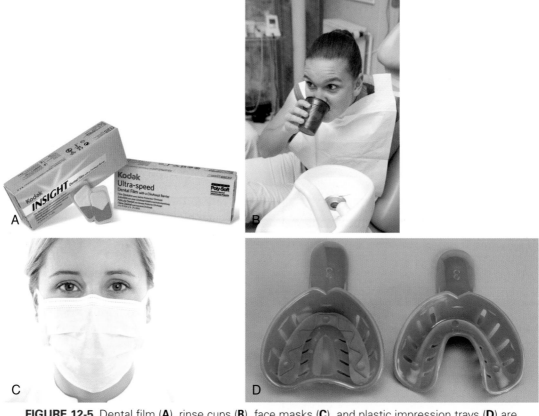

FIGURE 12-5 Dental film (**A**), rinse cups (**B**), face masks (**C**), and plastic impression trays (**D**) are all examples of consumable supplies. (**A,** Courtesy Carestream Health, Rochester, NY. **B,** Copyright © 2013 PeterTG, iStock.com. **C,** Copyright © 2009 AngiePhotos, iStock.com. **D,** Boyd LRB: *Dental instruments: a pocket guide*, ed 5, St Louis, 2015, Elsevier.)

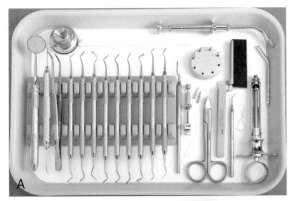

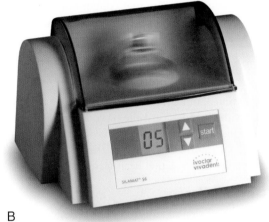

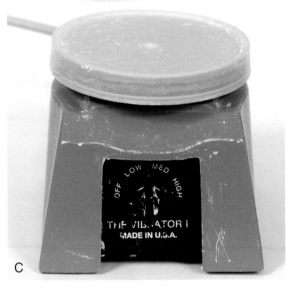

FIGURE 12-6 Dental instruments (**A**), an amalgamator (**B**), and a vibrator for the dental laboratory (**C**) are all examples of nonconsumable supplies. (**A** and **C**, Boyd LRB: *Dental instruments: a pocket guide*, ed 5, St Louis, 2015, Elsevier. **B**, Courtesy Ivoclar Vivadent, Inc., Amherst, NY.)

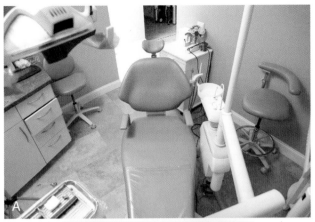

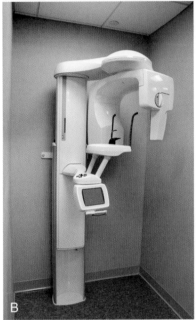

FIGURE 12-7 The dental chair and treatment room furniture (**A**) and all dental imaging units (**B**) are examples of major equipment. (**A**, Copyright © 2014 IPGGutenbergUKLtd, iStock. com. **B**, Copyright © 2008 lutherhill, iStock.com.)

SELECTING AND ORDERING SUPPLIES, PRODUCTS, AND EQUIPMENT

Selecting Supplies and Products

Supplies and *products* are terms that are sometimes interchangeable. For the purpose of this discussion, **supplies** are defined as consumable goods that are used in support of dental treatment. Examples include infection control supplies, paper towels, 2 × 2 gauze, disposable suction tips, mixing sticks, and business office supplies. **Products** are defined as materials used in direct patient care. They include dental materials and dental therapeutics.

The first step in the ordering process is to decide which supplies and products will be used. Some supplies are generic and do not require research before their purchase. Other products, such as restorative materials, require that the dental healthcare team research them before a decision is made as to which ones to use.

By attending trade shows and dental conventions, members of the dental healthcare team are able to speak with several different vendors. Each manufacturer has representatives available to answer questions and to demonstrate the correct application and use of products.

Networking is one of the most valuable sources of information. Information can be exchanged through study clubs, membership in professional organizations, and continuing education programs. These organizations help members of the dental healthcare team to reach their own conclusions by providing a wide range of opinions and shared experiences.

Manufacturers and vendors of dental products send representatives (detail persons) into the field (individual dental practices) to introduce new products. During their visit to the dental practice, they explain the intended usage, instruct the dental healthcare team, and answer questions about the products they represent.

COMMON TERMS ASSOCIATED WITH ORDERING SUPPLIES AND PRODUCTS

Manufacturer: Company that produces goods.

Vendor: Company that sells goods.

Consumer: Company or person who uses goods.

ADA approved: Products that have been tested and meet the standards of the American Dental Association (ADA Seal).

Dental supply house: Company that sells several different manufacturers' goods (supplies, products, and equipment).

Brand name: Manufactured supplies and products that are identified by a specific given name (registered trademark).

Generic name: Name of a product that is based on its composition—not the brand name. For example, *aspirin* is the generic name of a drug—not the brand name.

Dental salesperson: A representative for a dental supply house who visits dental practices for the purpose of selling supplies and products (also known as a "sales rep").

Direct sales: A process of ordering supplies by going directly to the manufacturer or by going to an online distributer (such as Amazon).

Purchasing Major Equipment

The purchasing of major equipment is time consuming and involves large sums of money. The cost of a dental chair ranges from $5000 to $20,000. When new equipment is needed, several factors must be considered:

- What is the budget (how much can be spent)?
- What features must be present (what is the minimal function)?
- What features would be advantageous (would like to have but are not necessary)?
- What features should not be included (would not consider even if they were free)?

The dentist and other team members should attend trade shows or dental conventions, where they can meet with several different manufacturers with samples of their equipment. Once a decision on the manufacturer is made, it may be necessary to shop for the best price and service.

Manufacturers usually do not sell directly to individual dental practices. Instead, equipment must be purchased through a supply house. This is similar to purchasing a new automobile. After you decide on the make and model of the automobile, you must purchase it through an authorized dealer. The price of the automobile will be competitive and you must decide which dealer will give you the best price and service.

Once major equipment has been purchased and installed, a file must be set up that contains all vital information about the equipment. This information includes equipment name and manufacturer, owner's manuals, maintenance schedules, serial and model numbers, date and price of purchase, and telephone numbers for technical assistance.

Information about equipment can be organized for quick reference with an index card file, Rolodex, or computerized database. This information is needed when someone calls for service and technical assistance and should be easy to access by any member of the dental healthcare team.

Selecting the Vendor

Several different dental supply houses are generally available. Small local supply houses are tailored to the individual needs of their clients and are personally involved in local community projects (somewhat like an extended family). Other types of supply houses include regional, national, and international organizations. Each type has its advantages and disadvantages. The choice may be determined by the individual needs of each dental practice. It is not necessary to purchase all of your supplies and products from the same dental supplier. Individual suppliers may not provide all of the products you use or may not offer the best price.

Supplies can be ordered through a sales representative from the supply house or by placing orders through a catalog service. The method of ordering will be determined by the dental practice and both systems have advantages and disadvantages. Most often, it is best to use more than one type of supply house.

CATALOG ORDERING

Advantages	Disadvantages
Lower prices	Very little personal service
Large selection	Limited technical support
Easy to compare several products while browsing through the catalog	Takes time to complete order forms
Direct online computer service	Returns require packaging and reshipping

SUPPLY HOUSE SERVICES

Advantages	Disadvantages
Personal service	Higher prices (although some are very competitive)
Technical support	Shipping can be slower
Share knowledge about specific products and feedback about what other offices are using (networking)	Selection of products is limited
Know your ordering pattern	No comparison shopping with catalogs
Know your preferences in supplies and products	
Advise on quantities to be ordered	

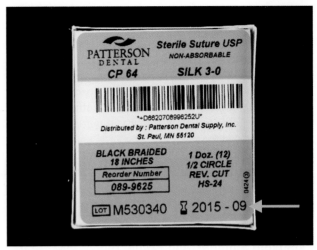

FIGURE 12-8 Certain products with limited shelf lives are marked with expiration dates (*arrow*). (Courtesy Patterson Dental, St. Paul, Minn.)

Dental supply houses that use sales representatives typically schedule their representatives to visit dental practices weekly or biweekly. The use of sales representatives can be advantageous, depending on the nature of the product. When representatives visit the office, they provide more than an opportunity to place an order. They also provide valuable information concerning new products and specials they are running and they can help to determine the quantity of items you need to purchase. The type of service required by the dental practice varies from office to office.

Similar to retail services, dental services may be provided in varying degrees. Depending on the type of service, the products needed, and the budget constraints, each service has advantages and disadvantages. Therefore it is up to each dental practice to decide on the type of service needed, to consider the costs of products, and to determine the amount of time it is willing or able to spend on ordering supplies and products.

Information to Consider Before Placing an Order

Before placing an order for supplies and products, you must consider several factors. Following is a list of questions that should be answered before orders are placed.

1. *What is the shelf life of the product?* The shelf life is the length of time that a product will continue to meet the manufacturer's specifications for use. After a certain amount of time, x-ray film will become foggy and will not produce diagnostically clear radiographs, anesthetic will not be as effective, and chemical compositions will change. Products that have a shelf life will have an expiration date printed on the box or container (Figure 12-8). The length of time before a product expires varies from product to product. When ordering, you should know the expected shelf life and not order more than can be used in the prescribed time. Caution should be exercised when ordering specials on products that are known to have a shelf life. Companies will place products on sale because they want to sell them before the expiration date. This type of sale is an advantage to the dental practice only if all of the product can be used before the expiration date is reached.

2. *What are the storage requirements?* The amount of available storage space is also a factor to consider when one is determining the quantity of a product to be ordered. If space is limited, it is not advisable to order large quantities. Health and safety codes may dictate where supplies can be stored safely. It is not safe to store combustible materials close to a heat source or in an area that can become very warm. Additionally, some products have very specific storage requirements, such as cool dry places, refrigerators, or dark areas.

3. *Will technology change before the product is used?* Because of rapid changes in research and technology, it is best not to order large quantities of products that are constantly being changed and updated.

4. *Has the product been tried and tested in the office?* Many products remain on the shelf because the dentist and staff did not research the product sufficiently. It is sometimes difficult to use new products because they require training in their proper manipulation and application. In most cases, it is awkward to change from one product to another. If a change is going to be successful, the dental healthcare team must be patient and expect that it will take time to learn to use the new product efficiently.

5. *Will information provided in printed material change before a new order can be used up?* When ordering stationery and other printed forms, make sure that no changes in the information printed will occur before a new order is placed.

6. *What is the return policy?* When trying new products, check with the dental representative to clarify your options if the product fails to live up to its claims or if the dentist decides that it is not in the patients' best interests to use the product. Some companies provide sample kits that contain a few applications of a product so that the

dentist can try the material before purchasing a larger amount. Other companies will trade the product for a different one if it does not meet the needs and expectations of the dentist.

7. *Is it economically advisable to invest in a large-quantity order?* Before expending money for a year's supply of something, check other options. Is a sufficient amount of money going to be saved that will not be better spent elsewhere?

> **❗ REMEMBER**
>
> All products used in direct patient care should meet the standards established by the American Dental Association.

Receiving Supplies and Products

After you have received supplies and products, the next step is to verify your order. Included with all orders are packing slips. These slips are used by the vendor to verify that the goods you ordered have been packaged (Figure 12-9). It is not uncommon to receive more than one box or package. If you have placed a large order, the goods will arrive in several boxes. Usually the labels on the boxes indicate the total number of boxes shipped and the individual number of the box. For example, you have placed a large order and the shipping company delivers four boxes. When you check the labels, you notice that they indicate that a total of five boxes were shipped. To help determine which box you are missing, check each of

the labels for the box number. For example, after checking labels, you can account for box 1 of 5, box 3 of 5, box 4 of 5, and box 5 of 5. You can then assume that box 2 is missing.

Most shipping companies have very sophisticated methods of tracking their shipments. They can tell you what time the box left the warehouse, was loaded on a plane or truck, and was delivered. Because of their tracking systems, they will be able to locate your missing box and give you an estimated time of arrival.

PROCEDURES

Steps in Accepting Shipments

1. Sign for the shipment.
2. Check for the correct number of boxes or items shipped.
3. Inventory the contents of each box and verify them with the shipping invoice.
4. Check the invoice against your original order.
5. File the shipping invoice, which will be used to verify the billing statement.
6. Record any backordered supplies.
7. File any new Occupational Safety and Health Administration (OSHA) Safety Data Sheets (SDSs) that are needed.
8. Enter the quantities of the new supplies into the inventory control system via a data communications device (barcode) or manually enter the data into the inventory management system (IMS).
9. Place supplies in the appropriate storage areas.

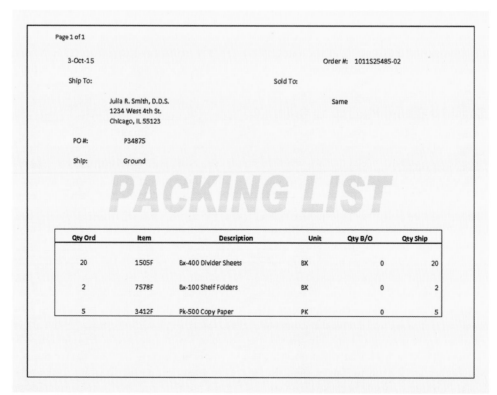

FIGURE 12-9 Each product order is accompanied by a packing list so that the office staff can verify the contents and quantities in the order.

Storage Areas

Areas where supplies and products will be stored are determined by several factors. The chemical composition of certain products will determine what type of storage environment they require. Accessibility is also important: How often is the product used? Is it stored near the area where it will be used? Can it be safely removed from the area (considering its weight and height)? These are all factors that must be considered before supplies and products are stored.

Another consideration is how easily a supply or product can be located. If supplies are not stored in a common area, a method of locating the supply must be established. To assist in the location of supplies, a master list is established. The list can be organized alphabetically or divided into broad categories. Once the desired supply is located on the list, directions to where it is stored can be followed. With this type of organization, all storage areas can be easily accessed by any member of the dental healthcare team.

When a large storage room is used, shelves should be marked and supplies arranged in a way that can be understood easily by all members of the dental healthcare team (Figure 12-10). If the room is large and the design does not allow for categorizing supplies, a master list should be posted that states what supplies are located in the storage area and where they are located.

> **! REMEMBER**
>
> Make sure that storage areas comply with Occupational Safety and Health Administration (OSHA) regulations.

OCCUPATIONAL SAFETY AND HEALTH ADMINISTRATION (OSHA)

It is the responsibility of the employer to instruct each and every employee about all areas of safety. The Occupational Safety and Health Administration (OSHA) mandates that a protocol be established that alerts employees to health hazards and instructs them about the proper ways to perform their assigned duties safely. A written hazard communication program must be maintained by the employer and annual training sessions should be held. Each employee must know the following:

- Which chemicals are hazardous
- What risk is involved when working with specific chemicals
- How to use the chemicals safely to minimize exposure
- How to handle the chemicals safely after an accident
- Where to find information about hazards (Safety Data Sheets)

For employees to gain this knowledge, they must be given product information. This information is communicated in the form of a Safety Data Sheet (SDS). The SDS is made available to the employer by the manufacturer of the product and is usually sent with the product when it is delivered. SDSs should be maintained in a notebook or in an electronic format that can be easily accessed by all employees. In addition, all product containers should be labeled with the proper warnings and information. It is the responsibility of the inventory manager to forward SDSs to the proper location when products are received. The complete hazard communication program for each dental practice will outline the established protocol, which must be followed by each employee.

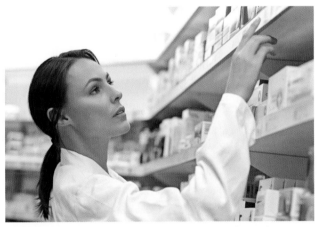

FIGURE 12-10 A central shelving location allows for proper ordering and easy location of supplies. (Copyright © 2015 Yuri_Arcurs, iStock.com.)

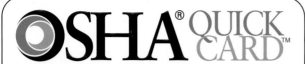

Hazard Communication
Safety Data Sheets

The Hazard Communication Standard (HCS) requires chemical manufacturers, distributors, or importers to provide Safety Data Sheets (SDSs) (formerly known as Material Safety Data Sheets or MSDSs) to communicate the hazards of hazardous chemical products. As of June 1, 2015, the HCS will require new SDSs to be in a uniform format, and include the section numbers, the headings, and associated information under the headings below:

Section 1, Identification includes product identifier; manufacturer or distributor name, address, phone number; emergency phone number; recommended use; restrictions on use.

Section 2, Hazard(s) identification includes all hazards regarding the chemical; required label elements.

Section 3, Composition/information on ingredients includes information on chemical ingredients; trade secret claims.

Section 4, First-aid measures includes important symptoms/effects, acute, delayed; required treatment.

Section 5, Fire-fighting measures lists suitable extinguishing techniques, equipment; chemical hazards from fire.

Section 6, Accidental release measures lists emergency procedures; protective equipment; proper methods of containment and cleanup.

Section 7, Handling and storage lists precautions for safe handling and storage, including incompatibilities.

(Continued on other side)

For more information:

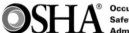
**Occupational
Safety and Health
Administration**
U.S Department of Labor
www.osha.gov (800) 321-OSHA (6742)

OSHA 3493-02 2012

Hazard Communication
Safety Data Sheets

Section 8, Exposure controls/personal protection lists OSHA's Permissible Exposure Limits (PELs); Threshold Limit Values (TLVs); appropriate engineering controls; personal protective equipment (PPE).

Section 9, Physical and chemical properties lists the chemical's characteristics.

Section 10, Stability and reactivity lists chemical stability and possibility of hazardous reactions.

Section 11, Toxicological information includes routes of exposure; related symptoms, acute and chronic effects; numerical measures of toxicity.

Section 12, Ecological information*

Section 13, Disposal considerations*

Section 14, Transport information*

Section 15, Regulatory information*

Section 16, Other information, includes the date of preparation or last revision.

*Note: Since other Agencies regulate this information, OSHA will not be enforcing Sections 12 through 15 (29 CFR 1910.1200(g)(2)).

Employers must ensure that SDSs are readily accessible to employees.
See Appendix D of 29 CFR 1910.1200 for a detailed description of SDS contents.

For more information:

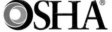
**Occupational
Safety and Health
Administration**
U.S Department of Labor
www.osha.gov (800) 321-OSHA (6742)

OSHA 3493-02 2012

OSHA Quick Card™ for Hazard Communication Safety Data Sheets. (From Occupational Safety and Health Administration, U.S. Department of Labor, www.osha.gov.)

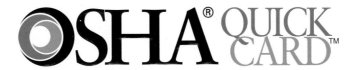

Hazard Communication Standard Labels

OSHA has updated the requirements for labeling of hazardous chemicals under its Hazard Communication Standard (HCS). As of June 1, 2015, all labels will be required to have pictograms, a signal word, hazard and precautionary statements, the product identifier, and supplier identification. A sample revised HCS label, identifying the required label elements, is shown below. Supplemental information can also be provided on the label as needed.

For more information:

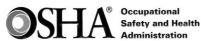

Occupational Safety and Health Administration

(800) 321-OSHA (6742)
www.osha.gov

SAMPLE LABEL

CODE_____
Product Name_____
} **Product Identifier**

Company Name_____
Street Address_____
City_____State_____
Postal Code_____Country_____
Emergency Phone Number_____
} **Supplier Identification**

Hazard Pictograms

Signal Word
Danger

Keep container tightly closed. Store in a cool, well-ventilated place that is locked.
Keep away from heat/sparks/open flame. No smoking.
Only use non-sparking tools.
Use explosion-proof electrical equipment.
Take precautionary measures against static discharge.
Ground and bond container and receiving equipment.
Do not breathe vapors.
Wear protective gloves.
Do not eat, drink or smoke when using this product.
Wash hands thoroughly after handling.
Dispose of in accordance with local, regional, national, international regulations as specified.

In case of Fire: use dry chemical (BC) or Carbon Dioxide (CO_2) fire extinguisher to extinguish.

First Aid
If exposed call Poison Center.
If on skin (or hair): Take off immediately any contaminated clothing. Rinse skin with water.

Precautionary Statements

Highly flammable liquid and vapor.
May cause liver and kidney damage.
} **Hazard Statements**

Supplemental Information

Directions for Use
_____
_____

Fill weight:_____ Lot Number:_____
Gross weight:_____ Fill Date:_____
Expiration Date:_____

OSHA 3492-02 2012

OSHA Quick Card™ for Hazard Communication Standard Labels. (From Occupational Safety and Health Administration, U.S. Department of Labor, www.osha.gov.)

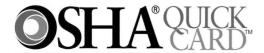

Hazard Communication Standard Pictogram

As of June 1, 2015, the Hazard Communication Standard (HCS) will require pictograms on labels to alert users of the chemical hazards to which they may be exposed. Each pictogram consists of a symbol on a white background framed within a red border and represents a distinct hazard(s). The pictogram on the label is determined by the chemical hazard classification.

HCS Pictograms and Hazards

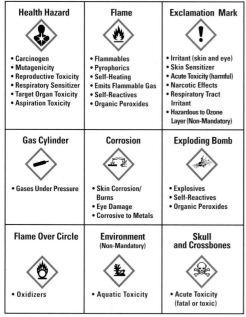

Health Hazard	Flame	Exclamation Mark
• Carcinogen • Mutagenicity • Reproductive Toxicity • Respiratory Sensitizer • Target Organ Toxicity • Aspiration Toxicity	• Flammables • Pyrophorics • Self-Heating • Emits Flammable Gas • Self-Reactives • Organic Peroxides	• Irritant (skin and eye) • Skin Sensitizer • Acute Toxicity (harmful) • Narcotic Effects • Respiratory Tract Irritant • Hazardous to Ozone Layer (Non-Mandatory)
Gas Cylinder	Corrosion	Exploding Bomb
• Gases Under Pressure	• Skin Corrosion/ Burns • Eye Damage • Corrosive to Metals	• Explosives • Self-Reactives • Organic Peroxides
Flame Over Circle	Environment (Non-Mandatory)	Skull and Crossbones
• Oxidizers	• Aquatic Toxicity	• Acute Toxicity (fatal or toxic)

For more information:

OSHA Occupational Safety and Health Administration
U.S. Department of Labor
www.osha.gov (800) 321-OSHA (6742)

OSHA 3491-02 2012

OSHA Quick Card™ for Hazard Communication Standard Pictogram. (From Occupational Safety and Health Administration, U.S. Department of Labor, www.osha.gov.)

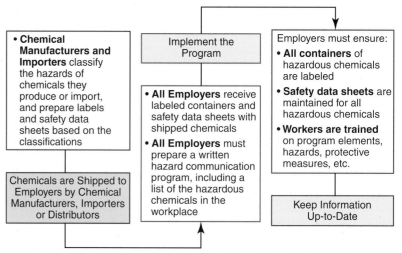

How hazard communication works. (From Occupational Safety and Health Administration, U.S. Department of Labor, www.osha.gov.)

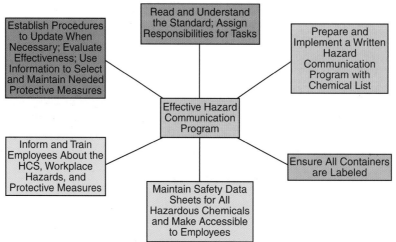

An effective hazard communication program (HCS). (From Occupational Safety and Health Administration, U.S. Department of Labor, www.osha.gov.)

KEY POINTS

- Ordering and managing supplies for the laboratory, business, and clinical areas in a dental practice requires organization, communication, and the cooperation of the entire dental healthcare team.
- Inventory management systems can be computerized or manual. Inventory systems use a variety of methods to identify when a product or supply needs to be ordered, who will place the order, and which vendor will fill the order.
- Elements of a good inventory management system include the following:
  - A qualified inventory manager
  - Identification of the supplies and products used in the dental practice
  - Proper storage
  - A master list of all supplies and products that provides their locations
  - Easy access to storage areas with clearly marked shelves
  - A clearly defined protocol for ordering
- Inventory includes supplies, products, and equipment. These items are purchased from vendors. The types of

vendors and delivery methods used will vary depending on the needs of the dental practice.
- All employers must prepare and implement a written hazard communication program that meets the following standards.
  - Provides a list of the hazardous chemicals in the workplace
  - Keeps labels on shipped containers and labels workplace containers where required
  - Provides easy access to Safety Data Sheets for all hazardous materials
  - Trains employees on the hazardous chemicals in their work area and when new hazards are introduced. Includes the requirements of the standard, hazards associated with chemicals used, appropriate protective measures, and where and how to obtain additional information.
  - Reviews the hazard communication program periodically to ensure that it is still working and meeting its objectives.

CAREER-READY PRACTICES

Career-Ready Practices activities are designed to provide students with experiences that can be "practiced" in preparation for skills needed on the job. In each of the following exercises, a variety of approaches may be used to address the problem, rather than "right" or "wrong" answers. Below each exercise, next to the compass icon, is a listing of suggested Career-Ready Practice numbers that correspond to the listing of 12 practices in the front of the text (see p. viii-ix); these practices provide suggestions for approaches to complete the exercise.

1. As the inventory manager, you have been given the task of researching a new IMS. Prepare a report that compares two or more systems. Identify the different elements of each system and make a recommendation based on your research.

 Career-Ready Practices

   7 *Employ valid and reliable research strategies.*
   4 *Communicate clearly, effectively, and with reason.*
   8 *Utilize critical thinking to make sense of problems and persevere in solving them.*

2. A sales representative informs you that his or her company is running a special on x-ray film. The film will be discounted 25% when you order 10 or more boxes. The current price of the film is $51 per box. You check your database and find that you currently have 8 boxes of film in stock. After reviewing your order history, you find that the office uses 3.5 boxes of film per month. You question the reason for the discount and the sales representative informs you that the expiration date on the film is 1 year from now.
   - What is the price for 12 boxes of film?
   - How long will it take to use the film you have in stock?
   - How many boxes of film are used in 1 year?
   - Should you take advantage of the sale?
   - If yes, how many boxes of film should you order?
   - What will be the total cost of your order?

 Career-Ready Practices

   2 *Apply appropriate academic and technical skills.*
   8 *Utilize critical thinking to make sense of problems and persevere in solving them.*
   5 *Consider the environmental, social, and economic impacts of decisions.*

13

Office Equipment

1. List the components of a dental practice information system and explain the function of each component.
2. Describe the features and functions of a telecommunication system and explain how they can be used in a modern dental practice.
3. Compare electronic and manual systems of intraoffice communications.
4. Identify office machines commonly found in a dental practice.
5. Describe an ideal business office environment and design an ergonomic workstation. Identify important elements and state their purpose.

INTRODUCTION

Business office equipment provides the tools and resources necessary to organize tasks and integrate many different functions into a seamless flow. A computer can perform many tasks using information that is maintained in a database with speed and accuracy. A telephone system integrated with a practice management software system can identify the patient and upload his or her information before the phone is answered. Cloud computing connects many devices together, from anywhere that there are Internet connections. Business office equipment is selected according to the needs of the staff and the dental practice. Equipment can be divided into two broad categories: equipment used to gather, transfer, and store information and equipment used to create a working environment that is safe, organized, and functional.

ELECTRONIC BUSINESS EQUIPMENT

The primary functions of the dental business office are collection, transmission, management, and storage of information. In a manual dental practice, the collection and processing of information require a variety of manual skills and tasks. Most dental practices in the twenty-first century gather similar information, which is then organized, processed, and stored with electronic technology supported by a computerized information system. An **information system** is a combination of equipment (hardware), **software**, data, personnel, and procedures for processing information. The functions of a computerized system are discussed in Chapter 7.

Hardware

Computer **hardware** is the physical part of the computer system. The hardware in a simple computer system includes the **central processing unit (CPU),** monitor, keyboard,

COMPONENTS OF AN INFORMATION SYSTEM

- Hardware
- Software
- Data
- Personnel
- Procedures

mouse, and printer (Figure 13-1). Additional hardware may include peripheral modems or routers; additional ports, such as a USB port for input and output; and scanners.

Central Processing Unit

The CPU is the main operating component of the hardware, or the brains of the computer. After data are entered through

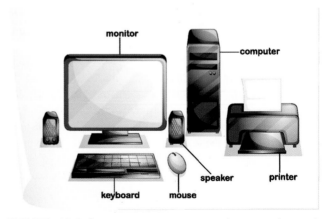

FIGURE 13-1 Computer system: central processing unit (CPU), monitor, keyboard, mouse, speakers, and printer. (Copyright © 2013 colematt, iStock.com. All rights reserved.)

an input device, the CPU processes the data and stores the information. When a command is given, the information can be transferred via an output device and transferred over a network or sent to a printer.

Common Input Devices

Input devices are peripheral pieces of hardware that transfer data into a computer system. Common input devices include the keyboard and the mouse. The keyboard, which is the most common type of input device, is similar in configuration to a typewriter. In addition, the keyboard may have a variety of function keys. These function keys are located at the top of the keyboard and are used to activate various functions of software applications. On the right side of many keyboards is a number pad that is configured in the same manner as a calculator. The number pad facilitates quick entry of numeric information. Directional arrows (right, left, up, or down) may also be located on the keyboard to permit scrolling (moving through information on the screen). In addition to the keyboard commands, a mouse can be used to activate commands. The mouse comes in a variety of styles.

Data can be transferred into the computer through a direct cable that connects one device to the other, such as a USB cable. These cables can be used to connect printers, download images from a camera or scanner, or update mobile devices. In addition, it is possible to connect devices to the computer via a wireless system.

Types of input devices found in a dental practice include the following:
- Audio conversation devices
- Barcode readers
- Biometrics (fingerprint scanners)
- Digital imaging (x-ray, cameras)
- Fingers (touchscreens)
- Graphic tablets
- Keyboard
- Microphone
- Mouse, touchpad, or other pointing device
- Optical Mark Reader (OMR)
- Pen or stylus
- Remote
- Scanners
- Tablets
- Video capture devices
- Webcam

Newer input devices include touchscreens (monitors) that are activated when the operator touches the screen. Tablets are portable computers that can be used by patients to enter data directly into the dental practice software system (Figure 13-2). Some systems are designed to receive data via voice command. The computer learns commands and activates functions when the voice message is received. Voice commands are hands free; this technology is extremely valuable when used in the clinical area. The type of input device can vary widely from office to office and is dependent on the type of equipment and technology being used.

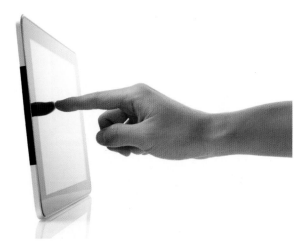

FIGURE 13-2 Virtual keyboard.

Common Output Devices

Several output devices are common to most computer systems: monitors, printers, and storage devices. These devices are used to transfer data out of the computer.

Monitors are designed for viewing information. A monitor is similar to a television screen. The sizes and shapes of monitors, as well as their resolutions, vary. High-quality monitors have a high level of color resolution (clear, bright picture). With special software, monitor screens can be activated by touch with a finger or a special wand. Touchscreens enable the monitor to act as an input device and an output device.

A printer is used to produce a hard copy of information stored in the CPU. In a dental practice, a printer is used to print reports, letters, and forms (insurance and statements).

Printers produce black ink and color printouts. Ink jet and laser printers are the most common types of printers. They use plain paper, produce a document of high visual quality, and can accommodate different sizes and weights of paper. The same printer can be used for insurance claims, billing statements, business letters, envelopes, and recall cards. All-in-one printers combine four additional functions in one machine. These units are printers, scanners, copiers, and fax machines and connect to the intranet, serving as both an input device and an output device (Figure 13-3).

Flash drives, also known as jump drives, thumb drives, pen drives, and USB keychain drives, are small data storage devices that can hold a few megabytes of data to several gigabytes of information (Figure 13-4, *A*). The purpose of these devices is to transfer data from one location to another. External hard drives hold more data and can be used as a means to back up information (Figure 13-4, *B*).

Software
Computer Networks

In the modern dental office there will be more than one computer terminal. To operate several computers at the same time and to share information, it is necessary to connect these workstations through a network. A computer network is a

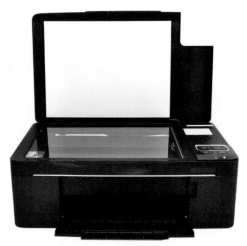

FIGURE 13-3 All-in-one printer, scanner, copier, and fax machine. (Copyright © 2012 vetkit, iStock.com. All rights reserved.)

system that allows computers to exchange information and data. Computer networks support applications such as practice management software, digital imaging, telecommunications, and access to the Internet. The network can be contained within the dental practice on a local area network (LAN) or may be part of a much larger network. The network can be connected by a wired system or a wireless system.

Servers

A network server is a computer that is used to store data. These servers can be located on the LAN or remote network servers can host them. Practice management software suites offer many electronic services, such as patient communications, web hosting, telecommunications, electronic insurance processing, electronic patient billing, integrated credit and debit card processing, accounting service, and more. All of these services require the use of shared data. The term *Cloud computing* is used to describe services that are hosted on a collection of servers (Figure 13-5). The Cloud provides the ability to access data and information from any device from any location that is connected to the Internet. The Cloud also serves as the backup for offsite storage of important data and information.

✚ HIPAA

Network and Data Storage

All networks and data storage (local, remote and cloud) must be secure and adhere to all federal regulations (Health Insurance Portability and Accountability Act of 1996 [HIPAA] and Health Information Technology for Economic and Clinical Health [HITECH] Act).

Operating System Software

Programs that allow the user to perform specialized tasks on the computer are called software. Operating system (OS) software provides the information needed for the computer

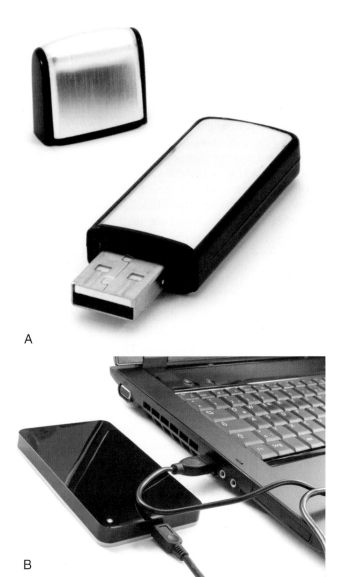

A

B

FIGURE 13-4 Flash (or jump) drives **(A)** and external hard drives **(B)** are both used to transfer moderate to large amounts of data from one location to another. **(A,** Copyright © 2007 AWSeebaran, iStock.com. All rights reserved. **B.** Copyright © 2010 IngaNielsen, iStock.com. All rights reserved.)

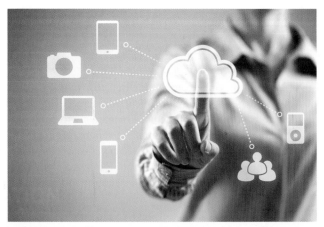

FIGURE 13-5 Cloud computing. (Copyright © 2015 Petar Chernaev, iStock.com. All rights reserved.)

to be able to function at any level and to run other programs or applications. The type of hardware and the function of the unit will determine the type of OS. Multiuser OSs allow multiple users to use the same computer at the same time and at different times. Multiprocessing OSs are capable of supporting and using more than one computer processer. Multitasking OSs allow multiple software processes to run at the same time. Multithreading OSs allow different parts of a software program to run concurrently.

Application Software

Application software is designed for specific tasks. Application software tasks include word processing, spreadsheets, databases, and graphics. Dental practice management software packages are combinations of application software and are designed to perform specific dental-related procedures (see Chapter 7 for more detailed information on dental-related procedures performed with a computer).

Data

Data are pieces of information. Both manual and computerized systems use the same information. For example, when new patients arrive at the dental practice, they are asked to complete several forms. Patient financial information is used to establish an account and process insurance. Medical alerts are identified and noted on the patient's clinical record (paper and electronic). Clinical information is used to establish a treatment plan. The manner in which the information is processed, organized, transmitted, and stored varies greatly between manual and electronic systems. Throughout this text, you have learned different ways in which information can be processed in manual and electronic systems.

Personnel

The number of people who will operate the information system varies depending on the size of the dental practice and the type of computer system used. Personnel who enter data are responsible for the accurate transfer of information. In a dental practice, the administrative dental assistant performs most of the information processing. In a large dental practice, networked computers (computers that share programs and information) may require a network manager. The duties of the manager are to maintain the system and to provide support for those who operate the system.

Procedures

For optimal use of an information system, it is necessary for personnel to know how to operate the equipment and use the application software. This knowledge can be obtained in training sessions, from the vendor's technicians, and from the user's manual. Office procedural manuals should outline the procedures and functions that are unique to the dental practice.

TELECOMMUNICATION

Telecommunication is the use of equipment to transfer information or to communicate among people over a distance.

In a dental practice, telecommunication methods include the telephone system (analog and Voice over Internet Protocol [VoIP]), mobile communications such as smartphones, and intraoffice communications.

Telephone Systems

VoIP is the technology that is most commonly used for telephone systems in dental offices. VoIP uses the Internet to receive and transmit calls. The equipment used to transmit the digital signals is typically housed with the service provider and the dental practice connects to the service via a modem. The equipment seen in the dental office is very similar to a traditional telephone system. VoIP technology allows the use of many features that are part of the day-to-day operations of the business office, such as:

- Computer-to-computer communications
- Mobile communications
- Voice mail
- Multiline telephone systems
- Automatic outgoing telephone messaging (confirmation of dental appointments)
- Conference calling
- Video conferencing
- Call forwarding
- Caller ID

Business telephone systems can be designed and customized to meet the needs of the individual business (Figure 13-6). A typical dental practice will have a multiline service. This service allows the dental practice to receive several calls at the same time.

The most visible component of a telephone system is the telephone unit. Basic components include the base unit and the handset. Located on the base unit are the keys used to activate the various functions. The handset contains the receiver and the transmitter. On cordless telephones, the handset is not connected to the base unit and will contain the same keys and functions as the base unit. Telephone units can be desk mounted or wall mounted.

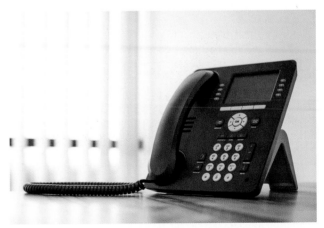

FIGURE 13-6 A multiline business telephone ensures that the dental office can receive several calls at the same time. (Copyright © 2014 Spiderstock, iStock.com. All rights reserved.)

Telephones are designed and programmed for several different tasks. A multiline telephone allows the user to access various lines simply by pressing a button. When a multiline telephone is used, it is very important to know how to answer, transfer, and place telephone calls (review the information in Chapter 3). The design of the system allows more than one call to be received or placed at the same time. In addition to multiple telephone lines, several telephone units can be placed conveniently throughout the dental practice.

COMPUTER TERMINOLOGY

Address: See URL.

Bit: A unit of information.

Bluetooth: This wireless technology enables communication between Bluetooth-compatible devices. It is used for short-range connections between desktop and laptop computers, digital cameras, scanners, cellular phones, mobile devices (smartphones, iPads, iTouch), and printers.

Browser: A program used to view hypertext (World Wide Web) pages, such as Internet Explorer or Firefox.

Byte: Small unit of storage; 8 bits; usually holds one character.

CD-ROM: Compact Disk Read-Only Memory storage medium that can hold 700 megabytes of information; usually used for large software programs. **CD-R** compact disk-recordable, **CD-RW** compact disk-rewritable.

Cloud computing: Term used to describe services over a network of servers (the Cloud) that enables the user to access programs and services from anywhere with Internet access.

CPU: Central processing unit; the brain of the computer; controls the other elements of the computer.

Database: A large, structured set of data; a file that contains numerous records with numerous fields.

Database management system: The software needed to establish and maintain the database and manage the stored information.

Domain name: The last component of a computer address; that is, com (commercial), edu (educational), gov (government).

Download: Transferring data from one computer to another.

EDI: Electronic Data Interchange; standardized method for transferring data between computer systems and networks.

E-mail: Electronic mail; messages passed from one computer to another over a network.

Export: To save information in a format that another program can read.

Field: One part of a record; several fields become a record; several records become a database.

File: An element of data storage; a single sequence of bytes.

Firewall: Software that prevents unauthorized persons from accessing certain parts of a program, database, or network.

Flash drives: Also known as jump drives, thumb drives, pen drives, and USB keychain drives; small data storage devices that can hold a few megabytes of data to several gigabytes of information. These devices have replaced other portable data storage mediums such as floppy disks and removable hard disks such as zip drives.

FTP: File transfer protocol; a protocol used to move software or data from one computer to another over a network.

Function key: Special key on the keyboard that is programmed to perform certain actions.

GUI: Graphical user interface; uses pictures and words to represent ideas.

Hard drive: A device (usually within the CPU) that reads and writes information.

Hardware: Physical parts of a computer; a fixed part of a computer.

HTML: HyperText Markup Language; the language used to write web pages.

HTTP: HyperText Transfer Protocol; this is the protocol used to transfer data over the World Wide Web. All website addresses begin with "http//".

HTTPS: HyperText Transport Protocol Secure; the same thing as HTTP but it uses a secure socket layer (SSL) for security purposes. Examples of sites that use HTTPS are banking and investment websites, e-commerce websites, and most websites that require a password and login.

Hypertext: Cross-reference or link; permits easy movement from one document to another.

Icon: A small picture used to represent a file or program in a GUI interface.

Import: To retrieve any text or other information created by one program and transfer it to another program.

Integrated software: Software that combines in one program a number of functions normally performed by separate programs.

Interface: The software that controls the interaction between the hardware and the user.

Internet: A network of computer networks encompassing the World Wide Web, FTP, Telnet, and many other protocols.

Intranet: A network, similar to the Internet, used within an organization with links to company information.

Keyboard: A hardware peripheral used to input data with the pressing of keys.

Kilobyte: 1024 bytes.

LAN: Local area network; a network of computers that are geographically close (e.g., in separate buildings) and can share information.

LCD: Liquid Crystal Display; LCDs are super-thin displays that are used in laptop computer screens and flat-panel monitors. Smaller LCDs are used in handheld TVs, personal data assistants (PDAs), and portable video game devices.

Listserv: An automatic mailing list; e-mail messages are automatically mailed to every subscriber.

Login: Procedure necessary to begin a computer session; usually requires an identification name or number and a password.

Megabyte: 1,048,576 bytes *or* 1024 kilobytes; enough storage to approximately equal a 600-page paperback book.

Modem: A hardware peripheral device used to connect one computer to another over a DSL or cable connection.

Monitor: A hardware device used to display information visually.

Mouse: A hardware peripheral device used to point to items on a monitor.

Network: A collection of computers that are connected.

Continued

COMPUTER TERMINOLOGY—cont'd

Network-enabled devices: A computer, server, router, printer, firewall, switch, input and output device, sensor, or hub that is connected to an Ethernet network or the Internet.

Operating system: The most basic level of software that interfaces with peripherals.

Password: A string of characters, usually chosen by the user, that must be entered before certain information can be accessed; provides a layer of security; often used to log in to a computer.

Peripheral: Any of a number of hardware devices connected to the CPU.

Protocol: A set of rules governing the transmission of data.

RAM: Random access memory; the type of storage that changes; when the computer is turned off, the RAM is erased.

Record: One part of a database; a collection of fields.

ROM: Read-only memory; the type of storage that cannot be changed, even when the computer is turned off.

Router: A networking device that forwards data packets between computer networks.

Server: A computer that delivers data to other computers linked on the same network.

Software: Instructions executed by a computer.

Spreadsheet: A program of rows and columns in which data can be manipulated.

Toolbar: A graphical representation of program activities; a row of icons used to perform tasks in a program.

Upload: To transfer information from a client computer to a host computer.

URL: Uniform resource locator; the address of a site on the World Wide Web; a standard way of locating objects on the Internet.

USB: Universal Serial Bus; the standard input and output port used to connect devices to computers.

VoIP: Voice over Internet Protocol; similar to a telephone connection over the Internet. The data are sent digitally, using the Internet Protocol (IP) instead of analog telephone lines. VoIP is also referred to as IP telephony, Internet telephony, and digital phone.

WAN: Wide area network; a network of computers that is geographically diverse (i.e., in different states or countries) and permits the sharing of information.

Wi-Fi: A wireless networking standard trademarked by the Wi-Fi Alliance. Wi-Fi allows computers and other devices to connect to wireless routers and therefore other systems on the network. If the router is connected to the Internet, devices connected to the wireless access point may also have Internet access.

Window: A screen in a software program that permits the user to view several programs at one time.

World Wide Web: A network of hypertext pages that is viewable by using browsers.

Features and Functions of Telephone Systems

- Answering machines and services automatically answer the telephone and deliver a message when an assistant is not available (during lunch hours or when the office is closed). Incoming callers are given information in the message. The system can be designed to be a message-only center or to accept incoming messages. The messages can be revived through a machine located in the dental office or through a service provider.

- Voice mail is a form of electronic message center. It is a method used to direct calls to individuals or departments. If the party is unavailable to answer the call, a message can be left in the voice mailbox. For example, a patient calls and has a question concerning insurance. The patient's call is forwarded to the insurance clerk. The insurance clerk has a message on her voice mail asking the patient to leave a message and saying that the call will be returned as soon as possible. Questions can be researched before the call is returned, which saves the insurance clerk and the patient time.

- A headset is a lightweight plastic earphone and microphone (Figure 13-7). When wearing a headset, the operator is able to move freely without the constraint of a handset. Headsets are attached to the base of the telephone with a long cord (typically 10 feet long); more advanced headsets are wireless. Having both hands free enables the operator to move to different locations, retrieve files, record information, use the computer, or make entries in the appointment book while talking on the telephone. An additional benefit is that the operator does not strain neck muscles by cradling the headset between the ear and the shoulder.

- Speaker phones can be used when a hands-free environment is needed or if a conference call is being conducted. During a conference call, a speaker phone is used so that everyone can hear and contribute to the conversation. Caution should be exercised if the conversation is confidential.

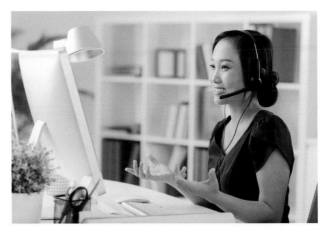

FIGURE 13-7 The headset allows the administrative dental assistant to move freely without the constraint of the phone cord. (Copyright © 2014 DragonImages, iStock.com. All rights reserved.)

- Speed dialing is a method of programming the telephone to dial telephone numbers automatically when a simple numeric code or telephone key is pressed. This feature is used to quickly access frequently called telephone numbers.
- Call forwarding allows the user to forward incoming telephone calls to another number or station.
- Intercom paging allows communication between different stations within the telephone system. For example, when the administrative dental assistant needs to speak to the assistant in the treatment area, the intercom is activated and communications are established.
- Call management is the feature of the telephone system that monitors and routes telephone calls. Incoming calls can be answered by a preprogrammed message that welcomes callers to the dental practice and gives them a selection of options. Callers can be transferred to different extensions or placed on hold to listen to music or recorded educational messages.
- Computer integration allows communication between a computer and a telephone. Telephone numbers can be dialed by computer automatically with the use of information in the computer database. The computer can initiate audio messages. These features can be part of an automated calling system to remind patients of appointments, overdue accounts, and so forth.
- Other individual features vary depending on the type of system and equipment used. These features include remote access to messages, programming features, security codes, voice mailboxes, and enhanced keypad functions.

Mobile Communication Devices

Mobile Telephones

Mobile phones, smartphones, or cellular telephones are wireless telephone systems that permit the receiving and sending of calls anywhere a signal can be received (Figure 13-8). Cellphones are extremely popular for both business and private use because they are small, can be carried easily in a pocket, and are always available. Smartphones are capable of functioning as a computer away from the office. These devices can

be used to access many functions of the dental practice such as e-mail, patient information, contact information, and mobile banking.

Fax Machines

Facsimile (fax) machines are used to transmit information quickly (Figure 13-9). A document can be sent and received in a matter of seconds over a telephone line and printed out. In a dental practice, a fax can be used to send patient information to insurance companies or to another professional. Care should be taken to ensure the confidentiality of the information being sent. If security cannot be confirmed, it is best to send confidential documents via regular mail.

A fax machine may use plain paper, produce color copies, double as a printer, or integrate with a computer system. Although the need to send documents via a fax has been drastically reduced by emerging technology, there still may be a need to use this type of technology occasionally.

INTRAOFFICE COMMUNICATIONS

Communication between members of the dental healthcare team is essential to the smooth operation of the practice. It is necessary for staff to send and receive messages during the day. For example, the administrative dental assistant may need to communicate with the clinical assistant when a patient arrives for treatment. Again, these communications can be manual, electronic, or a combination of the two.

Electronic Systems

Electronic communication systems include intraoffice memos in electronic form. Electronic memos are usually more secure than their paper counterparts because most computer systems require passwords before they can be accessed. Other forms of electronic communication systems are electronic schedulers, e-mail, text messaging, and intranets

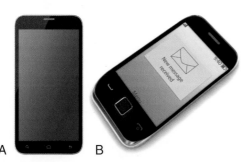

FIGURE 13-8 Mobile devices such as cellphones and various types of smartphones can be used to access many dental office functions, including e-mail, patient information, and mobile banking. (**A,** Copyright © 2014 alexsl, iStock.com. All rights reserved. **B,** Copyright © 2010 alexsl, iStock.com. All rights reserved.)

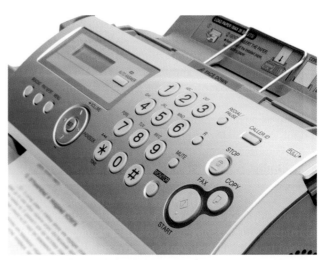

FIGURE 13-9 A facsimile (fax) machine is used to transmit information quickly, such as insurance claims information. (Copyright © 2010 wabeno, iStock.com. All rights reserved.)

(using instant messaging). Electronic schedulers provide a simple method of communication for the dental healthcare team. Members can tell, very quickly, where other members are and what they are doing. This enables someone to determine which of the other communication systems should be used to contact someone else. For example, if the hygienist is busy with a patient, the administrative dental assistant can use a system that provides one-way contact. However, if the hygienist is just in another part of the office, the administrative dental assistant can initiate two-way contact.

E-mail is becoming a more frequent tool for communicating internally, within the practice, and externally, with other companies or patients. E-mail is the most frequently used tool on the Internet because it provides a fast, simple form of communication from one person to another, who may or may not be at the computer when the message arrives. E-mail will sit in storage until the receiver is available. Intranets are becoming a more popular way to communicate information among entire staffs or companies. Intranets are similar to the Internet but are not accessible by people outside of an office. They provide a place for frequently needed information or for information needed by several people. Instead of sending everyone in the office a memo, users can place the memo on the intranet for everyone to view.

Unfortunately, no intraoffice communication system can work without the full support of all members of the team. If one person forgets to check his or her mailbox, voice mailbox, or e-mail or fails to respond to instant or text messaging, communication will not take place efficiently.

Manual Systems

Manual communication systems include intraoffice memos, voice mail, coded light systems (Figure 13-10), and intercoms. Paper intraoffice memos are a frequently used method of communication between departments. They enable team members who are not in the same place at the same time to communicate. Voice mail is another form of communication. It is often easier and faster to leave a voice mail message than to send a memo. Voice mail is also a more private method of conveying information. Coded light systems can be used to inform members of the team of basic information such as when a patient is ready for treatment or when additional help is needed. Complex communication cannot take place with coded lights. Intercoms provide an alternative form of communication whereby two-way conversations can take place. Remember to respect your patient's privacy. Intercoms should not be used to relay private information if someone else can overhear the conversation.

OFFICE MACHINES

Copiers can perform tasks of varying complexity depending on the model selected. A basic model is small enough to fit on a tabletop and can copy one document at a time in black ink. A more advanced copier can print multiple documents, collate and staple, print in color, and, in some cases, print directly from the computer, scan documents, and send documents via fax or e-mail.

Postage meters are used to weigh and calculate the correct postage for outgoing mail. These machines can process several pieces of mail quickly. Envelopes are run through the machine and the correct postage and a postmark are stamped on the envelope (Figure 13-11). Postage and postmarks can also be printed on labels and the labels applied to oversized envelopes and packages.

Credit card terminals are used to process credit card payments. A credit card is processed by being swiped through the terminal; information contained in the magnetic strip on the back of the credit card is read (Figure 13-12). The amount of the charge is keyed into the terminal's keypad and other information may be coded (according to the correct protocol). Data are electronically transmitted to the credit card company. After

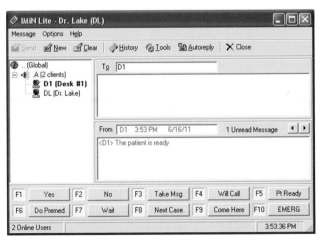

FIGURE 13-10 The DataMate IMiN Lite system is a type of instant messaging system that can be used by office staff members to communicate easily from various parts of the dental office. The IMiN screen here shows a message being transmitted from the business office to the treatment room. (IMiN screen capture courtesy JustWrks, Inc., www.justwrks.com.)

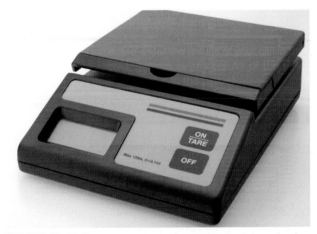

FIGURE 13-11 Postage meters are used to weigh and calculate postal charges for outgoing mail. (Copyright © 2008 didden, iStock.com. All rights reserved.)

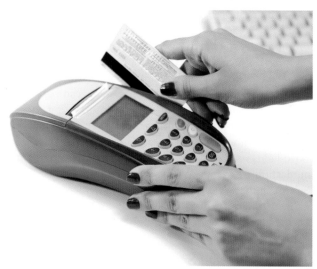

FIGURE 13-12 Credit card terminals are essential parts of the business aspect of a dental practice. They are used to capture and transmit credit card information for patients paying through this method. (Copyright © 2012 photobac, iStock .com. All rights reserved.)

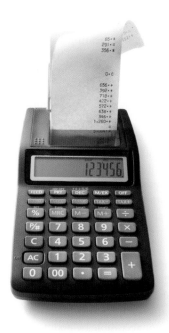

FIGURE 13-14 A printing calculator is useful in the dental office, as it is often larger than a standard version and provides a printout of all calculations. (Copyright © 2009 Floortje, iStock.com. All rights reserved.)

the company authorizes the transaction, a receipt is printed by the terminal and the money is deposited into the dental practice's account.

Electronic signature pads are devices that can be used to capture a patient's signature and transfer it to a computerized form (Figure 13-13). This is used in a paperless dental practice for forms and authorizations that require a signature.

Calculators used in a dental practice should be printing calculators (Figure 13-14). These are larger than nonprinting ones and they provide a printout of all calculations. This type of calculator has a keypad with numbers and function keys (for adding, subtracting, multiplying, and so forth).

BUSINESS OFFICE ENVIRONMENT

The dental practice environment should be organized, safe, and pleasant for those who work in the office and those who

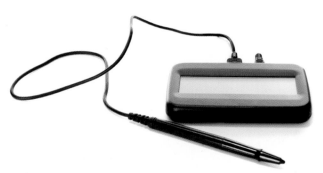

FIGURE 13-13 The electronic signature pad is becoming more common as part of the paperless dental office. It transmits a patient's signature electronically for forms and authorizations. (Copyright © 2013 McIninch, iStock.com. All rights reserved.)

patronize it. The organization of a dental practice business office is based on several factors, including the size of the business area, the number of rooms, the function of each area, the accessibility of the area by patients, the number of personnel working in the area, and the equipment used in the office.

Questions to Consider When Organizing a Business Office

How many workstations will be needed? It is necessary to know how many people are going to be working at one time. Workstations should be designed to accommodate the type of equipment (computer, telephone, and so forth) that will be housed there. For example, expanded counter space is needed when an appointment book is used instead of a computer scheduler. Assistants who complete forms and balance daysheets will need extra space to accommodate the size of these papers.

What type of equipment will be used? Types and specifications of equipment will determine how many electrical outlets and telephone lines are needed. Sizes and heights of counters should be configured to meet the specifications of the equipment.

What are the storage requirements? Storage equipment includes cabinets for supplies and filing cabinets for patient and business files. Workstations should include conveniently located drawers and cubicles for storage of items used often during the day.

What types of business office personnel will be hired? The types of business personnel (e.g., business manager, office manager, insurance clerk, bookkeeper, receptionist) to be

ANATOMY OF AN ERGONOMIC WORK STATION

WORKPLACE ENVIRONMENT
- Most important consideration is working comfortably and efficiently
- Sufficient desk area for keyboard, monitor, mouse, document holder, telephone, etc.
- Organize the area so that it reflects the way you use equipment
- Things you use most often should be within easiest reach
- Vary your tasks
- Take frequent breaks
- If area is shared, be sure all who use it can adjust everything to their needs
- Document holders same height and distance from monitor
- Adequate leg room
- Unobscured line of sight

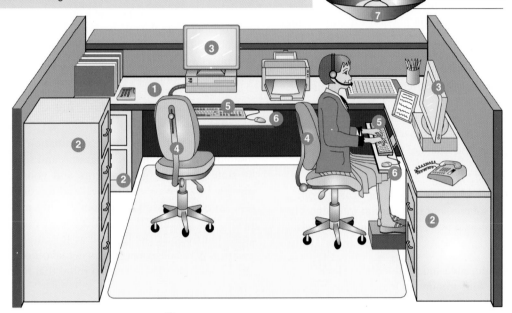

1 WORK SURFACE
- Proper height and angle
- Neutral postures
- Adjustable
- Standing—prevent slipping, adequate traction
- Sit/stand stools
- Anti-fatigue floor mats
- Darker, matte finishes are best

2 STORAGE AREAS
- Good body positions
- Reduce muscular forces
- Avoid excessive reach
- Heavy items between knee and shoulder height
- Frequently used storage closest to worker

3 VIDEO DISPLAY TERMINAL (VDT) [MONITOR]
- Position to minimize glare and reflections
- Top of screen is slightly below eye level
- Tilted slightly backward (less than 15 degrees)
- Distance from display 18-30 inches
- Perpendicular to windows
- Keep your head upright
- Set contrast and brightness
- Clean the screen (and your glasses)
- Anti-glare filters
- Adjustable monitor arm

4 CHAIRS
- Comfortable (padded seats that swivel)
- Back and seat are adjustable while seated
- Provide good back support (can add additional cushion if necessary)
- Adjustable arm support
- Back straight
- Knees slightly higher than chair bottom
- Thighs are horizontal
- Feet flat on the floor (use a footrest if necessary)
- Change positions occasionally

5 KEYBOARD
- Back should be lower than the front
- Rounded edges
- Wrist rests (sharp edges, neutral position) same height as front of keyboard
- Type properly; don't force your fingers to stretch to incorrect keystrokes

6 MOUSE
- Keep it on the same level as the keyboard or slightly above
- Keep wrist straight
- Do not stretch your arm; keep mouse within immediate reach
- Use the whole arm to move the mouse...not just the forearm

7 LIGHTING
- Less illumination for computer work
- Indirect lighting is best

AVOID THE FOLLOWING
Awkward posture
Can include reaching behind, twisting, working overhead, kneeling, bending and squatting. Deviation from ideal working posture can lead to fatigue, muscle tension and headaches. **Correct working posture**—arms at sides, elbows bent at approximately 90 degrees, forearms parallel to floor, wrists straight.

Repetitiveness
Judgment is based on frequency, speed, number of muscle groups used, required force. Not all people react to the same conditions, so carefully monitor your personal physical response to repetitiveness.

hired will determine the number of rooms or cubicles needed and the type of space they will require. Some areas will need to be more private than others.

Safety

The Occupational Safety and Health Administration (OSHA) is concerned with safety in the workplace. Safety concerns in a dental practice business office primarily involve equipment and ergonomics. Other considerations include background noise, lighting, temperature, and humidity.

Ergonomics

Ergonomics is the science of fitting the job to the worker. When the job does not match the physical capacity of the worker, work-related musculoskeletal disorders (WMSDs) can result. These injuries usually occur over a prolonged time. Research has revealed that all workers are at risk for WMSDs. In the business office, repeated movement (e.g., when one is using a computer keyboard or typewriter) may place the operator at risk for carpal tunnel syndrome. Placement of the keyboard, height of the chair, and other factors play an important role in the comfort and health of the operator.

Background Noise

In a dental practice, background noise can come from a number of different sources and may vary in intensity. The ambient sound level should not be higher than 55 decibels.

Lighting

It is crucial for a comfortable and productive workstation to have the correct type and amount of lighting. The optimal light level depends on the task at hand. The best level of illumination for people who use video display terminals (VDTs) as well as paper documents is 300 to 400 lux (30 to 40 foot-candles). If paper documents are not used, the level can be reduced to 200 lux.

To minimize screen glare, light from windows should be controlled by drapes, dark film, blinds, or louvers. Intense overhead lighting may also produce glare. In this case, louvers or screens for overhead lights may help. Filters for monitor screens may help to reduce reflections.

Temperature and Humidity

Most workers in an office environment find that they are comfortable when the relative humidity level is between 40% and 60%. Stable temperatures are important for computer systems as well as for people. Major temperature fluctuations can damage a computer.

The Americans with Disabilities Act

The Americans with Disabilities Act, signed into law on July 26, 1990, prohibits discrimination on the basis of disability in employment, programs, and services provided by state and local governments and goods and services provided by private companies, and in commercial facilities. Access to buildings and public offices must be easy and safe for all people. Dental offices must provide access for patients in wheelchairs as well as for employees with disabilities. When designing a new dental office or remodeling an old one, one should keep in mind that these regulations must be met.

▌KEY POINTS

- Office equipment helps the administrative dental assistant to organize tasks and saves time by integrating different types of procedures. Equipment can be divided into two broad categories: equipment used to gather, transfer, and store information and equipment used to create a work environment that is safe, organized, and functional.
- A computerized information system is a composite of equipment (hardware), software, data, personnel, and procedures for processing information.

- Telecommunication is the use of equipment to transfer information to or communicate with someone over a distance. In a dental practice, telecommunication includes the telephone system and intraoffice communications.
- The work environment should be organized, safe, and pleasant for those who work in the office and for those who patronize it.

▌CAREER-READY PRACTICES

Career-Ready Practices activities are designed to provide students with experiences that can be "practiced" in preparation for skills needed on the job. In each of the following exercises, a variety of approaches may be used to address the problem, rather than "right" or "wrong" answers. Below each exercise, next to the compass icon, is a listing of suggested Career-Ready Practice numbers that correspond to the listing of 12 practices in the front of the text (see p. viii-ix); these practices provide suggestions for approaches to complete the exercise.

1. At your last staff meeting the team decided it was time to look into a new telephone system and assigned you the task of researching different systems. Develop a set of questions you can use to guide your research.

 Career-Ready Practices
   11 *Use technology to enhance productivity.*
   5 *Consider the environmental, social, and economic impacts of decisions.*

7 *Employ valid and reliable research strategies.*

8 *Utilize critical thinking to make sense of problems and persevere in solving them.*

2. In a small group, compare your questions and decide on the set of questions that you will present to the team at your next staff meeting.

 Career-Ready Practices

4 *Communicate clearly, effectively, and with reason.*

2 *Apply appropriate academic and technical skills.*

12 *Work productively in teams while using cultural/global competence.*

PART IV

Managing Dental Office Finances

14 Financial Arrangement and Collection Procedures, 201

15 Dental Insurance Processing, 213

16 Bookkeeping Procedures: Accounts Payable, 235

17 Bookkeeping Procedures: Accounts Receivable, 258

Financial Arrangement and Collection Procedures

1. List the elements of a financial policy and discuss the qualifying factors for each of the elements.
2. Describe the different types of financial policies and explain how they can be applied in a dental practice and how they should be communicated to the patient.
3. State the purpose of managing accounts receivable, including:
   - Explain the role of the administrative dental assistant in managing accounts receivable

- Interpret aging reports
- Classify the five levels of the collection process
- Place a telephone collection call
- Process a collection letter
- Implement proper collection procedures

INTRODUCTION

The responsibility for collecting fees is shared by all members of the dental healthcare team. The team will establish the policies and then follow them. The administrative dental assistant has the most visible task (Figure 14-1). After a treatment plan has been drawn up, the administrative dental assistant will write the financial plan, present the plan to the patient, and then monitor compliance with the plan. If the plan is not followed, it is usually the administrative dental assistant who initiates collection procedures.

DESIGNING A FINANCIAL POLICY

Elements of a Financial Policy

- Community standards
- Practice philosophy
- Business principles

Community Standards

The community or area where the dental practice is located and the people served by the practice are factors in the financial policy. The policy in an affluent area will be different from that in an economically disadvantaged one. The types of dental insurance accepted are among the other factors considered in financial policy making. It is conceivable that practices that accept a variety of insurance plans and that treat people from different socioeconomic levels will have more than one payment plan option. These options are designed to meet the needs of the practice's patients while providing for the economic welfare of the employees and the dentist.

Practice Philosophy

The philosophy of the dental practice is described in its mission statement. The goals and objectives of the dental practice summarize the attitudes of the dentist and staff toward patient care and financial policy. This information is a component of the policy and procedure manual and is communicated to the patient in the dental practice's brochure.

Business Principles

A dental practice is a business and it must be run according to sound business principles. As a business, it is necessary to adhere to a strict business model and one of the most important business principles is the collection of fees for services. If these practices are not followed, the dental practice will soon be in deep financial trouble. A major roadblock to implementing sound practices is that those who work in the healthcare industry provide help to patients by being caring and understanding. Asking for money naturally makes us uncomfortable and healthcare workers are reluctant collectors. Many practices that tried to be a bank by financing dental treatment soon found that they were not good bankers. Accounts receivables were high and time was wasted in an effort to collect from patients. The patient also loses because he or she cannot come back to the office to continue treatment. An accountant or business manager can provide valuable financial information and can set guidelines that must be followed.

FINANCIAL POLICIES

The dental practice of the twenty-first century is faced with many challenges. Dentists must constantly strive to improve the quality of dental care, provide for their employees, and meet the expectations of their patients. For dentists to meet these challenges, they must be flexible in the types of financial plans they provide to their patients. They may need

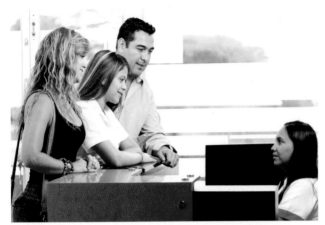

FIGURE 14-1 The administrative dental assistant has the most visible task in the fee collection process: asking the patient for payment. (Copyright © 2012 angelima, iStock .com. All rights reserved.)

to customize financial plans to meet the needs of each patient while practicing prudent business strategies.

Payment in Full

The payment in full policy requires that the patient pay in full after each visit. Payment may be given in the form of cash, check, or credit card. Payment in full plans are beneficial to the dental practice because they provide a constant cash flow. For this type of financial policy to be successful, you must follow several steps:

- Inform patients of the expected amount to pay in advance of treatment. Patients should always know the estimated fee for each dental visit. This information can be given when they call for their appointment or it can be outlined in the treatment plan.
- Be direct in asking for payment: "Ms. King, the fee for today's visit is $234.00."
- Know your patients: If they have insurance and according to their policy the insurance company should be billed first, ask for the patient's portion: "Ms. King, the fee for today is $234.00. I will bill your insurance company. According to our records, your company will pay 80% of the fee, leaving a balance of $46.80, which is due from you today."
- When patients are unprepared to pay, be prepared to offer alternatives such as the use of a credit card or apply for a third-party payment plan. When all else fails, give them a walkout statement (itemized list of charges) and a return envelope and instruct them to send the payment as soon as possible.
- Offer cash discounts to patients who pay for a treatment plan in advance of the treatment. This policy is attractive to those who view the discount (5% or less) as a savings.

Insurance Billing

Insurance billing plans are considered types of payment plans that have established policies that must be followed.

Some dental practices will bill the insurance company first and then bill the patient for the balance. Again, it is very important that patients understand the process and that they are made aware of the approximate balance they will be paying. When the balance is going to be large, a financial payment plan can be drawn up and patients can start paying their portion before the work is completed.

Copayment represents that portion of the dental treatment fee for which the patient is responsible. For example, some insurance policies state that the patient will pay a $10 copayment for each visit. These fees should be considered due and payable at the time service is provided. Other insurance policies clearly outline the patient portion for each procedure. These charges should be discussed with the patient before treatment is begun and financial arrangements are made.

Extended Payment Plans

When it is necessary to allow payments for treatment over time, several different methods can be used to set up extended payment plans. In-house payment plans (budget plans) are established by the dental practice. A contract is drawn up and the proper forms are completed (Figure 14-2). A payment coupon book may be given to the patient or a computerized statement system can generate monthly bills for the agreed-on amount.

A variation of the payment plan is the divided payment plan. In this plan, payments are divided according to the length of treatment. For example, one third of the balance is due at the beginning of treatment, one third at the midpoint of treatment, and the balance at the completion of treatment.

Third-Party Finance Plans

Because there has been a need for good business practices in the collection of dental fees, third-party outsourcing has been on the rise. Currently many different companies provide financing options for the payment of dental fees as well as other healthcare charges that are not typically covered by insurance. A third-party company will provide special payment plans via credit extension. This allows the patient to pay over time. The payments are made directly to the third-party company, freeing the dental office from managing and collecting payment for dental services. Typically a patient will apply for a loan through a company and the terms of the loan will range from interest-free loans to extended payment plans with an interest charged. These services are not free to the dental office. The company will charge a percentage to the dental practice (3% or higher depending on the type and term of the loan). A dental practice will need to consider the cost and determine if this is the best option. However, considering the time generally spent in collection of accounts receivable and the amount of money that is lost in most cases, this option will more than pay for itself over time.

Typically, the financial application is completed in the dental office and is sent to the third-party company for approval. The company will then approve the application for a preset amount. Some companies issue a credit card that can be used only in the dental practice. Each time the patient receives treatment, the credit card is activated and the charges are recorded. The advantage of this service is that the dental practice does not have to manage the account and the third-party company assumes the risk for collecting the charges.

Credit Cards

Credit card payments are considered cash payments. Each time the patient receives treatment, the charge is posted to the credit card via an electronic modem (as in, for example, a department store). The discounted payment is deposited directly into the practice's account.

Financial Policy Communications

Once financial policies are created, they must be communicated to the patient. Patient communication begins at the first time a patient calls the office to ask for information or to make an appointment. Office policy can be delivered tactfully to the patient without discomfort to the administrative dental assistant. Verbal information should be followed by a written statement. This can be accomplished by sending the patient a copy of the practice's brochure.

When a treatment plan is completed, it is the responsibility of the administrative dental assistant to complete a financial plan. This plan can be written on a simple form that illustrates the work to be performed, the fee for each service, and the desired method of payment (Figure 14-3).

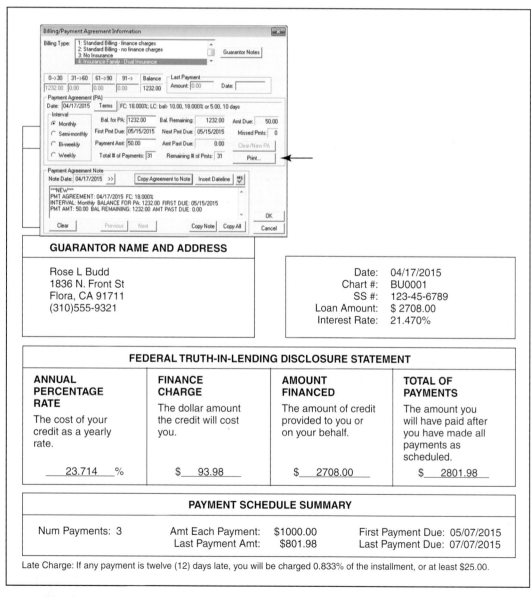

GUARANTOR NAME AND ADDRESS

Rose L Budd
1836 N. Front St
Flora, CA 91711
(310)555-9321

Date:	04/17/2015
Chart #:	BU0001
SS #:	123-45-6789
Loan Amount:	$ 2708.00
Interest Rate:	21.470%

FEDERAL TRUTH-IN-LENDING DISCLOSURE STATEMENT

ANNUAL PERCENTAGE RATE	FINANCE CHARGE	AMOUNT FINANCED	TOTAL OF PAYMENTS
The cost of your credit as a yearly rate.	The dollar amount the credit will cost you.	The amount of credit provided to you or on your behalf.	The amount you will have paid after you have made all payments as scheduled.
23.714 %	$ 93.98	$ 2708.00	$ 2801.98

PAYMENT SCHEDULE SUMMARY

Num Payments: 3	Amt Each Payment: $1000.00	First Payment Due: 05/07/2015
	Last Payment Amt: $801.98	Last Payment Due: 07/07/2015

Late Charge: If any payment is twelve (12) days late, you will be charged 0.833% of the installment, or at least $25.00.

A

FIGURE 14-2 A, Financial arrangement form and truth-in-lending statement on an electronic system.

Canyon View Dental Associates
4546 North Avery Way
Canyon View, CA 91783
Telephone (987) 654-3210

| 3 | 2 | 6 | 5 | 7 | 0 |

PATIENT NUMBER

PATIENT'S NAME ___*Budd*___ ___*Rose*___ ___*L*___
                    Last   First   Initial

I ___*Rose*___ have had my treatment plan and options explained to me and hereby authorize this treatment to be performed by Dr. ___*Mary Edwards*___

Patient's Signature ___*Rose L Budd*___ Date ___*7-23-15*___
(Parent or Guardian MUST sign if patient is a minor)

I also understand that the cost of this treatment is as follows and that the method of paying for the same will be:

Total (Partial) estimate of treatment	$	*2708.00*
Less:		
Initial Payment	—	*1000.00*
Insurance Estimate if Applicable	—	*1000.00*
Other _____	—	*Ø*
Balance of Estimate Due	$	*708.00*

Terms: Monthly Payment $ *236.00* over a *3* month period.

PLEASE CONTACT THE BUSINESS OFFICE IF YOU ARE UNABLE TO MEET YOUR FINANCIAL OBLIGATION

The truth in lending Law enacted in 1969 serves to inform the borrowers and installment purchasers of the true Annual Interest charged on the amounts financed. This law applies to this office whenever the office extends the courtesy of Installment Payments to our patients, even when no finance charge is made.

The signatures below indicate a mutual understanding of the ESTIMATE for treatment and the acceptable schedule of payment as noted.

Today's Date ___*7-23-15*___   ___*Rose L Budd*___
                                 Signature of Responsible Party

___*Sharon Williams*___
Financial Advisor   Phone Number

Note: THIS IS AN ESTIMATE ONLY, if treatment plan should change please request an amended estimate should it not be offered by our staff. This estimate is valid for 90 days from the date above IF treatment has not begun within that period. A patient's voluntary termination of treatment makes this agreement invalid.

FINANCIAL ARRANGEMENTS

B

FIGURE 14-2, cont'd B, Financial arrangement form and truth-in-lending statement on a manual system. (Dentrix screen capture courtesy Henry Shein Practice Solutions, American Fork, Utah.)

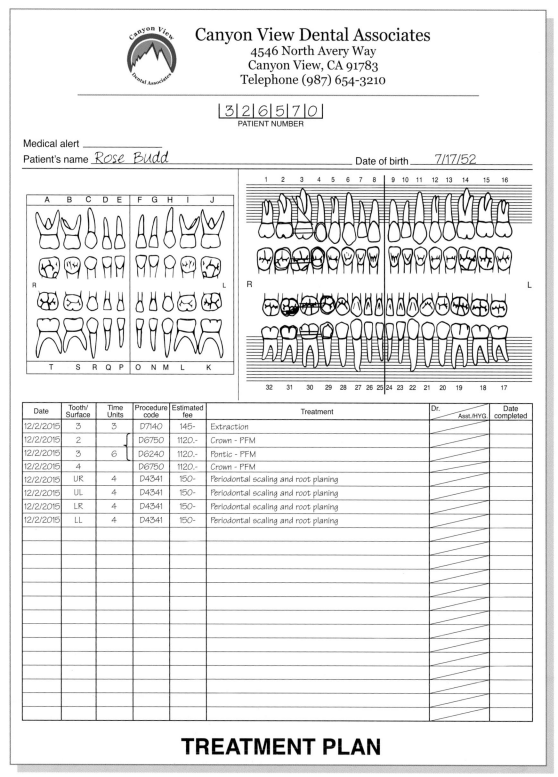

Canyon View Dental Associates
4546 North Avery Way
Canyon View, CA 91783
Telephone (987) 654-3210

| 3 | 2 | 6 | 5 | 7 | 0 |
PATIENT NUMBER

Medical alert _____

Patient's name *Rose Budd* _____ Date of birth ___ 7/17/52 ___

Date	Tooth/ Surface	Time Units	Procedure code	Estimated fee	Treatment	Dr. Asst./HYG.	Date completed
12/2/2015	3	3	D7140	145-	Extraction		
12/2/2015	2		D6750	1120.-	Crown - PFM		
12/2/2015	3	6	D6240	1120.-	Pontic - PFM		
12/2/2015	4		D6750	1120.-	Crown - PFM		
12/2/2015	UR	4	D4341	150-	Periodontal scaling and root planing		
12/2/2015	UL	4	D4341	150-	Periodontal scaling and root planing		
12/2/2015	LR	4	D4341	150-	Periodontal scaling and root planing		
12/2/2015	LL	4	D4341	150-	Periodontal scaling and root planing		

TREATMENT PLAN

FIGURE 14-3 The treatment plan clearly states the treatment and associated fees.

MANAGING ACCOUNTS RECEIVABLE

Accounts receivable represents the amount of money patients owe the dental practice for services rendered. The dentist, accountant, or business manager will set a limit on the amount of money that can be outstanding. When the dollar amount exceeds the limit, a careful analysis of the system should be conducted. This analysis will reveal areas that need to be strengthened to keep the accounts within budget. Several steps must be followed in managing and controlling the accounts receivable.

Gather Financial Data

> **! REMEMBER**
>
> Patient information can be gathered and stored in a variety of methods depending on the system used by the dental practice.

Financial information is obtained when the patient completes the patient registration form (Figure 14-4). As discussed in Chapter 8, this document lists who is financially responsible for the account and pertinent insurance and employment information. It may be necessary to determine who is financially responsible for a child whose parents are

Canyon View Dental Associates
4546 North Avery Way
Canyon View, CA 91783
Telephone (987) 654-3210

Thank you for selecting our dental healthcare team!
We always strive to provide you with the best possible dental care.
To help us meet all your dental healthcare needs, please fill out this form completely.
Please let us know if you have any questions.

Patient Information (CONFIDENTIAL)

Patient # _326570_
Soc. Sec. # _123-45-6789_
Date _7/1/2015_

Name _Rose L Budd_ Birthdate _7/17/52_ Home Phone _555-4321_
Address _1836 N Front Street_ City _Flora_ State _CA_ Zip _91771_
Check Appropriate Box: ☐ Minor ☒ Single ☐ Married ☐ Divorced ☐ Widowed ☐ Separated
Patient's or Parent's Employer _Town Bank_ Work Phone _555-3210_
Business Address _123 S Business Way_ City _____ State ____ Zip _____
Spouse or Parent's Name _____ Employer _____ Work Phone _____
If Patient is a Student, Name of School/College _____ City _____ State ____ Zip _____
Whom May We Thank for Referring you? _____
Person to Contact in Case of Emergency _Evelyn Jones_ Phone _____

Responsible Party

Name of Person Responsible for this Account _Rose L Budd_ Relationship to Patient _Self_
Address _1836 N Front Street_ Home Phone _555-4321_
Driver's License # _M3205167_ Birthdate _7/17/52_ Financial Information _____
Employer _Town Bank_ Work Phone _555-3210_
Is this Person Currently a Patient in our Office? ☐ Yes ☐ No Cell Phone _____
Email Address _R.L.Budd@townbank.com_

Insurance Information

Name of Insured _Rose Budd_ Relationship to Patient _Self_
Birthdate _7/17/52_ Social Security # _123-45-6789_ Date Employed _____
Name of Employer _Town Bank_ Work Phone _555-3210_
Address of Employer _123 S Business Way_ City _____ State ____ Zip _____
Insurance Company _Blue Cross_ Group # _____ Union or Local # _____
Ins. Co. Address _1116 Form St._ City _Los Angeles_ State _CA_ Zip _91110_
How Much is your Deductible? _____ How much have you met? _____ Max. Annual Benefit _____

DO YOU HAVE ANY ADDITIONAL INSURANCE? ☐ Yes ☒ NO   IF YES, COMPLETE THE FOLLOWING

Name of Insured _____ Relationship to Patient _____
Birthdate _____ Social Security # _____ Date Employed _____
Name of Employer _____ Work Phone _____
Address of Employer _____ City _____ State ____ Zip _____
Insurance Company _____ Group # _____ Union or Local # _____
Ins. Co. Address _____ City _____ State ____ Zip _____
How Much is your Deductible? _____ How much have you met? _____ Max. Annual Benefit _____

I attest to the accuracy of the information on this page.
Patient's or guardian's signature _____ Date _____

REGISTRATION

FIGURE 14-4 The patient registration form used to gather contact and financial information.

divorced. This can be a complicated process and the situation should be thoroughly researched before a determination is made. When another parent or guardian is responsible, that person must be contacted to complete the financial portion of the registration form. The responsible party will need to be informed of the treatment and must authorize any payment plan before treatment is begun.

Credit reports are another tool used to gather credit information. These reports list the names of all creditors, all amounts owed, and payment history. Accounts that have been turned over for collection or a legal judgment are identified. Credit reports are available through a credit reporting agency and can be used by the dental practice to determine payment patterns.

> **! REMEMBER**
>
> Patients must give permission before reports are requested from the credit reporting agency.

Prepare a Treatment Plan

A treatment plan is an outline of the treatment that the dentist has recommended and the patient has agreed to (see Figure 14-3). The administrative dental assistant is responsible for preparing the written treatment plan (manual or computerized). The assistant will present the written plan to the patient and discuss financial arrangements.

Payment Plans

Payment plans are confidential and should be discussed in a quiet area away from distractions. Once the plan has been presented, the administrative dental assistant will discuss the payment options with the patient or responsible party. After the patient and the administrative dental assistant agree on the payment plan, the appropriate paperwork can be

prepared, such as truth-in-lending statements (see Figure 14-2), budget plan payment coupons, and contracts.

Billing Statements

Billing statements are monthly accounts of business transactions. They contain important information and must be easy for the patient to understand. These statements should include the following (Figure 14-5):

- Date of each transaction (payments, charges, and adjustments)
- Name of the patient associated with each transaction
- Description of each transaction in terms that the patient will understand
- List of fees for each transaction
- Current balance for the account
- Statement of patient's balance

The statement should look professional yet attractive and should include a return envelope. Information provided in the statement should be consistent with previous financial information given to the patient. The budget plan payment due must match the agreed-on amount. Insurance transactions must match the information sent to the patient from the insurance company (in Explanation of Benefits forms). Transactions and amounts should also be the same as those recorded on the walkout statement given to the patient at the end of the appointment.

Billing cycles are used to process monthly statements in batches. For example, practice statements are divided into four batches and one batch is generated and mailed during each week of the month. Statements will have information printed on the back summarizing the payment policy. If interest is charged, the correct legal statement must be included to notify the patient of the interest rate and whom they should contact if there is a problem.

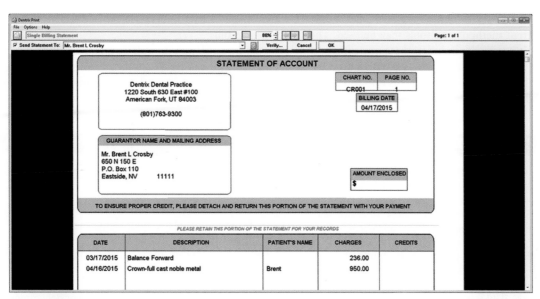

FIGURE 14-5 A sample billing statement shows a balance forward for treatment this patient already received. (Dentrix form courtesy Henry Schein Practice Solutions, American Fork, Utah.)

Monitor the Accounts Receivable Report

It is a prudent business practice to monitor the accounts receivable. Several different elements should be checked each month. The dentist, business manager, or accountant will put a limit on the amount of money that can be owed to the dental practice. When the accounts receivable exceeds the limit, the accounts must be reviewed and areas that need attention must be identified (reports can reveal these areas).

Budget plan reports indicate patients who have failed to make a payment (or to make a full payment). Insurance reports indicate when payments have not been received, allowing the assistant to follow up on unpaid claims. Insurance reports also identify treatments that have not been billed to the insurance company, prompting the assistant to submit a claim.

Account aging reports analyze the length of time that has elapsed since a charge was made. Traditionally, accounts are current if the money has not been owed for more than 30 days and the patient has not received the first statement. Periods of 30 days, 60 days, and 90 days are used to indicate the length of time that money has been owed. Statistics show that money loses value over time. The inability of the dental practice to use the money for salaries or to meet the obligations of the accounts payable (money owed by the dental practice) places a financial burden on the dental practice and prevents financial growth.

WHAT WOULD YOU DO?

You have just met with the accountant; he tells you that the accounts receivable is high. What ideas do you have to help reduce the amount of money owed to the dental practice? What can you do to control new charges? What can be done to collect money that has been owed for more than 2 months?

Collection Process

When it becomes necessary to remind a patient that a payment is due, different methods and tools may be used. The collection process is a series of reminders that payment is past due. At each step, a different strategy is used with a different level of intensity. The objective of the process is to collect the payment from the patient.

Level One: "Friendly Reminders"

The first level of the collection process is the "friendly reminder." Several methods are available for reminding patients that their payments have not been received. If a computerized billing method is used, reminder notices can be printed directly on the billing statement. These reminders will vary according to the length of time the account is past due. The system automatically ages the accounts and includes the correct phrase on the statement. When a manual system is used, a variety of stickers or stamps can be placed on the statement.

LEVEL ONE COLLECTION REMINDERS

- Don't delay further; your payment of $75.00 was due last month.
- Now is the time to take care of this balance of $34.00.
- Prompt payments for your regular dental checkups are appreciated.
- Don't delay. Please pay $123.00 today for last month's recall cleaning and exam.
- Have you overlooked this balance due? You agreed to send a check for $90.00 following your recall appointment.
- Remember that you agreed to pay for your dental exam and cleaning 30 days following your appointment.
- We took your word in good faith; you promised to pay the remaining $100.00 for your crown within 60 days.
- We are counting on you to pay the remaining balance of $120.00 due for dental services rendered on January 10th.
- If there is any reason for not paying this balance of $89.00, please contact us. Thank you.

From Dietz E: *SmartPractice: the complete dental letter handbook: your fingertip resource for practice communication*, Phoenix, 1989, Semantodontics.

Level Two: "Telephone Reminders"

If the bill remains unpaid for a period of two billing cycles or the patient has not followed the agreed-on payment plan, a telephone reminder is necessary. It has been proven that telephone reminders are more effective than letters or repeated bills.

Before a telephone call is made, review and become familiar with the legal aspects of contacting a patient concerning a debt that is owed. Consult the Fair Debt Collection Practices Act.

FAIR DEBT COLLECTION GUIDELINES

When and how can you contact a debtor?
Calls cannot be made before 8 AM or after 9 PM, unless directed by the debtor. Calls can be made to the responsible party at home or at work (unless the employer disapproves). Contact can be made in person or by mail, telephone, and e-mail.

What type of debt collection practice is prohibited?
Harassment: You may not harass, oppress, or abuse anyone. For example, you may not:
- Use threats of violence or harm against the person, property, or reputation

- Publish a list of consumers who refuse to pay their debts (except to a credit bureau)
- Use obscene or profane language
- Repeatedly use the telephone to annoy someone
- Telephone people without identifying yourself
- Advertise debts

False statements: You may not use any false statements when collecting a debt. For example, debt collectors may not:
- Use a false name
- Falsely imply that they are attorneys or government representatives

Continued

FAIR DEBT COLLECTION GUIDELINES—cont'd

What type of debt collection practice is prohibited?—cont'd

- Falsely imply that the debtor has committed a crime
- Falsely represent that they operate or work for a credit bureau
- Misrepresent the amount of the debt
- Misrepresent the involvement of an attorney in collecting the debt
- Indicate that papers being sent are legal forms when they are not
- Indicate that papers being sent are not legal forms when they are
- Send anything that looks like an official document from a court or government agency when it is not
- Give false credit information to anyone

Threats: You may not threaten to do something unless it is legal and you really intend to do it. For example, you may not state that:

- They will be arrested if they do not pay
- You will seize, garnish, attach, or sell their property or wages, unless the collection agency or creditor intends to do so and it is legal to do so

- Actions, such as a lawsuit, will be taken, which legally may not be taken or which you do not intend to take

Unfair practices: Collectors may not engage in unfair practices when they try to collect a debt. For example, collectors may not:

- Collect any amount greater than the debt, unless allowed by law
- Deposit a postdated check prematurely
- Make the debtor accept collect calls or pay for telegrams
- Take or threaten to take the debtor's property, unless this can be done legally
- Contact the debtor by postcard

Who can be contacted?

The only person who can be contacted is the person or persons legally responsible for the account. If you are trying to locate patients, you can call a third party but you cannot reveal that you are trying to reach them because of a debt they owe. You can usually contact them only one time.

Level Three: "The Collection Letter"

Collection letters are another method of reminding patients that their accounts are past due. A collection letter should be short, concise, and to the point (review letter writing in Chapter 4).

Letters can be generated automatically by a computer system or personally typed. Letters should never be sent from the dental practice without the approval of the dentist, accountant, or business manager. The dentist, business manager, or administrative dental assistant can sign the letter. When someone other than the dentist signs the letter, identify the signer, state his or her position, and identify the name of the dental practice.

The tone of the letter should increase in intensity as time goes on. Letters should be sent in stages: Begin the first letter in a pleasing tone and increase the intensity in later letters (Figure 14-6).

Level Four: "The Ultimatum"

The final attempt by the dental practice to collect on an overdue account will also include a letter of increased intensity (see Figure 14-6). The letter will give the patient one more chance to pay the balance before the account is turned over to a collection agency or a claim is filed in Small Claims Court. The letter should clearly outline what will happen if the account is not paid within 10 days. The letter should be sent using a carrier who provides delivery certification. This will document that the patient received or refused the letter.

There will be times when patients move and do not inform the dental practice of their new addresses. Steps can be taken to locate them. This procedure is referred to as **skip tracing.**

- Use envelopes with the words "address correction requested" below the return address. This will prompt the postal service to send a notice with the patient's new address.

- Call the patient's old telephone number; a forwarding number may be available.
- Contact the patient's friend or relative (from information on the patient's registration form).
- Contact the patient at work. The employer may be able to answer questions or relay messages.
- Send a certified letter and request a return receipt. Use a plain envelope without a return address (patients who are trying to avoid you will not know who sent the letter).

Level Five: "Turning the Account Over to Collections"

After you have tried all other methods of collecting the amount due and have not succeeded, your last resort is to turn the account over for collection. Collection agencies take over the process and collect a fee from the dental practice. The fee is a portion of the account, normally 30% to 50% of the balance due.

Accounts turned over to collection agencies should still be collectable. If a collection agency is used, it should be a reputable agency with a record of receiving payment. You can check on an agency's reputation by calling the Chamber of Commerce or the Better Business Bureau. Check with the local dental society and talk with other professionals. Professional organizations that monitor collection agencies include the National Retail Credit Association and the Associated Credit Bureau of America. Select a collection agency that follows the same ethical standards that the dental practice does.

Once the account is turned over to the agency, the agency controls the collection process. Payments can be made directly to the agency and then a percentage is forwarded to the dental practice. The agency will provide monthly statements and keep the dental practice up to date on any progress. The agency should consult with the dental practice before turning the account over for legal action.

Canyon View Dental Associates
4546 North Avery Way
Canyon View, California
Telephone (987) 654-3210

April 11, 2016

Ms. Jennifer Lyons
1256 Roanoke Avenue
Canyon View, CA 91787

Dear Ms. Lyons:

Two months ago you agreed to pay your account by the 15th of April. Our contract was based on two things: (1) your word that you would pay as agreed and (2) your ability to pay the total bill of $456.00.

You'll have to agree that we have kept our part of the agreement. Now, please keep your part by sending a check for the full amount of $456.00 within the next week.

We have enclosed a self-addressed, postage-paid envelope for your convenience.

Yours truly,

Cliff Usher
Business Manager, Canyon View Dental Associate

CPU: sw
Enclosure

A

Canyon View Dental Associates
4546 North Avery Way
Canyon View, California
Telephone (987) 654-3210

April 11, 2016

Mr. James Spencer
1198 Berry Drive
Canyon View, CA 91787

Dear Mr. Spencer:

We recently reviewed your financial status and were surprised by your lack of response to our numerous attempts to collect final payment for treatment you received November 11, 2015.

According to our records, your remaining balance of $221.00 has now accumulated interest of $25.00. Please check your records and contact us immediately if they do not match ours, so we can correct any discrepancy.

If your records agree with ours, we regard this as a very serious situation. We certainly do not wish to be forced to seek other recourse to collect the money owed. We want to communicate with you. But if we do not hear from you within 10 days, we will turn your account over to a collection agency.

Sincerely yours,

Cliff Usher
Business Manager, Canyon View Dental Associates

CPU: sw

B

FIGURE 14-6 A, Collection letter, moderate intensity. **B,** Collection letter used as an ultimatum. (Modified from Dietz E: *SmartPractice: the complete dental letter handbook: your fingertip resource for practice communications*, Phoenix, 1989, Semantodontics.)

The use of a collection agency may cause additional problems for the dental practice. Patients may become irritated and alienate themselves and their family from the dental practice. Some patients will use this as an excuse to bring alleged charges of malpractice against the dental practice. Before turning accounts over to collection agencies or taking additional legal action, such as filing a lawsuit, make every effort to resolve the problem.

Use tact and diplomacy when discussing delinquent accounts with patients. Try to make arrangements with them by setting up a realistic financial plan.

Try to find outside financing that will help the patient to spread out payments over a longer period.

Use final letters and notices to warn the patient that further action, such as a small claims suit or a collection agency, will be used if the account is not settled. Give the patient time to respond, generally 10 days. Be prepared to follow through with the action if your demands are not met.

After the account is turned over, cooperate with the agency and notify someone at the agency if the patient contacts you to make payment arrangements.

Roadblocks to Effective Collections

There may be several reasons for poor or ineffective payments. It is important to identify the reason and to take action to correct the problem.

Patient attitudes and excuses can sometimes prevent effective collections. The patient may become defensive and angry when asked for payment. Common excuses for not paying a dental bill include the following:
- "I can wait to make this payment; dentists don't report late payments to credit agencies."
- "The doctor makes plenty of money. I will send only $20 a month."
- "It won't matter that I have not paid; the dentist has to see me to complete the work."

PROCEDURES

Steps in Placing Collection Calls

1. *Plan the call.* Obtain the patient's clinical record, insurance information, and billing statement. If collection calls (or letters) have been made in the past, review your notes. Follow the correct protocol.
2. *Plan your questions.* Phrase questions in a way that will get you the answers you want. Open-ended questions are the best form to use because they require a person to provide specific information: "When can we expect to receive your payment? Is there a reason for the delay of your payment?" Closed-ended questions require only a yes or no answer: "Will you send a payment?" When the patient responds "yes," you still do not know how much will be sent and when.
3. *Place the call.* Select a time of day when you can place the call without interruptions. Know the name of the responsible party. When the call is answered, identify yourself and the name of the dental practice. Use a confident, professional voice. With your best professional voice, state the reason you are calling, pause, and give the patient a chance to respond before you continue. Remember, you will get better results with a voice that is professional, friendly, and sincere. Never sound timid, angry, embarrassed, annoyed, or rushed: "Hello, Mr. Jones, this is Diane from Canyon View

Dental. I am calling about the balance due for Susie's dental treatment."
4. *Be prepared to resolve the problem.* This may take some creative planning but remember that the end result is to collect the money. You may find that the patient is having some financial difficulties and cannot send you the full amount; set up a payment plan instead. When the current payment plan is not working, renegotiate it. When patients owe the dentist money, they are not likely to continue with their scheduled treatment. Sometimes, they are embarrassed and will seek treatment elsewhere. During collection calls, it is not unusual for patients to become angry (this is a defensive reaction). It is important that you remain calm and professional.
5. *Review what is expected.* At the conclusion of the call, summarize what has been said and clearly state the expected outcome: "Thank you for taking the time to work out a new payment plan. I will expect your payment of $75 by Monday and then $75 by the 15th of each month until the balance is paid."
6. *Record what is expected.* Enter the results of your call in the patient's clinical record. Summarize the results of the telephone call in a letter and mail it to the patient.

TIMETABLE FOR COLLECTION LEVELS

- 0–30 days: Send statements, process insurance claims, monitor budget plans.
- 30–60 days: Level One: Use a friendly reminder on statements.
- 60–90 days: Level Two: Follow up with a telephone call. Identify the problem and provide a solution. Notify the patient in writing, summarizing the results of the telephone call.
- 90–120 days: Level Three: Send a collection letter and follow up with a telephone call.
- Beyond 120 days: Level Four: Send a letter, giving the patient an ultimatum.

No response to letter or the patient does not follow through with payment promises: Level Five: Turn the account over for collection or file a suit in Small Claims Court. Time intervals may vary, depending on the policies of the dental practice.

The following excuses should not be accepted:
- "I will pay the bill in full when all of the work is completed" or "I will pay the bill when I get my tax return." Tactfully explain the office payment policy. If the patient does not accept the financial policy, do not schedule a next appointment.
- "Let me talk to the dentist; he is an old friend." Explain that the dentist has given you the responsibility of making the financial arrangements. When patients demand to speak with the dentist, ask them to wait while you see if the dentist is available to speak with them. Tell the dentist the situation and have the dentist tell the patient that you are in charge. This formally returns control to you.

Sometimes, even the attitudes of the dental healthcare team can hamper effective collections. Some examples of this include:
- "I don't think he can pay the bill, so I won't ask and embarrass him."

- "I hate to ask for money. I hope she pays the bill after the insurance company pays."
- "I am the dentist. I will let someone else worry about collecting the money."
- "I don't have time to write letters and make telephone calls; there are other things that need to be done first."
- "I know he has a lot of money. He will pay his account. I will just send him a statement."
- "I don't have time to write an aging report; it will just have to wait."

Even though these are natural feelings, you should make sure that they do not prevent you from performing this aspect of the job. Keep in mind that if collections are done with a professional attitude, you do not have to be mean or insulting.

KEY POINTS

- When designing financial policies, consider the community's standards, the practice's philosophy, and sound business principles.
- Types of financial policies include payment in full at the time of service, insurance billing, and extended payment plans.
- Managing accounts receivable includes gathering financial data, preparing treatment plans, making financial arrangements, and monitoring accounts receivable reports.

- Collection procedures are a series of reminders that payment is past due. The objective of the process is to collect payment from the patient. There are five levels:
  - Level One: Friendly reminder
  - Level Two: Telephone reminders
  - Level Three: Collection letter
  - Level Four: The ultimatum
  - Level Five: Turning the account over for collection

CAREER-READY PRACTICES

Career-Ready Practices activities are designed to provide students with experiences that can be "practiced" in preparation for skills needed on the job. In each of the following exercises, a variety of approaches may be used to address the problem, rather than "right" or "wrong" answers. Below each exercise, next to the compass icon, is a listing of suggested Career-Ready Practice numbers that correspond to the listing of 12 practices in the front of the text (see p. viii-ix); these practices provide suggestions for approaches to complete the exercise.

1. Consider the elements of a financial policy and outline the practices you would initiate to serve the dental patients in your community.

 Career-Ready Practices
- 5 *Consider the environmental, social, and economic impacts of decisions.*
- 7 *Employ valid and reliable research strategies.*
- 8 *Utilize critical thinking to make sense of problems and persevere in solving them.*

2. In small groups, discuss the policies you have each outlined and develop a group policy. Identify the demographics of

your community and the type of dental practice (general practice or dental specialty). Present your written policy to the larger group and explain how you will manage the policy and what makes it a sound business practice.

 Career-Ready Practices
- 12 *Work productively in teams while using cultural/global competence.*
- 9 *Model integrity, ethical leadership, and effective management.*
- 5 *Consider the environmental, social, and economic impacts of decisions.*

3. In your groups, develop a script that will help assistants when presenting treatment plans, explaining financial options, and asking for payment. To practice your scripts, mix the groups and take turns being the patient and the assistant.

 Career-Ready Practices
- 4 *Communicate clearly, effectively, and with reason.*
- 6 *Demonstrate creativity and innovation.*
- 9 *Model integrity, ethical leadership, and effective management.*

Dental Insurance Processing

INTRODUCTION

In the early days of dentistry, payment for dental treatment was arranged between the dentist and the patient. As dentistry progressed into a complex healthcare delivery system with a wide range of treatment options, the need for financial assistance was recognized. In the middle of the twentieth century, dental insurance was offered as a method of supplementing payment for dental treatment.

During the latter part of the twentieth century, dentistry changed rapidly. The changes provided more comprehensive dental care, including preventive dentistry, advanced techniques for restorative dentistry, prosthodontics, orthodontics, dental implants, periodontics, and corrective surgical procedures. The dental insurance industry made changes to meet the new needs of policyholders. In addition to changes in dental treatment, the types of dental insurance changed. These changes expanded the scope of coverage and the delivery system. Today, employers and policyholders have a wide range of policy choices and can customize their coverage to meet their financial needs.

Whether only a few or many insurance claims are processed, the fundamental duties are the same. In a small dental practice, the administrative dental assistant may be in charge of the insurance process, along with several other assigned duties. In large dental practices, one or more insurance assistants may be responsible for processing insurance claims.

Before successfully processing a dental claim form, the administrative dental assistant must understand the types of dental insurance coverage available, insurance terminology (a glossary is provided later in this chapter), and how to correctly code dental procedures. In addition, a clear-cut policy must be in place that outlines the requirements of the dental practice in relation to insurance billing, the patient's responsibilities, and the dental practice's responsibilities. It is extremely important, as it is in all phases of dental treatment, that patients have a clear and concise understanding of the treatment, what the insurance company will pay, and what their portion of the payment will be before any treatment is begun.

TYPES OF DENTAL INSURANCE

Dental benefits are determined by the type of dental insurance policy and the extent of the coverage. Insurance coverage is calculated with specifications outlined in the insurance contract. Insurance contracts are between the carrier (insurance company), the purchaser of the insurance (group; in most cases, employers), and the subscriber (individual or employee). Insurance policies are purchased for the subscriber and additional coverage may be extended to the subscriber's dependents (spouse and children).

Insurance plans can be divided into several very broad categories. These categories are based on the types of coverage and the methods by which the dental office is paid.

Fee for Service

Fee for service is a method of payment that compensates the dentist according to individual services and procedures. Reimbursement is determined by established fee schedules.

Usual, Customary, and Reasonable Plans

Dental insurance companies establish fee schedules on the basis of a variety of information. The fee schedules in **usual, customary, and reasonable (UCR) plans** are based on the following criteria: **usual fee**, the fee the dentist uses most often for a given dental service; **customary fee**, the fee determined by the third-party administrator from actual fees

213

submitted for specific dental services; and **reasonable fee**, a determination by the third-party administrator that a particular service for a given procedure has been modified to take into consideration unusual complications. This fee may vary from the dentist's usual fee and the administrator's customary fee. UCR fee schedules are calculated with distinct demographic information and criteria. Insurance companies survey dental practices within a geographic location and determine the average fee charged for each procedure code. Using this information, they establish a fee schedule. Each

insurance company has its own criteria and method by which it determines the UCR fee.

Some insurance contracts require participating dentists to file a fee schedule. A review of the fee schedule determines whether the fees fall within the established UCR fee range. If the schedule is accepted, it will become the established fee schedule for that dental practice. If the fees do not fall within the established UCR, the schedule is not accepted and is returned to the dentist for revision. Once the fee schedule has been established, it becomes the basis for reimbursement from that insurance company.

DENTAL INSURANCE TERMINOLOGY

Accepted Fee: The dollar amount that has been agreed to by the dentist and the insurance carrier as payment in full (including the patient portion).

Administrator: A person or group of persons who represents dental benefits plans for the purpose of negotiating and managing contracts with dental service providers.

Allowable Charges: The maximum amount paid for each procedure.

Application Service Provider: Web-based practice management software that includes the electronic claims submissions and is on a hosted server.

Assignment of Benefits: Authorization given by the subscriber or patient to a dental benefit plan, directing the insurer to make payment for dental benefits directly to the providing dentist.

Attending Dentist's Statement: The form used by the dentist to request payment of services (dental claim form) from the dental benefit plan.

Audit: A method used by third parties to check the accuracy of dental claim forms by comparing patient clinical records with information submitted on the dental claim form.

Balance Billing: Billing the patient for the difference between the amount paid by the dental benefits plan and the fee charged by the dentist (according to the specification of the dental benefits plan contract).

Benefit Payment: The amount of the total bill paid by the dental benefits plan.

Benefit Service: A service that will be paid for by the dental benefits plan.

Birthday Rule: A method used to determine which parent is considered the primary provider of dental coverage. The rule simply states that the parent whose birth date comes first in the year is the primary provider. The gender rule states that the father is always the primary provider. These rulings are outlined in each individual insurance contract.

Cafeteria Plan: A menu of benefit programs provided by the employer that gives patients several plans from which to choose. Most plans include basic coverage paid for by the employer with additional benefit plan costs being shared by the employer and the employee.

Capitation: A contract with a dental benefits plan that stipulates that payment will be made to the dentist per capita (per patient).

Claim: Also known as the Attending Dentist's Statement. Claims are a method used to request payment or authorization for treatment. Each claim provides necessary information about the patient, treating dentist, and treatment.

Claims Payment Fraud: Changing or manipulating information (by a dental benefits plan) on a dental claim form that results in a lower benefit being paid to the treating dentist (intentionally falsifying information and services).

Claims Reporting Fraud: Changing or manipulating information (by the dentist) on a dental claim form that results in a higher benefit being paid by the dental benefits plan (intentionally falsifying information and services).

Closed Panel: Panels are groups of dental providers who are under contract with third parties to provide dental services. Patients who receive benefits from the dental benefits plan must seek dental services only from members of the panel. Contracts also limit the number of panel members (dental providers) in a specified geographic area.

Code on Dental Procedures and Nomenclature (CDT Code): Code set adapted under the Administrative Simplification provisions of the Health Insurance Portability and Accountability Act of 1996 (HIPAA) used to identify dental procedures. The Code is a listing of a five-digit code set and a description of the dental service. The CDT Code is published by the American Dental Association (ADA).

Consolidated Omnibus Budget Reconciliation Act (COBRA): Legislation that mandates guaranteed medical and dental coverage for a period of 18 months after the loss of group benefits coverage. Individuals are given the option of purchasing their own coverage at a group rate under special COBRA contracts.

Contract Benefit Level: The percentage of the maximum contract allowance that an insurance carrier will pay after the deductible has been satisfied.

Contracted Dentist: A dentist who has a contract with an insurance carrier to participate in its network. The dentist agrees to accept the predetermined fees as payment in full for services rendered to an enrollee of the network. Also referred to as Participating Dentist, Network Dentist, or Contracting Dentist.

Contracted Fee: The fee for each single procedure that a contracted dentist has agreed to accept as payment in full for covered services provided to a network enrollee.

Coordination of Benefits (COB): A system that coordinates the benefits of two or more insurance policies. The total benefits paid should not be more than 100% of the original service fee.

Copayment: The portion of the service fee that remains after payment is made by the dental benefits plan.

Corporate Dentistry: Dental facilities that are owned and operated by companies for the purpose of providing dental care to their employees and dependents.

Covered Charges: Allowable services outlined in dental benefits plan contracts, fee schedules, or tables of allowance, provided by the dental provider and paid for, in whole or part, by the third-party dental benefits plan.

Current Procedural Terminology (CPT Codes): CPT-4 standardized list of codes and procedures developed by the American Medical Association (AMA) for the purpose of consistency in reporting medical treatment and services. It is the standard code under HIPAA.

Deductible: The service fee that the patient is responsible for paying before the third party will consider payment of additional services. The deductible may be payable annually, during a lifetime, or as a family.

Dental Benefit Plan: Provides dental service to an enrollee in exchange for a fixed, periodic payment made in advance of the dental service. Such plans often include the use of deductibles, coinsurance, and maximums to control the cost of the program to the purchaser.

Dental Benefit Program: Dental benefit plan being offered to the enrollees by the sponsor.

Dental Insurance: A method of financial assistance (provided by a dental benefits service) that helps to pay for specified procedures and services concerning dental disease and accidental injury to the oral structure.

Dental Service Corporation: A legally formed, not-for-profit organization that contracts with dental providers for the sole purpose of providing dental care (e.g., Delta Dental Plans and Blue Cross/Blue Shield).

Dependents: Persons who are covered under another person's dental benefits policy, including but not limited to spouses and children. The terms of dependent coverage are stated in the dental benefits contract for each coverage group.

Direct Reimbursement: A plan that allows an organization to be self-funded for the purpose of providing dental benefits. The plan is administered by the individual provider or by an outside organization for the purpose of processing claims and distributing service benefit payments. These plans allow the patient to seek dental care and treatment at a facility of their choice and in most states this is not yet regulated by the insurance commission.

Downcoding: A method of changing a reported benefits code by third-party payers to reflect a lower cost for the procedure.

Dual Choice Program: An insurance policy (benefit plan) that provides the eligible individual the choice of an alternative dental benefit program or a traditional dental benefit program.

E-Claims Service Provider: Stand-alone electronic claims processing hosted by an outside vendor. These solutions allow the dental practice to submit all of its insurance claims electronically and provides the practice with the benefits of using electronic data interchange without having to invest in a complete practice management system.

Eligibility Date: The effective date of dental coverage.

Established Patient: Patient who has received dental care recently.

Exclusions: The option in a dental benefits program to exclude dental services and procedures (as outlined in the patient contract book).

Exclusive Provider Organization (EPO): A dental benefit plan or program that will cover dental services only if they are provided by an institutional or professional provider with whom the dental benefit plan has a contract.

Expiration Date: Date on which the patient is no longer eligible for dental benefits based on expiration of the dental contract or termination of the patient's employment.

Family Deductible: A deductible that can be satisfied when combined deductibles of the family have been met. This deductible will be less than the total of the individual family members' deductibles.

Fee for Service: Dental benefits paid for each dental service or procedure performed by the dental practitioner, instead of payment that is salary based or capitation based.

Fee Schedule: A list of charges for dental services and procedures established by the dentist or a dental benefits provider and mutually agreed on.

Franchise Dentistry: A method of providing dental care under a common name, with regional or national advertising, contract agreements with dental benefits providers, and financial and managerial support.

Health Insurance Portability and Accountability Act of 1996 (HIPAA): A federal law that requires all health plans, healthcare clearinghouses, and providers of healthcare who transmit protected health information (PHI) electronically to use a standard transaction code set. The official code set for dental services is the *Code for Dental Procedures and Nomenclature,* published by the ADA.

Health Maintenance Organization (HMO): A healthcare delivery system with a network of providers who will accept payment for services on a per capita basis or a limited fee schedule. The purpose of the HMO is to contain costs through control of services provided. Patients who are enrolled in an HMO must seek dental treatment from the assigned provider. The period of time that a patient must stay with the provider varies according to the individual contract. Usually patients cannot change providers without authorization from the HMO.

Incentive Program: The copayment percentage changes when patients follow a preset standard of treatment. For example, a dental benefits plan may offer new enrollees a 70%–30% copayment arrangement for the first year of coverage (with the patient responsible for 30%). If the patient receives preventive care at set intervals during the first year, the dental benefits plan will increase the insurance company's copayment percentage to 80%–20% in the following year (with the patient responsible for 20%). The increase will continue as long as the patient follows the preset standard of treatment. If the patient fails to follow the standard, the copayment percentage will revert backward (although never to be lower than the original ratio).

Indemnity Plan: Dental benefits plan that uses a schedule of allowance, table of allowance, or reasonable and customary fee schedule as the basis of payment calculation.

Individual Practice Association (IPA): Legally formed organization that enters into contracts with dental benefits plans to provide services to the dental benefit plans' enrollees. The IPA is composed of individual dental practitioners.

Insured: A person who has enrolled with an insurer (third party) to provide payment for dental services and procedures.

Insurer: The third party (not the dentist or the patient) that assumes the responsibility for payment of dental services and procedures for enrollees in the program.

Continued

DENTAL INSURANCE TERMINOLOGY—cont'd

International Classification of Disease (ICD): ICD-10 HIPAA code set used for diagnoses and procedures codes used in medical and dental claim transactions.

Least Expensive Alternative Treatment (LEAT): A provision in dental benefits plans that allows payment for dental services and procedures to be based on the least expensive treatment available. For example, a patient chooses to have a composite restorative material placed in a posterior tooth. The dental benefits plan will base payment on the least expensive restorative material, amalgam. The patient is responsible for the difference in payment.

Managed Care: A method employed by some benefits plans designed to contain the costs of healthcare, including limitations in access to care (enrollees are assigned healthcare providers), covered services and procedures, and reimbursement amounts.

Maximum Allowance: The total amount of specific dental benefits (dollars) that will be paid toward dental services and procedures. Maximums are determined by the provisions of individual group contracts.

Maximum Benefit: The total amount of dental benefits that will be paid for an individual or family for the purpose of dental services and procedures. This amount is determined by the individual group contract and may be a yearly maximum or a lifetime maximum.

Maximum Fee Schedule: The total acceptable fee for a dental service or procedure that can be charged by a dental provider under a specific dental benefits plan (e.g., preset fee schedules that have been accepted by the dental provider and the dental benefits plan).

Necessary Treatment: Dental services and procedures that have been established by the dental professional as necessary for the purpose of restoring or maintaining a patient's oral health. Treatment is based on established standards of the dental profession.

Nonduplication of Benefits: This applies if a subscriber is covered by more than one benefit plan. In the case of dual coverage, the subscriber will never receive payment for more than 100% of the covered benefit.

Nonparticipating Dentist: A dental professional who is not under contract with a dental benefits plan to provide dental services and procedures to enrollees.

Open Enrollment: A period during the year when a member of a dental benefits program has the option of selecting the type of coverage and the provider of dental services.

Open Panel: A type of dental benefits plan in which any licensed dentist can participate. The enrollee (insured) can seek treatment from any licensed dentist, with benefits being paid to the enrollee or to the dentist. The dentist may accept or refuse any enrollee.

Out-of-pocket: An amount the patient is responsible for paying, such as coinsurance or copayments, deductibles, and costs above the annual maximum.

Overbilling: Fraudulent practice of not disclosing the waiver of patient copayment to benefits plan organizations.

Overcoding: Billing dental benefits plans for higher-paying procedures than the service or procedure that was actually performed.

Participating Dentist: A dentist who has contracted with a dental benefits organization to provide dental care to specific enrollees.

Payer: Insurance companies, dental benefits plans, or dental plan sponsors (direct reimbursement, unions) that make payments on behalf of patients.

Preauthorization: Confirmation by a dental benefits plan that a pretreatment plan has been authorized for payment according to the patient's group policy.

Precertification: Confirmation by a dental benefits plan that a patient is eligible to receive treatment according to the provision of the contract.

Predetermination: A process in which a dentist submits a pretreatment plan and documentation to a dental benefits plan organization for approval. The dental benefits plan organization will establish the patient's eligibility for payment of the procedure and will approve the fees to be charged according to the patient's contract. The document returned by the payer will state the benefit that will be paid, limitations if any, and the amounts of the copayment and deductible. Some contracts mandate that all treatments over a set dollar amount require predetermination.

Preexisting Condition: A clause in most dental benefits plans that limits coverage for conditions that existed before the patient enrolled in the benefits plan.

Preferred Provider Organization (PPO): A contract between a dental benefits plan organization and a provider of dental care that states that, in return for the referral of dental patients, the dentist will provide services and procedures at a reduced fee or according to a preestablished fee schedule. The purposes of this contract are to cut costs for the dental benefits plan organization and to provide a patient base for the dental professional.

Prefiling of Fees: A procedure in which a dental professional files a fee schedule with the dental benefits plan organization for the purpose of receiving preauthorization of fees. If the fee schedule is accepted by the dental benefits plan organization, it will be the basis for coverage of enrolled patients. If an enrollee is charged a fee higher than that on file, the difference is not allowed and cannot be charged to the enrollee.

Subscriber: The holder of the dental benefits (insurance). Usually, this is the person whose name is on the policy and additional coverage is extended to the spouse and children. Other terms used to describe the subscriber are *enrollee, insured,* and *certificate holder.*

Systematized Nomenclature of Dentistry (SNODENT): A combination of medical (SNOMED) conditions and dental conditions used to define dental diseases in an electronic environment. The use of these codes enables the dentist to describe conditions and other factors that relate to a given diagnosis in a standard language. These common codes will be required in electronic health records (EHRs).

Table of Allowances: A list of the services and procedures that will be paid by the dental benefits plan, with a dollar amount assigned to each procedure. Tables of allowances are also referred to as *schedules of allowances* and *indemnity schedules.*

Third Party: A group or organization that has the capacity to collect insurance premiums, accept financial risk, and pay dental claims (the patient is the first party and the healthcare provider is the second party). Also known as the *administrative agent, carrier, insurer,* or *underwriter,* the third party also performs other administrative services.

Usual, Customary, and Reasonable (UCR) Plan: A dental plan that uses the following criteria to establish a fee schedule: **usual fee,** the fee the dentist uses most often for a given dental service; **customary fee,** the fee determined by the third-party administrator from actual submitted fees for specific dental services; and **reasonable fee,** a determination by the third-party administrator that a particular service for a given procedure has been modified to take into consideration unusual complications. This fee may vary from the dentist's usual fee and the administrator's customary fee.

Table of Allowances

Tables of allowances, schedules of allowances, and indemnity schedules are lists of procedures covered by an insurance company and their respective dollar amounts. These fees are the same for all dentists, regardless of location. The dental practice submits the dental practice fee for service and reimbursement is calculated with the amount listed on the table of allowances. The difference between the fees is charged to the patient.

Fixed Fee Schedule

Government assistance programs and other programs establish a fixed fee schedule. These fee schedules include preestablished fees that are charged by all dentists, regardless of geographic area. If the usual fee charged by the dental practice is higher than the fixed fee, the difference between fees cannot be charged to the patient.

Capitation Programs

Capitation programs are programs in which the dental practice is paid a set amount for each patient who is enrolled in the program. Payment is made for each enrolled patient, regardless of whether he or she receives treatment. In addition to the monthly fee paid to the dentist under some contracts, the dentist can charge the patient a copayment. Copayments apply to each visit and may be applied to designated procedures.

Closed Panel Programs

Closed panel programs are programs that dictate to patients where they can receive their dental treatment. Under closed panel programs, dentists and dental entities enter into an agreement to provide services for a select group of patients. Contracts for closed panel programs are limited to a preset number in a geographic area. This limitation provides a larger patient pool for those dental practices or entities with contracts.

Another type of closed panel program is provided by large corporations that provide dental clinics for their employees and families. The dentist and the dental auxiliary are employees of the corporation.

Franchise Dentistry

Franchise dentistry is a method that allows a corporation (formed by a dentist or other entity) to own several dental practices (most states have very specific regulations and laws dealing with the ownership of medical and dental practices). The benefits of this type of dental practice are a common name and the means for a large advertising budget. Some franchise dental practices offer supplemental dental insurance to their patients to pay that portion of the fee that is not paid by their primary dental insurance. This type of insurance pays only when the patient is seen in one of the franchise dental practices. Dentists and staff members work for the corporation.

Direct Reimbursement

Direct reimbursement is a method of payment that bypasses an insurance company and pays fees directly from a fund established by an employer.

Preferred Provider Organization

The preferred provider organization (PPO) is a plan that establishes a list of dentists who have a contract with the insurance company. The contract states that the dentist will use only the fee schedule preapproved by the third party (insurance company). In exchange for the fixed fee schedule, the third party places the dentist's name on the preferred list, thus supplying a patient base for the dental office.

Patients who belong to PPOs have the option of receiving treatment from approved providers or from a dentist outside of the program. When a nonmember dentist performs treatment, the fee schedule is different and may result in a greater out-of-pocket expense for the patient.

Two variations of the PPO are exclusive provider organization (EPO) and point of service. In the EPO the patient is restricted to only those dentists who are members of the plan's network. If a patient chooses to go outside the network, he or she will not be reimbursed for services. Some plans do offer an exception for emergency treatment and treatment outside the service area. A point of service plan has a different fee schedule for network providers and nonnetwork providers.

Health Maintenance Organization

A health maintenance organization (HMO) accepts responsibility for payment of dental procedures and services for its members. Members enter into HMOs for the purpose of having all of their medical or dental fees covered. Members of HMOs can receive treatment only from assigned dentists. If they receive treatment outside of the HMO, the fees are not covered and become the responsibility of the patient. Patients are assigned contract HMO dentists and cannot make changes easily. Each month, the HMO sends the dental practice a roster of patients. The dental practice is paid a capitation for each patient on the roster.

Additional payment for treatment or a copayment is collected for covered expenses according to the individual contract. When an HMO patient is seen, the dental practice is required to submit an encounter claim form to the HMO. Supplemental payment to the dental practice is made according to services rendered. Patients may be required to pay a copayment at the time of the appointment. Copayments may be assessed according to a visit charge or for individual services. Each group has a different protocol for the collection of copayments and the filing of encounter forms.

Managed Care

Managed care is a program that is designed to contain the costs of dental procedures and services. This is accomplished by restricting the types and frequencies of procedures and services, preestablishing where a patient may seek dental care (contract dentist or dental entities), and controlling fee schedules.

Individual Practice Association

An individual practice association (IPA) is an organization that has been legally established by a group of dentists to enter into third-party contracts. The objective of the association is to work collectively to secure third-party contracts. The IPA usually consists of a small staff and an administrator.

Union Trust Funds

Union trust funds administer the distribution of their members' benefits. They are not insurance companies and are not mandated to follow the same rules as insurance companies. They establish their own fee schedules (table of allowances) that outline the amount of money paid for each procedure. Depending on the type of contract and on the program offered by the union, payment may be made from a fee for service, PPO, or capitation program.

OTHER TYPES OF INSURANCE COVERAGE

Secondary Coverage

Often, patients have more than one insurance plan to cover their dental expenses. This occurs when a husband and wife both have insurance coverage and the spouse is included in the policy. The person who is the patient is the primary carrier and the spouse is the secondary carrier. The primary carrier is always billed before the secondary carrier. The patient does not have the option to determine who is going to be the primary carrier.

Secondary coverage for children is determined by the gender rule or the birthday rule. The gender rule determines the primary and secondary coverage of the child by assigning primary coverage to the father and secondary coverage to the mother. The birthday rule designates primary coverage to the parent whose birthday comes first in the year. Coverage can become very confusing when stepparents and parents with custody have dental insurance. It is advisable to check with the third-party carrier to help determine who is considered primary.

Once the primary carrier pays, the secondary company is billed. When billing the secondary insurance company, send the same information that is contained in the first claim. In addition to the information asked on the dental claim form, a copy of the explanation of benefits (EOB) is attached. The secondary insurance company will not pay more than the balance that was not paid by the primary carrier. It is hoped that the secondary carrier will pay the full amount not paid by the primary carrier. Because of stipulations in some insurance policies, this is not always the case and care should be taken not to imply to the patient that the full amount will be paid by the carrier. Patients with dual coverage (primary and secondary coverage) should check with their carriers before treatment if they have any questions regarding the amounts that will be paid.

Government Assistance

Government assistance programs are administered by the U.S. government and by state and local governments. Special filing procedures and dental claim forms are used. Check with each state to determine available programs and correct protocols. Insurance companies that process claims hold seminars on how to file.

Workers' Compensation

Workers' compensation programs cover employees who sustain dental injuries while working; these cases require special handling and authorization. Patients who have a work-related claim also must provide billing information. It is wise to contact the insurance carrier and receive clear instructions before any work is begun.

Auto Accidents

Similar to workers' compensation cases, cases involving auto accidents and auto insurance must be handled according to specific procedures. These must be determined before any treatment is provided.

Other Accidents

Some claims can be processed through medical insurance instead of dental insurance. Be sure that you understand all procedures involved before treatment is begun.

INSURANCE CLAIMS PROCESSING

Because of the large number of dental claims processed by dental practices, it has become a full-time task in some practices to work with insurance claims. When a patient arrives for the first time, it is the task of the administrative dental assistant to determine insurance coverage. A process should be developed to help the assistant gather all needed information quickly and efficiently. A number of methods have been established to organize this process. The administrative dental assistant can use the database within the practice management system or manually retrieve the demographic information from the patient's dental record. Once the demographic information has been gathered, the next step is to determine the patient's insurance eligibility and coverage. When the treatment has been completed, the claim is then processed and filed with the insurance carrier for payment.

Collecting Information and Determining Benefits

Before processing claims, it is necessary to collect all of the information needed to complete the claim form. The patient will provide the demographic information when he or she completes the patient registration form. The data from the form will be entered into the practice management system or be located (see Anatomy of a Dental Registration Form in Chapter 8) in the patient's paper dental record. Demographic information will include the patient's name, address, date of birth, and relationship to the insurance policy holder. In addition to the demographic information of the patient, the patient record will need to include the demographic information about the policyholder, including employer, name of the insurance provider, group identification number, and if there is any additional insurance coverage. The administrative dental assistant will use the demographic and insurance information to determine eligibility and coverage. When determining benefits and coverage for patients, insurance providers use the following terms and conditions.

Maximum Coverage

Maximum coverage is the total dollar amount that an insurance company will pay during a year. It is important to determine when the year begins and ends. Most companies use a calendar year but some use a fiscal year, which can be any 12-month period.

Deductible

Most patients must pay a set dollar amount toward treatment each year (the deductible) before the third party will consider payment for additional services. This deductible may be payable annually, during a lifetime, or as a family.

Percentage of Payment

Not all services are covered by insurance at the same percentages. Preventive procedures and services are covered at higher percentages than restorative and prosthetic services. It is very important to determine how each percentage is calculated (different percentages may be used to calculate different categories of service). The percentage of coverage is determined by the provisions of each insurance group and varies from group to group and from company to company. Some insurance policies have provisions that pay services at a higher percentage if the patient has followed the established protocol for preventive care. For example, during the first year the patient is covered, the insurance company may pay 70% of expenses. If the patient is seen in the dental practice for routine preventive care during the year, the policy can increase to 80% coverage for the second year. This type of coverage is referred to as an incentive program. Each year that the patient receives the approved type and frequency of preventive care, the per-

centage is raised, until he or she is covered at 100%. If the patient does not follow the guidelines, the percentage is dropped (although never below the original amount).

Copayment

A copayment is the portion of the fee that the patient is responsible to pay. For HMO and PPO policyholders this may be a set fee that is paid at each visit; for example, there may be a $25.00 copayment that the patient is responsible to pay each appointment. A copayment can also be the portion (or percentage) of the fee that is the responsibility of the patient to pay. With the use of electronic verification and real-time reporting by insurance providers or third-party services, this portion can be determined easily at each visit. When the patient's copayment is known and verified at the time of the appointment, the fee can be collected at each visit. This process eliminates billing the patient after the insurance provider pays, thus saving time and money for the dental practice.

Limitation to Coverage

To keep the costs of dental insurance down, most companies establish limitations to coverage. They will pay for basic dental services but any work that is considered more than basic is limited or is not a covered benefit. For example, if a patient wants to have porcelain crowns placed on posterior teeth, an insurance company may determine that the teeth can be restored with metal crowns (the use of porcelain crowns on posterior teeth is considered cosmetic). Patients who choose porcelain over metal are responsible for the difference in fees. These types of limitations must be discussed with patients before dental treatment is begun.

Eligibility

Sometimes, the administrative dental assistant will have to determine eligibility by contacting the insurance carrier and asking for verification. Most insurance providers and third-party services have the capability of providing the information electronically and in real time. Eligibility can refer to the employer, patient, or dependent. It is not uncommon for employers to change their dental coverage yearly. A family who had dental coverage last year may have a different carrier this year as well as different benefits. It is prudent to check eligibility often.

Preauthorization or Pretreatment

When a treatment exceeds a specified dollar amount or if there is any question about the amount of coverage, it is wise to submit a pretreatment form (a requirement of some third-party carriers). Once pretreatment approval has been obtained, a financial plan can be established between the dentist and the patient. When submitting electronic requests either to the insurance provider directly or through a third-party service, the information is often transmitted in a matter of minutes.

It is important to remember that the estimated amount of coverage is just that, an estimate. Some companies give an estimate of coverage and do not check the eligibility of the patient. Before actual treatment is begun, check with the insurance company and reconfirm that the patient is eligible for the treatment. Insurance companies calculate eligibility on a monthly basis. Eligibility is determined by the payment of policy premiums, continued employment, and remaining benefits. If any of these conditions have changed between the time the original claim was submitted for authorization and the date of actual treatment, the third-party carrier may no longer be liable for payment for treatment.

ADVANTAGES OF PRETREATMENT ESTIMATES

- Helps to determine how best to plan treatment and maximize patient benefits. For example, the treatment may be done in segments, over weeks, months, or years.
- Provides benefit information that helps the dental practice and the patient to formulate a payment plan.

! REMEMBER

There should be no surprises: All work and financial responsibility must be disclosed before treatment.

Electronically Submitted Forms

Electronically submitted forms contain the same information as a paper dental claim form, except that they are "mailed" via electronic transfer. When documentation of dental services is ready to be submitted to an insurance company for payment or preauthorization, the software program will prepare the electronic dental claim form. If supporting documents are required, such as digital radiographic images, scanned documents, photographs, letters, and intraoral images, these are attached electronically and included with the dental claim form. There are many different insurance companies and protocols vary for the submission of electronic dental claim forms; thus electronic formatting of the submitted claims is required. There are several options available to organize and process claims electronically, such as practice management systems, application service providers, e-claims service providers, and individual insurance providers. Each type of processing service will follow the same basic method in transmitting electronic claims and must follow all Health Insurance Portability and Accountability Act of 1996 (HIPAA) standards. Electronic claims are first sent to a clearinghouse that translates the submitted electronic claim and supporting documents to the required protocol that is used by the insurance company's computers. Although this sounds like a very difficult and time-consuming job, the process is very rapid because it is done electronically. Claims can be sent electronically from the office to the clearinghouse and translated and forwarded to the insurance company within seconds.

When supporting documents are requested for electronically submitted claims and they cannot be attached electronically (e.g., radiographs, models), the documents are assigned an identification number and mailed to the insurance company.

The turnaround time (amount of time it takes to pay a claim) is much longer for paper claims than for electronic claims. All paper claims must first be opened in the mail room. From the mail room, claims are scanned and entered into a computer databank or placed on microfiche (for the purpose of storage). They are then transferred to the claim center, where they are processed by insurance clerks. The turnaround time for a paper claim is about 1 week. Electronically submitted claims can be turned around in 1 to 2 days. Additional turnaround time can be avoided if the dental practice participates in a direct deposit program. Direct deposits are made from the insurance company into the checking account of the dental practice. Documentation is then forwarded to the dental practice to complete the bookkeeping process.

Practice Management Systems

Many of the practice management systems provide the capability of processing insurance claim forms. The process begins when the information is entered in the system, through manual data entry by the administrative dental assistant; directly by the patient; or using a combination of patient entry, office entry, and direct input by the insurance carrier. Along with the data required to process each individual claim, such as patient information, employer information, and insurance information, the system will automatically code the claim. Insurance codes are stored in a database and upgraded when needed. When treatment is completed or pretreatment is requested, the practice management system will collect the date from multiple databases and correctly complete the dental or medical claim form. By taking advantage of these applications the administrative dental assistant will save substantial time. The system will be able to verify eligibility, submit claims, track claim status, electronically deposit claim payments, and attach digital images (x-rays, periodontal charting, intraoral images, and documentation).

Application Service Providers

Application service providers are web-based practice management software applications that allow the dental practice to run various applications from a hosted system. These applications may interface directly with the practice management system or can be used independently. The advantage of this type of system is that it allows the dental practice to use only the functions that it needs and it is hosted and maintained by an outside vendor.

E-Claims Service Providers

E-claims service providers are companies that provide stand-alone electronic claims solutions. These companies act as a clearinghouse to process dental claims, check on patient eligibility and benefits, and provide claim status. They also provide the ability to attach digital images and documentation. In many cases these companies act as a bridge between your practice management systems to safely transmit e-claims, patient statements, and credit and debit card processing.

Insurance Provider Claims Processing

Individual insurance providers also provide the capability to process e-claims. They provide tools for the submission of claims and digital attachments, pretreatment estimates, and verification of eligibility. These services will vary from provider to provider and the administrative dental assistant will have to batch and submit claims that are covered only by the provider. This may be an option for the dental practice that produces a small number of claims or provides services that are covered by only a few insurance providers.

Benefits of Electronic Claims Processing and Management

Dental providers

- Real-time coverage verification and eligibility reporting
- Access benefits summaries and details
- Fewer rejected claims
- Faster payments and improved cash flow
- Reduced administrative costs
- Improved case acceptance and patient relationships
- Improved insurance provider relationships
- Track claim status and provide activity reports

Insurance provider

- Receives cleaner claims, reducing claim-handling costs
- Drastically reduces call center volume and costs by providing online real-time claim status and eligibility
- Reduces administrative costs by delivering electronic EOB information to dental providers
- Clearinghouse reviews claims and validates prior to sending to insurance provider, ensuring that claims are routed to the correct provider

✚ HIPAA

E-claims Service Provider Certification

Health Insurance Portability and Accountability Act of 1996 (HIPAA) certification is required for all electronic submission and processing of dental claims. Companies that process and transmit claims have to follow all regulations outlined in the HIPAA regulations and be certified.

Paper Dental Claim Forms

Paper dental claim forms are generated by computer and printed in the office or are typewritten by the administrative dental assistant and sent from the dental office to the correct carrier via mail. The forms used should be approved by the American Dental Association (ADA) and the third-party carrier.

Superbills and Encounter Forms

Superbills and encounter forms are used to communicate the same type of information contained on a dental insurance claim form. Each superbill or encounter form contains patient information, subscriber information, billing dentist information, and signatures for assignment of benefits and release of information. The purpose of the superbill is to consolidate several different functions of the business office on one form. It provides a means by which to communicate what treatment procedures were completed and a method to track treatment (with routing slips); it is helpful in controlling the posting of dental procedures and services. It is also a quick method of supplying the patient with needed insurance information because the patient can use the superbill to bill the insurance company directly for services. Superbills are designed to be used with computer software programs and in manual posting systems (e.g., pegboard; Figure 15-1).

Encounter forms are used by third-party carriers for reporting of services rendered to policyholders. These forms are similar to superbills and are preprinted for manual or computerized billing. The configuration of the information varies from carrier to carrier. Superbills and encounter forms are typically forms that consist of multiple copies for the patient, the dentist, and the insurance carrier.

When superbills and encounter forms are ordered for the first time, all dentist billing information and the codes to be included on the preprinted forms must be supplied. Most companies will help the dental practice to design superbills and encounter forms that best meet its requirements.

INSURANCE PAYMENTS

Insurance payments can be made in one of two ways. The dental practice can enroll in automatic deposit. This service, when available, processes claims and deposits the payment as quickly as a few minutes or up to a maximum of a day or two, increasing the cash flow of the dental practice. When checks

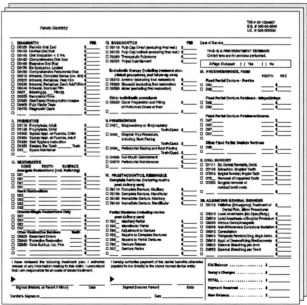

FIGURE 15-1 Example of a superbill to be completed manually. (Courtesy Patterson Office Supplies, Champaign, Ill.)

are sent to the dental practice in the form of a voucher, they are attached to an EOB form. Whether the check is deposited directly or mailed to the office, an EOB is provided. EOBs identify the name of the patient and the group number or other identification number. Depending on the type of insurance and stipulations outlined in an insurance contract, the EOB may contain an adjustment of any fee charged that was over the allowed amount. Normally, the EOB is self-explanatory regarding the breakdown of payment. The total fee is listed, including the amount the insurance company pays and the amount the patient must pay.

Some companies list several patients on a single voucher and care must be taken to post each patient correctly. Once the payment has been received, checked, and posted, the final step in the tracking system is completed. If a manual system is used, an entry is made in the insurance log or the claim is pulled from the file and stapled to the EOB.

INSURANCE TRACKING SYSTEMS

The objective of an insurance tracking system is to monitor the status of insurance claims. It is easy to overlook unpaid claims if they are forgotten. It is important to remember that the amount of money that flows through the dental practice depends on the amount of money that is billed to insurance companies. Each day a claim goes unpaid, the dental practice loses money. Develop a routine that is easy to follow and take the time to work the system. This will improve cash flow.

PROCEDURES

Steps in a Manual Insurance Tracking System

1. Place a copy of the dental claim form in a file for the month in which the claim was generated. Each claim filed during a given month is kept in a single file.
2. When payment is received, the copy of the claim is pulled from the file and stapled to the explanation of benefits (EOB). If the claim has a secondary carrier, the information can be entered on the claim and forwarded to the second insurance carrier for payment. A copy of the secondary claim is placed in the insurance file for the current month.
3. After 1 month, review any remaining claims for that month. If necessary, track the claim and determine why it has not been paid. After 2 months, further tracking is necessary. Claims should never remain in the file for longer than 2 months without the assistant's knowledge. Sometimes payment has been delayed because some information is missing. When additional information is sent, a notation should be made directly on the original dental claim form and in the patient's clinical record.
4. Place all paid claims in a file for the month in which the claim is paid (chronological filing system). These files can be stored in an area with easy access in case they are needed during the year. If EOBs must be checked, they can be located easily by the date of payment. After 1 year, these files can be placed in permanent storage. Check the established recommendations for the amount of time that this type of record must be kept.

Computerized systems that process claims produce electronic forms for submission. Tracking is done through the computer. Once a claim has been marked for submission, it is placed in a databank. Reports can be generated that identify the patient, amount of the claim, date filed, and date paid. Processing reports in the same manner as used in the manual system allows the administrative dental assistant to track all claims (Figure 15-2).

HELPFUL HINTS TO MANAGE INSURANCE PROCESSING

- Know the details of each insurance group, such as coverage, deductibles, limitations, and special handling instructions.
- Use the tools provided by insurance providers or third-party services to verify coverage quickly and efficiently.
- Know the details of contracts with insurance companies for preferred provider organizations (PPOs) and health maintenance organizations (HMOs).
- Use the appropriate fee schedule for each company (make sure the patient is charged the same fee that is submitted to the insurance company).
- Check each claim for accuracy. Procedures not listed will not be paid. If information is missing or the claim is not sent to the correct address, payment will be delayed.
- Develop a tracking system. Computer software programs will include functions to track the insurance billing from the time the claim is generated to the time it is paid. Sophisticated programs will also generate reports to identify unpaid claims or treatments that have not been billed.
- Work the tracking system to follow up on unpaid claims.
- Use the tracking system to identify work that has been authorized but not completed.
- Do not keep copies of dental claim forms in the clinical record. Copies of claims and explanations of benefits (EOBs) should be kept in a separate file.

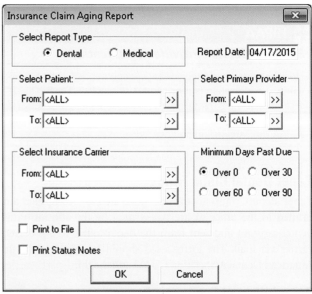

FIGURE 15-2 The Insurance Claim Aging Report quickly and easily locates outstanding insurance claim payments. (Dentrix screen capture courtesy Henry Schein Practice Solutions, American Fork, Utah.)

COMPLETING A DENTAL CLAIM FORM

There are two basic ways to file a dental claim form: The first is to mail the form (paper copy) directly to the insurance company and the second is to send the claim electronically. When a paper dental claim form is submitted, the form will be generated electronically or manually. The electronically prepared form will be generated by a software program, printed, and prepared for submission. The administrative dental assistant will check the dental claim form for completeness, obtain the necessary signatures, and attach documentation if required. When it is necessary for the administrative dental assistant to complete the dental claim form, he or she must enter the information on an approved claim form. It is the responsibility of the assistant to know how to complete the dental claim form correctly. This requires an understanding of what information, including coding, goes in each of the 58 specific data items on the form.

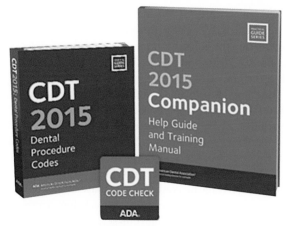

FIGURE 15-3 *CDT 2015 Dental Procedure Codes and CDT 2015 Companion on Dental Coding.* (Courtesy American Dental Association, Chicago, Ill.)

DOS AND DON'TS FOR SUBMITTING CLAIMS

Do Use
- A laser printer with black ink (if not transmitting electronically)
- A 10-point font and all capital letters (use a serif font such as Times New Roman or Courier)
- Eight-digit dates with no spaces, slashes, or dashes (for example, 05162016 for May 16, 2016)
- Standard size paper (8.5 × 11 inches) for claims and written documentation
- Fees with decimal points (for example, 200.00, not 200)

Don't Use
- Free form text—text that is not applicable to the data field; for example, writing the name of the tooth instead of the number or letter of the tooth
- Ditto marks or arrows to indicate duplicate information
- Stray marks in spaces that should be left blank
- Lines outside of boxes or writing on top of lines
- Correction fluid or a highlighter pen
- More than one font style on a claim

INSURANCE CODING

Current Dental Terminology, CDT-2015, is published by the ADA and is recognized by the federal government as the standard for reporting dental services in compliance with HIPAA (Figure 15-3). The first list of procedures was produced in 1969 and the Code Revision Committee (CRC) has made revisions and additions to the Code on an ongoing basis. This committee comprises members of the ADA and representatives from major health insurance plans and government programs.

Although the primary use of the *CDT-2015* is to identify and define the various transactions codes, it also contains information useful to the dental healthcare team in the

compilation of dental claim forms. The *CDT-2015* is cross-referenced, so it is easy to locate a procedure numerically by procedure code or alphabetically by procedure nomenclature in addition to the full description of the procedure code and nomenclature. Each time the Code is revised and updated, a section of the manual is used to identify and explain the new and revised codes. The first section of the manual contains the Code on Dental Procedures and Nomenclature (the Code). This section of the manual divides procedure codes into 12 categories (Table 15-1). Procedure codes are identified by a five-digit alphanumeric code, constituting the only approved coding system for the submission of dental claim forms that cannot be changed. The first digit of the code will be *D*, which identifies the code as a dental service code. The second digit describes the category and the remaining digits describe the nature of the procedure or service. For example, code D1110 is interpreted as follows: The first digit (letter), D, indicates a dental service. The second digit, 1, indicates a preventive procedure or service (see Table 15-1). The last three digits identify the procedure or service performed. After each dental procedure code is a

TABLE 15-1	**CDT-2015 Categories**	
I.	Diagnostic	D0100-D0999
II.	Preventive	D1000-D1999
III.	Restorative	D2000-D2999
IV.	Endodontics	D3000-D3999
V.	Periodontics	D4000-D4999
VI.	Prosthodontics, Removable	D5000-D58999
VII.	Maxillofacial Prosthetics	D59900-D5999
VIII.	Implant Services	D6000-D6199
IX.	Prosthodontics, Fixed	D6200-D6999
X.	Oral & Maxillofacial Surgery	D7000-D7999
XI.	Orthodontics	D8000-D8999
XII.	Adjunctive General Services	D9000-D9999

brief literal definition. This definition is referred to as the **nomenclature**. When the procedure is defined on a dental claim form, the nomenclature can be abbreviated. When necessary, a written narrative of the dental procedure may follow the nomenclature.

The most current CDT Manual is used to code dental claims. When claims are processed manually, it is the responsibility of the insurance clerk to enter correct codes by referencing the CDT Manual. This procedure requires that the insurance clerk be familiar with the outline of the Manual. When claims are processed electronically, the code is entered in the computer database by the developer of the software or the insurance clerk. When a procedure is coded and entered during transaction posting, the software converts the transaction code to the proper CDT code. When a dental claim is generated or printed electronically, the proper CDT code will appear. It is the responsibility of the administrative dental assistant to check the accuracy of the codes to ensure that the correct conversion has taken place.

The Systematized Nomenclature of Dentistry (SNODENT) is a combination of medical (SNOMED) conditions and dental conditions used to define dental diseases in an electronic environment. SNODENT is a comprehensive coding system used to identify diseases, diagnoses, anatomy, conditions, morphology, and social factors that may affect the outcomes of diagnosis and treatment. The use of these codes enables the dentist to describe conditions and other factors that relate to a given diagnosis. When fully implemented, the electronic health record (EHR) will be a more comprehensive patient history containing a patient's medical and dental history (from multiple providers) that can be used to improve quality, safety, and efficiency; reduce health disparities; engage patients and families; improve care coordination; provide information to be used in research and public health; and maintain privacy and security of the patient's health information. Currently, the use of SNODENT codes is optional in dentistry but when EHR mandates go into place around 2016, it is believed that a revised set of SNODENT codes will be used.

CODE FACTS

- In dentistry, CDT Procedure Codes are the codes used to report dental services.
- Dental specialists who submit medical claims use Physicians Procedures (CPT) codes to report medical procedures.
- The HIPAA Standard Diagnostic Code set for all transactions will be the ICD-10 (effective October 2015).
  - ICD-10-CM: used in medicine and dentistry
  - ICD-10-PCS: used in hospitals only
- ICD-10-CM codes will be used in the presence of a systemic condition that necessitates particular oral health services. The ICD-10 code can be reported on the American Dental Association (ADA) 2012 dental claim form or a medical claim form (depending on the requirements of the insurance carrier). (See Anatomy of a Dental Claim Form, boxes 29a, 34, and 34a.)

The International Classification of Diseases (ICD) is a set of codes used worldwide to classify medical diagnoses and inpatient procedures. ICD codes are primarily used for patient health records, provider reimbursement, and public health reporting and monitoring.

The primary purpose of using ICD-10 codes is to provide additional information that gives a better picture of why a procedure is necessary. For example, some insurance companies will cover an additional prophylaxis if certain systemic medical conditions, such as pregnancy, diabetes, chronic heart disease, and certain cancer treatments, exist. For example, the patient is diabetic and is eligible for an additional prophylaxis per year therefore you would code the claim using CDT code *D1110–prophylaxis, adult* and *ICD-10, E08.630 Diabetes due to underlying condition with periodontal disease.* By using the ICD-10 code, you have provided the documentation required by the insurance company without having to provide extensive written documentation.

Documentation Needed for Insurance Processing

Most claims submitted will not need documentation but for some procedures supporting documentation such as x-rays or charts help the insurance provider to determine if treatment is covered under the patient's benefit plan. For example, a consultant reviews a preoperative x-ray of a tooth to determine if the contractual criterion for a cast crown has been met. The contract may state that in order for a crown to be a covered benefit, so much tooth structure has been lost due to caries or fracture that a direct amalgam or resin restoration would not be an adequate restoration.

Each insurance provider has its own regulations and policies for documentation. The following are a sampling of common procedures that may require documentation.

When to Send X-Rays

- Restorative procedures such as crowns, laboratory processed (D2710-D2794) and core buildup, including any pins (D2950).
- Implant services, Implant supported prosthetics (D6055-D6077)
- Prosthodontics, Fixed partial denture retainers–crowns (D6710-D6794)

When to Send Periodontal Charting

- Osseous and other periodontal surgery procedures (D4210-D4212, D4240-D4245, and D4260-D4278)

When to Send a Narrative Report

- Hard and soft tissue biopsies (D7285-D7286)

The ADA Dental Claim Form (Figure 15-4) is accepted by all insurance carriers in submitting dental treatment for preauthorization and payment. The form is organized into 10 related sections and has a total of 58 data items (see Anatomy

ADA American Dental Association® **Dental Claim Form**

HEADER INFORMATION

1. Type of Transaction (Mark all applicable boxes)

☐ Statement of Actual Services   ☐ Request for Predetermination/Preauthorization

☐ EPSDT / Title XIX

2. Predetermination/Preauthorization Number

INSURANCE COMPANY/DENTAL BENEFIT PLAN INFORMATION

3. Company/Plan Name, Address, City, State, Zip Code

OTHER COVERAGE (Mark applicable box and complete items 5-11. If none, leave blank.)

4. Dental? ☐   Medical? ☐   (If both, complete 5-11 for dental only.)

5. Name of Policyholder/Subscriber in #4 (Last, First, Middle Initial, Suffix)

6. Date of Birth (MM/DD/CCYY)   7. Gender ☐ M ☐ F   8. Policyholder/Subscriber ID (SSN or ID#)

9. Plan/Group Number   10. Patient's Relationship to Person named in #5 ☐ Self ☐ Spouse ☐ Dependent ☐ Other

11. Other Insurance Company/Dental Benefit Plan Name, Address, City, State, Zip Code

POLICYHOLDER/SUBSCRIBER INFORMATION (For Insurance Company Named in #3)

12. Policyholder/Subscriber Name (Last, First, Middle Initial, Suffix), Address, City, State, Zip Code

13. Date of Birth (MM/DD/CCYY)   14. Gender ☐ M ☐ F   15. Policyholder/Subscriber ID (SSN or ID#)

16. Plan/Group Number   17. Employer Name

PATIENT INFORMATION

18. Relationship to Policyholder/Subscriber in #12 Above ☐ Self ☐ Spouse ☐ Dependent Child ☐ Other   19. Reserved For Future Use

20. Name (Last, First, Middle Initial, Suffix), Address, City, State, Zip Code

21. Date of Birth (MM/DD/CCYY)   22. Gender ☐ M ☐ F   23. Patient ID/Account # (Assigned by Dentist)

RECORD OF SERVICES PROVIDED

	24. Procedure Date (MM/DD/CCYY)	25. Area of Oral Cavity	26. Tooth System	27. Tooth Number(s) or Letter(s)	28. Tooth Surface	29. Procedure Code	29a. Diag. Pointer	29b. Qty.	30. Description	31. Fee
1										
2										
3										
4										
5										
6										
7										
8										
9										
10										

33. Missing Teeth Information   (Place an "X" on each missing tooth.)

1 2 3 4 5 6 7 8 9 10 11 12 13 14 15 16

32 31 30 29 28 27 26 25 24 23 22 21 20 19 18 17

34. Diagnosis Code List Qualifier ☐   (ICD-9 = B; ICD-10 = AB)

34a. Diagnosis Code(s)   A _____   C _____

(Primary diagnosis in "A")   B _____   D _____

31a. Other Fee(s)

32. Total Fee

35. Remarks

AUTHORIZATIONS

36. I have been informed of the treatment plan and associated fees. I agree to be responsible for all charges for dental services and materials not paid by my dental benefit plan, unless prohibited by law, or the treating dentist or dental practice has a contractual agreement with my plan prohibiting all or a portion of such charges. To the extent permitted by law, I consent to your use and disclosure of my protected health information to carry out payment activities in connection with this claim.

X _____
Patient/Guardian Signature   Date

37. I hereby authorize and direct payment of the dental benefits otherwise payable to me, directly to the below named dentist or dental entity.

X _____
Subscriber Signature   Date

BILLING DENTIST OR DENTAL ENTITY (Leave blank if dentist or dental entity is not submitting claim on behalf of the patient or insured/subscriber.)

48. Name, Address, City, State, Zip Code

49. NPI   50. License Number   51. SSN or TIN

52. Phone Number ( ) -   52a. Additional Provider ID

ANCILLARY CLAIM/TREATMENT INFORMATION

38. Place of Treatment ☐ (e.g. 11=office; 22=O/P Hospital) (Use "Place of Service Codes for Professional Claims")   39. Enclosures (Y or N) ☐

40. Is Treatment for Orthodontics? ☐ No (Skip 41-42) ☐ Yes (Complete 41-42)   41. Date Appliance Placed (MM/DD/CCYY)

42. Months of Treatment Remaining   43. Replacement of Prosthesis ☐ No ☐ Yes (Complete 44)   44. Date of Prior Placement (MM/DD/CCYY)

45. Treatment Resulting from

☐ Occupational illness/injury   ☐ Auto accident   ☐ Other accident

46. Date of Accident (MM/DD/CCYY)   47. Auto Accident State

TREATING DENTIST AND TREATMENT LOCATION INFORMATION

53. I hereby certify that the procedures as indicated by date are in progress (for procedures that require multiple visits) or have been completed.

X _____
Signed (Treating Dentist)   Date

54. NPI   55. License Number

56. Address, City, State, Zip Code   56a. Provider Specialty Code

57. Phone Number ( ) -   58. Additional Provider ID

©2012 American Dental Association
J430D (Same as ADA Dental Claim Form – J430, J431, J432, J433, J434)

To reorder call 800.947.4746
or go online at adacatalog.org

FIGURE 15-4 The American Dental Association dental claim form. (Copyright © 2012 American Dental Association, Chicago, Ill.)

of a Dental Claim Form for detailed information on each of the data items).

❗ REMEMBER

Incorrect coding that causes an overpayment of services is an act of fraud.

✚ HIPAA

Electronic Transactions and Code Sets

Code on Dental Procedures and Nomenclature lists the code sets that are recognized by the Health Insurance Portability and Accountability Act of 1996 (HIPAA) for the electronic submission of dental claims.

✚ HIPAA

Privacy Rule

The patient authorizes release of protected health information (PHI) to the insurance company for the purpose of processing the insurance claim.

HIPAA

National Provider Identifier (NPI)

Beginning as early as May 23, 2005, providers were eligible to apply for their NPI. All entities covered by the Health Insurance Portability and Accountability Act of 1996 (HIPAA) were required to use NPIs by the compliance dates: May 23, 2007, for most groups and May 23, 2008, for small health plans. The personal NPI is the only allowable identifier (accepted by all insurance companies and third-party payers) and must be included on all claims submissions.

The NPI replaced other identifying numbers used in electronic claims submission such as:
- Medicaid
- Blue Cross and Blue Shield

- Unique Physician Identification Number (UPIN)
- Civilian Health and Medical Program of the Uniformed Services (CHAMPUS)

The NPI *did not* replace the following numbers, which are used for purposes other than general identification:
- Social Security
- Drug Enforcement Administration (DEA)
- Taxpayer Identification
- Taxonomy
- State license

ANATOMY OF A DENTAL CLAIM FORM

ADA American Dental Association® **Dental Claim Form**

HEADER INFORMATION

1. Type of Transaction (Mark all applicable boxes)
   - ☒ Statement of Actual Services
   - ☐ Request for Predetermination/Preauthorization ①
   - ☐ EPSDT/Title XIX

2. Predetermination/Preauthorization Number ②

HEADER INFORMATION (1,2)
The header contains information about the type of transaction; statement of actual treatment; predetermination/preauthorization; Early and Periodic Screening, Diagnosis and Treatment program (EPSDT); and the predetermination/preauthorization number.

① **Type of Transaction (Mark all applicable boxes):**
Statement of Actual Services: This box is checked when the services listed have been completed.
Request for Predetermination/Preauthorization: This box is used to request an estimate of dental benefits before treatment begins. Some insurance carriers ask that all treatment for a specified procedure or dollar amount be submitted. It is best to have complete information about the insurance coverage before treatment is started in order to make financial arrangements with the patient. **REMEMBER**: *There should be no surprises — insurance coverage and patient financial responsibility must be disclosed and agreed upon before treatment begins.*

CAUTION: Pre-estimate figures are not a guarantee of payment by the insurance carrier. The final payment may change due to previous unpaid claims and current enrollment status of the patient.
EPSDT/Title XIX: This box is checked if the patient is part of a *special* program through the Early and Periodic Screening, Diagnosis, and Treatment Program.

② **Predetermination/Preauthorization Number:** This box is used when a claim has been previously preauthorized and you are now submitting it for payment. The preauthorization number will be provided by the insurance company.

INSURANCE COMPANY/DENTAL BENEFIT PLAN INFORMATION

3. Company/Plan Name, Address, City, State, Zip Code

Cigna ③
P.O. Box 467
Denver CO 76452

INSURANCE COMPANY/DENTAL BENEFIT PLAN INFORMATION (3)
This section contains information about the insurance company or the third party payer. If the patient is covered by more than one insurance company, the primary insurance company information is entered in this section.

③ **Company/Plan Name, Address, City, State, Zip Code:** This item must always be completed. The information is provided by the patient and will be used to mail the insurance claim form to the insurance company. If the patient is covered by more than one insurance plan, this information will

be for the primary carrier. **REMEMBER:** *Each insurance company may have several different offices that process claims. Check the patient's insurance identification card for the correct billing address.*

OTHER COVERAGE (Mark applicable box and complete items 5-11. If none, leave blank.)

4. Dental? ☒ Medical? ☐ (If both, complete items 5-11 for dental only.) ④

5. Name of Policyholder/Subscriber in #4 (Last, First, Middle Initial, Suffix)
⑤ Rogers, Doris

6. Date of Birth (MM/DD/CCYY) ⑥ 12/02/1960

7. Gender ⑦ ☐ M ☒ F

8. Policyholder/Subscriber ID (SSN or ID#) 63224 ⑧

9. Plan/Group Number ⑨ 63467

10. Patient's Relationship to Person Named in #5 ☐ Self ☐ Spouse ☒ Dependent ☐ Other ⑩

11. Other Insurance Company/Dental Benefit Plan Name, Address, City, State, Zip Code
Delta Dental ⑪
P.O. Box 3333
San Francisco CA 90234

(Portions of claim form shown Copyright © 2012 American Dental Association, Chicago, Ill. All rights reserved. Reprinted with permission.)

Text continued on page 232

ANATOMY OF A DENTAL CLAIM FORM (cont'd)

OTHER COVERAGE (4-11)

This section describes additional insurance coverage information. This may include additional dental or medical insurance coverage. The purpose of this section is to help the insurance company determine whether there is additional insurance and the need for coordination of benefits.

④ Other Dental or Medical Coverage?
Mark the type of coverage (Dental or Medical) the patient has under any other dental or medical plan. When either box is checked, complete Items 5-11. If neither of the boxes is marked leave 5-11 blank. Note: if both Dental and Medical are marked, enter information about the dental benefit plan in 5-11.

⑤ Name of Policyholder/Subscriber in #4 (Last, First, Middle Initial, Suffix): In this box you will identify the person who has additional dental or medical insurance. The additional coverage could be through a spouse, domestic partner or, if a child, through both parents. In some cases the secondary coverage could be through a second policy of the patient.

⑥ Date of Birth (MM/DD/CCYY): The birth date entered pertains to the person identified in Item 5. Enter the full date (eight digits): two for the month, two for the day of the month, and four for the year.

⑦ Gender: Enter the gender for the person identified in Item 5.

⑧ Policyholder/Subscriber ID (SSN or ID#): Enter the number that has been assigned to the subscriber (Item 5) by the insurance carrier. **REMEMBER:** *You must use the number issued by the insurance company. The use of the SSN may not be permitted as an identifier in some states.*

⑨ Plan/Group Number: Enter the group plan or policy number of the person in Item 5. This number will be on the patient's insurance card.

⑩ Patient's Relationship to Person Named in #5: Enter the relationship between the person identified in Item 5 and the patient.

⑪ Other Insurance Company/Dental Benefit Plan Name, Address, City, State, Zip Code: Enter the information for the insurance carrier of the person identified in Item 5.

POLICYHOLDER/SUBSCRIBER INFORMATION (For Insurance Company Named in #3)

12. Policyholder/Subscriber Name (Last, First, Middle Initial, Suffix), Address, City, State, Zip Code

Rogers, Donald S
8176 Hillside Drive
Riverville CA 90070　⑫

13. Date of Birth (MM/DD/CCYY)	14. Gender ⑭	15. Policyholder/Subscriber ID (SSN or ID#)
⑬ 02/08/1967	☒ M ☐ F	⑮ 01234

16. Plan/Group Number	17. Employer Name
43216 ⑯	Riverville Police Department ⑰

POLICYHOLDER/SUBSCRIBER INFORMATION (12-17)

This section contains information about the insured person (policyholder/subscriber), who may or may not be the dental patient.

⑫ Policyholder/Subscriber Name (Last, First, Middle Initial, Suffix), Address, City, State, Zip Code: Enter the full name and address of the policyholder/subscriber (employee).

⑬ Date of Birth (MM/DD/CCYY): This is the birth date of the insured, identified in item #12 (this may or may not be the patient). Enter the full date (eight digits): two for the month, two for the day of the month, and four for the year.

⑭ Gender: This information applies to the insured, identified in item #12 (who may or may not be the patient).

⑮ Policyholder/Subscriber ID (SSN or ID#): Enter the assigned identifier issued by the insurance company. This information will be located on the patient's insurance identification card.

⑯ Plan/Group Number: Enter the plan or group number of the primary insurance company. This information will be located on the patient's insurance identification card.

⑰ Employer Name: If applicable, enter the name of the insured's employer.

Continued

ANATOMY OF A DENTAL CLAIM FORM (cont'd)

PATIENT INFORMATION

18. Relationship to Policyholder/Subscriber in #12 Above ⑱
☐ Self   ☐ Spouse   ☒ Dependent Child   ☐ Other

19. Reserved For Future Use ⑲

20. Name (Last, First, Middle Initial, Suffix), Address, City, State, Zip Code

Rogers, Jason
8176 Hillside Drive ⑳
Riverville CA 90070

21. Date of Birth (MM/DD/CCYY)	22. Gender ㉒	23. Patient ID/Account # (Assigned by Dentist)
㉑ 03/12/2000	☒ M ☐ F	㉓ R349877

PATIENT INFORMATION (18-23)
This section contains information about the patient.

⑱ **Relationship to Policyholder/Subscriber in #12 Above:**
Check the box that identifies the relationship of the policyholder/subscriber to the patient. If the patient is also the insured, check the "Self" box and skip to item #23.

⑲ **Reserved for Future Use:**
Leave blank.

⑳ **Name (Last, First, Middle Initial, Suffix), Address, City, State, Zip Code:** Enter the complete name of the patient.

㉑ **Date of Birth (MM/DD/CCYY):**
This is the birth date of the patient identified in item 20. Enter the full date (total of eight digits): two for the month, two for the day of the month, and four for the year.

㉒ **Gender:**
This information applies to the patient.

㉓ **Patient ID/Account # (Assigned by Dentist):**
Enter the patient ID# that has been assigned by the dental practice (this is not required to process the claim).

RECORD OF SERVICES PROVIDED

	24. Procedure Date (MM/DD/CCYY)	25. Area of Oral Cavity	26. Tooth System	27. Tooth Number(s) or Letter(s)	28. Tooth Surface	29. Procedure Code	29a. Diag. Pointer	29b. Qty.	30. Description	31. Fee
1	12/10/2015	10				D0220			**Periapical First Film**	$62.00
2	12/10/2015	20		㉗	㉘	D0230			**Additional Film**	$36.00
3	12/10/2015	00				D1110	A		**Prophylaxis - Adult**	$121.00
4	12/18/2015		JP	2	MO	D2150			**Amalgam**	$105.00
5	12/18/2015		JP	7		D2720			**Crown-Resin /High Noble**	$861.00
6		㉕								
7	㉔		㉖			㉙	㉙a	㉙b	㉚	㉛
8										
9										
10										

33. Missing Teeth Information (Place an "X" on each missing tooth) ㉝

☒ 2 3 4 5 6 7 8 9 10 11 12 13 14 15 ☒
☒ 31 30 29 28 27 26 25 24 23 22 21 20 19 18 ☒

34. Diagnosis Code List Qualifier A|B (ICD-9 = B; ICD-10 = AB) ㉞

34a. Diagnosis Code(s) ㉞a   A E08.630 ___   C ___
(Primary diagnosis in "A")   B ___   D ___

31a. Other Fee(s) ㉛a

32. Total Fee $1185.00 ㉜

35. Remarks ㉟

RECORD OF SERVICES PROVIDED (24-35)
This section records information about each of the services being submitted for payment or predetermination/preauthorization (do not enter dates for predetermination/preauthorization).

NOTE: Items 24-31 apply to each dental service and will be repeated if multiple services are being billed. There is space for 10 services on each dental claim form; if additional space is needed it will be necessary to complete additional claim forms. Each additional claim form will need to be fully completed (all information will be repeated on the second claim form).

㉔ **Procedure Date (MM/DD/CCYY):**
Enter the date for each completed procedure. Enter the full date (eight digits): two for the month, two for the day of the month, and four for the year. If the claim is for preauthorization the date is left blank.
Remember: You **cannot** combine "actual services" and a request for "predetermination/preauthorization" on the same dental claim form.

㉕ **Area of Oral Cavity:** The use of this data item will depend on the type of service or procedure being reported. You will not need to complete this item if:
- The procedure requires the identification of a tooth number, or a range of teeth.
- The procedure identifies a specific area. For example, complete denture—mandibular
- The procedure does not relate to any portion of the oral cavity. For example, sedation/general anesthesia.

Two-digit Codes Used to Identify Specific Areas of the Oral Cavity	
Code	**Area of Oral Cavity**
00	Entire oral cavity
01	Maxillary arch
02	Mandibular arch
10	Upper right quadrant
20	Upper left quadrant
30	Lower left quadrant
40	Lower right quadrant

ANATOMY OF A DENTAL CLAIM FORM (cont'd)

26 **Tooth System:** Enter "JP" when the tooth designation system being used is the ADA's Universal/National Tooth Designation System (1-32 for permanent dentition and A-T for primary dentition). Enter "JO" when using the International Standards Organization System (see Chapter 2 for full details of the various tooth designation systems).

27 **Tooth Number(s) or Letter(s):** Enter the number or range of numbers that applies to the procedure. If the procedure does not involve a specific tooth or range of teeth leave item #27 blank.
REMEMBER: *If the same procedure has been completed more than one time, each repeated procedure will have to be entered on a separate line.* When entering a range of teeth numbers (and it is appropriate to enter them on the same line) the teeth numbers can be separated with a comma, for example: 2,3,5, or for a continual range of numbers 3-6.

28 **Tooth Surface:** When a procedure requires that the tooth surface be identified, the following is a list of the single abbreviations (see Chapter 2 for a complete list of tooth surfaces)

Surface	Code
Buccal	B
Distal	D
Facial (or Labial)	F
Incisal	I
Lingual	L
Mesial	M
Occlusal	O

29 **Procedure Code:** Enter the appropriate procedure code found in the latest version of the *Code on Dental Procedures and Nomenclature.*

29a **Diagnosis Code Pointer:** This box is used to 'point' to the ICD-10 diagnosis code(s) in 34a that are applicable to the dental procedure. List the primary diagnosis pointer first.

29b **Quantity:** This box identifies the quantity or the number of times (01-99) the procedure identified in box 29 is delivered to the patient on the date of service shown in box 24.

30 **Description:** Briefly describe the service. You can abbreviate the description. CAUTION: Use standard abbreviations that are common with dental terminology.

31 **Fee:** Enter the full fee charges by the dentist.

31a **Other Fee(s):** Enter any other charges applicable to dental services provided that must be reported, such as state tax and other charges imposed by regulatory agencies.

32 **Total Fee:** The sum of fees from line #31 and #31a

33 **Missing Teeth Information:** Chart missing teeth when reporting periodontal, prosthodontic (fixed and removable), or implant procedures.

34 **Diagnosis Code List Qualifies:** Enter the appropriate code to identify the source of the diagnosis code. AB=ICD-10CM. This code will provide additional information that will give a better picture of why a procedure is necessary.

34a **Diagnosis Code(s):** Enter the primary ICD-10CM code in A and additional applicable codes in B-D

35 **Remarks:** Enter additional information for procedure codes that require a report, or when you believe additional information will help in the processing of the claim (for example, the amount the primary carrier paid on the claim).

AUTHORIZATIONS

36. I have been informed of the treatment plan and associated fees. I agree to be responsible for all charges for dental services and materials not paid by my dental benefit plan, unless prohibited by law, or the treating dentist or dental practice has a contractual agreement with my plan prohibiting all or a portion of such charges. To the extent permitted by law, I consent to your use and disclosure of my protected health information to carry out payment activities in connection with this claim.

X _Jason Rogers_ **36** _12-18-15_
Patient/Guardian signature   Date

37. I hereby authorize and direct payment of the dental benefits otherwise payable to me, directly to the below named dentist or dental entity.

X _Donald Rogers_ **37** _12-18-15_
Subscriber signature   Date

AUTHORIZATIONS (36,37)
This section requests the signature of the patient or guardian stating consent to the treatment plan, acceptance of financial responsibility, and permission to release protected health information (PHI) to the insurance company or third party payer. In addition, the subscriber signs to authorize the insurance company to send payment for treatment directly to the dentist or dental business entity

36 **Patient Consent:** The patient, or patient's parent, caretaker, guardian, or other individual as appropriate under state law, must sign the form stating that they have been informed of the treatment, accept financial responsibility, and have established a professional relationship with the dentist for the delivery of dental health care.

37 **Signature of Policyholder/Subscriber:** The signature and date, or signature on file, is required when the policyholder/subscriber wishes to have benefits paid directly to the dentist.

Continued

ANATOMY OF A DENTAL CLAIM FORM (cont'd)

ANCILLARY CLAIM/TREATMENT INFORMATION

38. Place of Treatment 11 (e.g. 11=office; 22=O/P Hospital (Use "Place of Service Codes for Professional Claims") 38	39. Enclosures (Y or N) 39 Y
40. Is Treatment for Orthodontics? 40 ☒ No (Skip 41-42) ☐ Yes (Complete 41-42)	41. Date Appliance Placed (MM/DD/CCYY) 41
42. Months of Treatment Remaining 42	43. Replacement of Prosthesis 43 ☒ No ☐ Yes (Complete 44)	44. Date of Prior Placement (MM/DD/CCYY) 44
45. Treatment Resulting from 45 ☐ Occupational illness/injury ☐ Auto accident ☐ Other accident	
46. Date of Accident (MM/DD/CCYY) 46	47. Auto Accident State 47

ANCILLARY CLAIM/TREATMENT INFORMATION (38-47)
This section contains additional information needed by the insurance company or third party payer to determine patient coverage.

38 Place of Treatment:
Enter the 2-digit HIPAA standard code for Professional Claims
11-Office, 12-Home, 21-Inpatient Hospital, 22-Outpaitent Hospital,
31-Skilled Nursing Facility, 32-Nursing Facility
For a complete list search CMS Place of Service Codes

39 Number of Enclosures (00 to 99):
Place a "Y" in the box if enclosures, such as radiographs, digital images, or models are included with the claims submission. Place a "N" in the box if there are no enclosures.

40 Is Treatment for Orthodontics?:
No (Skip 41 and 42): If the treatment is not for orthodontics check the box and skip to item #43.
Yes (Complete 41 and 42): If this box is checked you will need to complete data items 41 and 42.

41 Date Appliance Placed (MM/DD/CCYY):
Indicate the date an orthodontic appliance was placed. This information should also be reported in this section for later orthodontic visits.

42 Months of Treatment Remaining:
Enter the estimated number of months required to complete the orthodontic treatment.

43 Replacement of Prosthesis?:
This item applies to crowns and all fixed or removable prostheses (bridges and dentures). There are three statements to guide in the completion of the item.
1. If the claim **does not involve a prosthetic restoration**, *mark the box NO* and proceed to item #45.
2. If the claim is the **initial placement** of a crown or a fixed or removable prosthesis, *mark the box NO* and proceed to item #45.
3. If the patient **previously had these teeth replaced** by a crown or a fixed or removable prosthesis, *mark the box YES* and complete item #44.

44 Date of Prior Placement (MM/DD/CCYY):
Enter the date of the prior placement of the crown or the fixed or removable prosthesis.

45 Treatment Resulting From:
If the dental treatment is the result of an accident or injury, check the applicable box and complete items #46 and #47. If the dental treatment is not the result of an accident or injury, this item does not apply; proceed to item #48.

46 Date of Accident (MM/DD/CCYY):
Enter the date of the accident or injury.

47 Auto Accident State:
If the accident was an auto accident (item #45), enter the state in which the auto accident occurred. If not an auto accident, leave item #47 blank.

BILLING DENTIST OR DENTAL ENTITY (Leave blank if dentist or dental entity is not submitting claim on behalf of the patient or insured/subscriber.)

48. Name, Address, City, State, Zip Code 48
Canyon View Dental
4546 North Avery Way
Canyon View CA 91783

49. NPI 49 DDS34569	50. License Number 50 CA123567	51. SSN or TIN 51 95-7689321
52. Phone Number (000) 555-8976 52		52a. Additional Provider ID 52a

If the patient is submitting the dental claim form directly and has not signed item #37, do not complete items 48-52.

©2012 American Dental Association
J430D (Same as ADA Dental Claim Form – J430, J431, J432, J433, J434)

BILLING DENTIST OR DENTAL ENTITY (48-52)
This section provides information about the individual dentist or dental entity that is submitting the claim for payment. The information may or may not pertain to the treating dentist. This section will not be completed if the patient is submitting the claim directly to the insurance company for payment.

48 Name, Address, City, State, and Zip Code:
Enter the information of the billing dentist or dental entity.

49 NPI:
Enter the provider identifier assigned to the billing dentist or dental entity. This number **is not** an SSN or TIN number. The identifier is assigned by the insurance company or third party payer. This item can be left blank if an identifier has not been assigned.

ANATOMY OF A DENTAL CLAIM FORM (cont'd)

50 **License Number:**
Enter the license number of the billing dentist. If a dental entity is entered in item #48, leave this item blank.

51 **SSN or TIN:**
1. If the billing dentist is an individual (unincorporated) enter the SSN or TIN.
2. Enter the TIN if the individual dentist is incorporated or billing for an incorporated dental entity.
3. Enter the TIN if the billing dentist or dental entity is a group practice or dental clinic.

52 **Phone Number:**
Enter the business phone number of the billing dentist or dental entity.

52a **Additional Provider ID:**
Enter any additional provider identifiers for the dentist or dental entry.

TREATING DENTIST AND TREATMENT LOCATION INFORMATION

53. I hereby certify that the procedures as indicated by date are in progress (for procedures that require multiple visits) or have been completed.

X _Mary Edwards_ **53**   _12-18-2015_
Signed (Treating Dentist)   Date

54. NPI DDS89765 **54**	55. License Number CA123567 **55**
56. Address, City, State, Zip Code **56** **4546 North Avery Way** **Canyon View CA 91783**	57. Provider Specialty Code **1123G001X** **56a**
57. Phone Number **(000) 555-8976** **57**	58. Additional Provider ID **12230000X** **58**

To reorder call 800.947.4746
or go online at adacatalog.org

TREATING DENTIST AND TREATMENT LOCATION INFORMATION (53-58)
The information in this section pertains to the dentist who has provided treatment.

53 **Certification:**
Have the treating dentist (can be different from the billing dentist) sign the certification statement. By signing the certification the treating dentist is verifying the following that the procedures and services listed on the claim have been completed or are in progress.

54 **NPI:** Enter the provider identifier assigned to the treating dentist. This number is not an SSN or TIN number. The identifier is assigned by the insurance company or third party payer. This item can be left blank if an identifier has not been assigned.

55 **License Number:**
Enter the license number of the treating dentist.

56 **Address, City, State, and Zip Code:**
Enter the mailing address of the treating dentist.

56a **Provider Specialty Code:**
Enter the number that identifies the treating dentist. The following list is a code set that has been assigned to members of the dental healthcare team. The code comes from the *Dental Service Providers'* section of the *Healthcare Providers Taxonomy Code* list used in all HIPAA transactions.

> The Provider Taxonomy is a unique alphanumeric code, ten characters in length. The code list is structured into three distinct "Levels" including Provider Type, Classification, and Area of Specialization. (See page 224.)

57 **Phone Number:**
Enter the business telephone number of the treating dentist.

58 **Additional Provider ID:**
Enter any additional provider identifiers for the treating dentist.

Dental Provider Taxonomy

Dental Providers
- Dental Assistant – **126800000X**
- Dental Hygienist – **124Q00000X**
- Dental Laboratory Technician – **126900000X**
- Dentist – **122300000X**
  - Dental Public Health – **1223D0001X**
  - Endodontics – **1223E0200X**
  - General Practice – **1223G0001X**

- Oral and Maxillofacial Pathology – **1223P0106X**
- Oral and Maxillofacial Radiology – **1223X0008X**
- Oral and Maxillofacial Surgery – **1223S0112X**
- Orthodontics and Dentofacial Orthopedics – **1223X0400X**
- Pediatric Dentistry – **1223P0221X**
- Periodontics – **1223P0300X**
- Prosthodontics – **1223P0700X**
- Denturist – **122400000X**

PROCEDURES

Steps in Processing a Dental Claim Form

1. *Obtain information from the patient.* Have the patient complete the registration form, and check for completeness. Also, photocopy and check the patient's insurance card. The card provides information such as an ID number, group number, and billing addresses for claims.
2. *Verify coverage* by contacting the insurance carrier, consulting an insurance information service, or using information in the practice management system.
3. *Discuss the coverage with the patient and determine the patient's portion.* Stress that the patient is responsible for the full amount if the insurance company does not pay. File the treatment plan for preauthorization if required by the patient or the insurance company.
4. *Complete the dental claim form.* If submitting a paper claim, complete the dental claim form for completed dental procedures (use the patient's chart to identify completed treatment). Check the form for accuracy and make sure that the correct codes have been used and that all treatments have been listed. When submitting electronic claims, confirm the dental procedures and make sure that all data items have been completed on the dental claim form (Figure 15-5).
5. *Include documentation* such as radiographs, oral images, models, or pocket measurements as requested by the insurance company. If you are not sure what needs to be included, check the insurance handbook, call the insurance company, or check with the insurance information service. When you submit electronically, follow the protocol of the insurance company for needed documentation.
6. *Record in the patient's clinical record* the date on which the claim was submitted and the treatment included.
7. *Record the information in a tracking system.* A tracking system helps to organize insurance information and provides a means for the administrative dental assistant to check on the status of claims.
8. *Post insurance payments and bill the patient for the balance.* If an adjustment must be made, it is done at this time. For example, a claim filed with Delta Dental is over the preset fee schedule for a prophylaxis. According to the contract, you cannot charge the patient the difference; therefore adjust the disallowed amount from the patient's balance.

> **! REMEMBER**
>
> You cannot write off the patient balance.

9. *Record the payment in your tracking system.* When a claim has been paid, it should be removed from the tracking system. Develop a method to flag claims that have both primary and secondary insurance carriers. It is necessary to enter the amount paid by the primary carrier before billing the secondary insurance.
10. *Follow up on any unpaid claims within 30 days of submission.* The purpose of the tracking system is to ensure that claims are not forgotten when they are not paid. The longer you wait to follow up, the longer it will take the dentist to receive a payment.

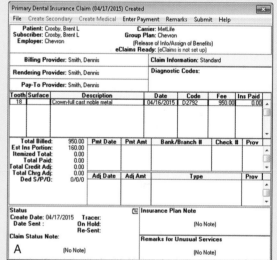

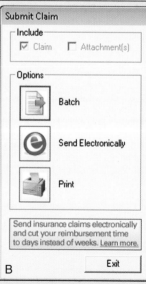

FIGURE 15-5 Electronic claims information can be completed easily in one place **(A)** and quickly submitted to the insurance company **(B)**. (Dentrix screen captures courtesy Henry Schein Practice Solutions, American Fork, Utah.)

> **! REMEMBER**
>
> The dentist has a legal and ethical obligation in the submission of dental claims. Review the ADA Principles of Ethics and Code of Professional Conduct, Advisory Opinions.

FRAUDULENT INSURANCE BILLING

No matter what the intention, when false information is given on a dental claim form, it becomes a concern to the dentist, the insurance carrier, and the patient. When a dental practice participates in a state or federally funded program it may be necessary to complete the Fraud, Waste and Abuse (FWA) training no later than December 31 of each year. The dental practice can complete this training through an authorized entity or develop its own training that meets the requirements of the Centers for Medicare and Medicaid Services (CMS). The ADA addresses this issue in section 5.B of its Principles of Ethics and Code of Professional Conduct, with official advisory opinions revised to April 2012.

Advisory Opinions
5.B. Representation of Fees
Dentists shall not represent the fees being charged for providing care in a false or misleading manner.

5.B.1. Waiver of Copayment
A dentist who accepts a third party* payment under a copayment plan as payment in full without disclosing to the third party* that the patient's payment portion will not be collected is engaged in overbilling. The essence of this ethical impropriety is deception and misrepresentation; an overbilling dentist makes it appear to the third party* that the charge to the patient for services rendered is higher than it actually is. (*A third party is any party to a dental prepayment contract that may collect premiums, assume financial risks, pay claims, and/or provide administrative services.)

5.B.2. Overbilling
It is unethical for a dentist to increase a fee to a patient solely because the patient is covered under a dental benefits plan.

5.B.3. Fee Differential
The fee for a patient without dental benefits shall be considered a dentist's full fee.** This is the fee that should be represented to all benefit carriers regardless of any negotiated fee discount. Payments accepted by a dentist under a governmentally funded program, a component or constituent dental society-sponsored access program, or a participating agreement entered into under a program with a third party shall not be considered or construed as evidence of overbilling in determining whether a charge to a patient, or to another third party* in behalf of a patient not covered under any of the aforecited programs constitutes overbilling under this section of the Code. (**A full fee is the fee for a service that is set by the dentist, which reflects the costs of providing the procedure and the value of the dentist's professional judgment.)

5.B.4. Treatment Dates
A dentist who submits a claim form to a third party* reporting incorrect treatment dates for the purpose of assisting a patient in obtaining benefits under a dental plan, which benefits would otherwise be disallowed, is engaged in making an unethical, false, or misleading representation to such third party.*

5.B.5. Dental Procedures
A dentist who incorrectly describes on a third party* claim form a dental procedure in order to receive a greater payment or reimbursement or incorrectly makes a non-covered procedure appear to be a covered procedure on such a claim is engaged in making an unethical, false, or misleading representation of such third party.*

5.B.6. Unnecessary Services
A dentist who recommends and performs unnecessary dental services or procedures is engaged in unethical conduct. The dentist's ethical obligation in this matter applies regardless of the type of practice arrangement or contractual obligations in which he or she provides patient care.

▮ KEY POINTS

- Dental insurance processing requires an understanding of different types of insurance coverage (insurance plans), insurance terminology, and effective insurance coding.
- Insurance coding is accomplished by referring to the current *CDT User's Manual*. This manual provides standardized claim forms, procedure codes, and nomenclature. The codes are divided into 12 categories and each category is subdivided into specific procedures.
- To determine each patient's insurance coverage, you must identify the insurance carrier and the details of the coverage, including
  - Maximum coverage
  - Type of deductible
  - Percentage of payment
  - Limitation to coverage
  - Eligibility
  - Preauthorization or pretreatment specifications
- Forms for filing insurance claims include paper claims (manually and computer generated), superbills, encounter forms, and electronically submitted forms. Manual and electronic tracking systems monitor the status of each claim. This helps the administrative dental assistant to locate and follow up on unpaid claims.
- A correctly completed dental claim form will contain all information requested in each data item. This information is taken from the patient's clinical chart (review the clinical chart in Chapter 8).

CAREER-READY PRACTICES

Career-Ready Practices activities are designed to provide students with experiences that can be "practiced" in preparation for skills needed on the job. In each of the following exercises, a variety of approaches may be used to address the problem, rather than "right" or "wrong" answers. Below each exercise, next to the compass icon, is a listing of suggested Career-Ready Practice numbers that correspond to the listing of 12 practices in the front of the text (see p. viii-ix); these practices provide suggestions for approaches to complete the exercise.

Based on the information given in the boxes below for Jason Rogers, complete the following exercise.

1. List the information you would place on the attending dentist's claim form in the following boxes: 8, 12, 18, 19, 20, 21, 22, 24, 28, 32, 38, and 39. The policy uses the birthday rule.

Career-Ready Practices
  2 Apply appropriate academic and technical skills.

PERSONAL INFORMATION

Birth date	3-12-1995
Soc. Sec. #	321-68-2173
Name	Jason Rogers
Sex	Male
Address	8176 Hillside Drive, Riverville, CA
Employer	Full-Time Student, UCLA

RESPONSIBLE PARTY

Name	Donald Rogers
Relationship to Patient	Father
Birth Date	2/8/1967
Address	8176 Hillside Drive, Riverville, CA
Employer	Riverville Police Department
Occupation	Captain
Work Phone	261-324-9111
Home Phone	261-483-6217

DENTAL INSURANCE INFORMATION

Name of Insured	Donald Rogers
Relationship to Patient	Father
Insurer's Birth Date	2/8/67
Soc. Sec. #	012-34-5678
Employer	Riverville Police Department
Date Employed	Jan. 1970
Occupation	Police Captain
Insurance Company	Northwest
Group #	43216
Employee Certificate #	7321456790
Ins. Co. Address	P.O. Box 467, Denver, CO
Max. Annual Benefit	$2000.00

ADDITIONAL DENTAL INSURANCE INFORMATION

Name of Insured	Doris Rogers
Relationship to Patient	Mother
Insurer's Birth Date	12/2/70
Soc. Sec. #	632-24-7654
Employer	Riverville School District
Date Employed	Sept. 1991
Occupation	Teacher
Insurance Company	Delta Dental
Group #	634567
Employee Certificate #	632-24-7654
Ins. Co. Address	P.O. Box 3333, San Francisco, CA
Max. Annual Benefit	$1500.00

TREATMENT

Date	Tooth and Surface	Treatment	Fee
2/10/16		3 Periapical x-rays	40.00
2/10/16	2 MO	Amalgam	92.00
2/10/16	3 O	Amalgam	81.00
2/10/16	4 MOD	Amalgam	108.00
2/24/16	8 MI	Composite	140.00
2/24/16	9 M	Composite	110.00
3/8/16	17	Extraction full bony impaction	195.00
3/3/16	18	Extraction partially bony	110.00

Bookkeeping Procedures: Accounts Payable

LEARNING OBJECTIVES

1. Describe the function of accounts payable.
2. Formulate a system to organize accounts payable.
3. Analyze the methods of check writing and state their functions.
4. Discuss steps to reconcile a bank statement and list the necessary information.

5. Discuss payroll, including the information needed for a payroll record, the calculation of payroll and necessary taxes, reporting of payroll, and payroll services.

INTRODUCTION

Accounts payable is a system by which all dental practice expenditures are organized, verified, and categorized. The system identifies when checks for bills (including payroll) are to be written, verifies charges, and categorizes expenditures. Other elements of the accounts payable system include reconciliation of the checking accounts and preparation of documents for the accountant.

ORGANIZING AN ACCOUNTS PAYABLE SYSTEM

1. Establish set dates each month when checks will be generated. Some payroll checks, payments to government agencies, and other types of payments have a specific date that they must be paid on or a penalty will be assessed. Monthly statements include a grace period; when a payment is received after the grace period, additional interest or late fees may be charged. Always allow ample time for the payment to be received and processed. When a check is sent via mail, it may take up to 10 days for the check to be received and processed. When bills are paid electronically, this time is significantly reduced.
2. Develop a system that categorizes unpaid bills according to the date on which the checks to pay the bills will be written. In a manual system, when a statement is received, check the due date and file the statement in the correct folder. When using an accounting software program, the information can be entered into the program.
3. Before statements are paid, verify postings (charges and payments) by comparing invoices with the statement. If errors are discovered, it is the responsibility of the administrative dental assistant to ensure that corrections are made.

4. Prepare checks using a computer check writing program or a manual check writing system.
5. Stamp the date paid on the statement and include the check number. File the paid statement in the appropriate file.
6. Categorize expenditures for use in accounting reports.

VERIFICATION OF EXPENDITURES

The accounts payable process begins when an invoice arrives in the office. An invoice is a list of purchased items and their charges. The supplier of the goods or service sends a detailed list of the items shipped or the service provided. The assistant who receives the order confirms that the items listed have been included in the shipment. Notations are made if an item has been placed on backorder or is not included in the shipment. Invoices are then placed in the appropriate file.

A statement is a list of the totals of all invoices. For example, a dental laboratory processes several different cases during the month. Each time a completed case is returned to the dental practice, an invoice is included. At the end of the month, the dental laboratory creates a statement that summarizes all invoices. When a statement arrives from the laboratory for payment, the envelope is opened and the statement removed, along with the return envelope. Invoices received throughout the month are used to verify charges posted on the statement. After all invoices are accounted for, they are stapled to the corresponding statement.

On the day that bills are to be paid, statements are removed from the file. A protocol may be established that outlines a process for paying bills. It may be the responsibility of the administrative dental assistant to organize statements and give them to the dentist or business manager for authorization.

CHECK WRITING

After approval has been received to pay a bill, the next step is to write the checks or authorize payment. An account can be paid in several different ways. Paper checks can be issued in different formats: computer printout or handwritten check. Bills can also be paid by a variety of electronic methods (credit cards, electronic checks, or direct payment).

Payment Authorization and Transfer

Checks authorize a bank to transfer funds from a particular account to another person or company. Checks are no longer limited to paper form. They now include digital and electronic authorizations to transfer funds from an account. Check writing, or payment authorization, can be done via telephone, computerized online service, automatic payment, credit card, and debit card. Although methods of authorizing payments vary, the method of documentation, or record keeping, remains the same. Transactions must be recorded, documented, and verified.

 FOOD FOR THOUGHT

The use of electronic payments raises several questions for the administrative dental assistant. Each question should be addressed with dental personnel and a proper protocol should be established. How is documentation completed to ensure that all transactions are recorded? Who is authorized to make electronic transfers? Does the vendor accept electronic transfers? What system is in place to check and double-check the activity on an account, to protect the dental practice from fraudulent activity? Before electronic transfers are made, these questions must be answered to protect the integrity of the dental practice and the administrative dental assistant.

Electronic Check Writing

Check writing software has eased the processes of writing, recording, categorizing, and reconciling checking accounts. These software programs perform the functions required by the pegboard check writing system, such as producing a check register or deposit slip and generating numerous reports (Figures 16-1 and 16-2). When it is time to write checks, the program can fill in such information as payee, amount of payment, and code for category. Payments can be identified as paper checks or electronic checks. Deposit and payment information is used to calculate the account balance. When a statement is returned from the bank, it is reconciled in a manner similar to that used for the manual reconciliation.

Making a Deposit

Deposits are no longer limited to paper copies or face-to-face bank transactions. Deposits can be made through an ATM by scanning the checks and paper currency. After the deposit has been scanned the ATM will produce a deposit slip, complete with images of the checks and a count of the currency. Another type of scanned deposit takes place in the dental office by scanning an image of the check and transmitting the information directly to the bank (currency still needs to be taken to the bank). Transferring money directly from one bank account to another is termed *direct deposits*. This is a common practice with insurance companies.

When items are taken to the bank to be deposited, a deposit slip must accompany them (Figure 16-3). The deposit slip (usually preprinted) identifies the account and includes the amount of money being deposited into the account. It is necessary to list the types of funds being deposited (coin, cash, or checks) and amounts of each type. When large amounts in coin are being deposited, it is necessary to wrap the coins first. Cash is separated according to denomination. Checks are listed separately. Some banks require that all checks must be listed and American Bankers Association (ABA) routing numbers included for identification; others accept adding machine tapes with individual checks listed. Follow your bank's protocol.

All deposit methods will have a process for verifying and reporting deposits. Keep all receipts in a file (electronic or paper) and compare them with the bank statement when that is received. This will help with bank account reconciliation and will provide documentation if a deposit is questioned.

Text continued on page 241

ANATOMY OF A CHECK

FRONT OF CHECK

1 **NAME OF THE PERSON OR COMPANY ISSUING THE CHECK**

Can include address and telephone number. **Caution: Do not give more information than necessary. Do not print drivers license number and Social Security number on the check. This information could be used to counterfeit checks and credit cards.**

2 **ABA BANK IDENTIFICATION NUMBER**

Number that identifies the name of the bank and the region where it is located.

3 **CHECK NUMBER**

Used for documentation and record keeping reference.

4 **DATE**

The day the check is authorized to be paid.

5 **PAY TO THE ORDER OF**

The name of the individual or company to whom the funds are to be paid (payee).

6 **PAY _____ DOLLARS_____**

The amount of funds to be paid written in words.

7 **AMOUNT**

The amount of funds to be paid written in numbers.

8 **NAME AND ADDRESS OF THE BANK ON WHICH THE FUNDS ARE DRAWN**

The bank who will authorize payment of the check.

9 **SIGNATURE**

Where authorized person who can draw funds from the account signs his or her name.

10 **MEMO LINE**

The reason the check was written.

11 **CODES**

Codes for electronic identification.

12 **BANK NUMBER CODE**

13 **CHECK NUMBER CODE**

14 **ACCOUNT NUMBER CODE**

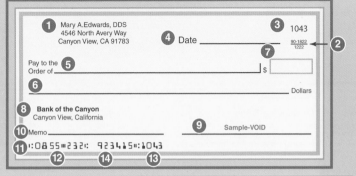

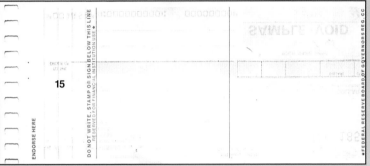

BACK OF CHECK

15 **ENDORSEMENT AREA**

Signature of payee (stamp or signature) and authorization to deposit funds into an account. Depending on the type of endorsement, different actions may occur. Restrictive endorsement contains special instructions (i.e., For Deposit Only). Endorsement in Full gives authorization for another person to receive funds (i.e., Pay to the order of ABC Dental Lab [followed by the signature of the original payee]). Blank endorsement contains the signature of the payee. When this type of endorsement is used, the check can be cashed by anyone (nonrestrictive). In almost all cases a restrictive signature should be used by a business (For Deposit Only), as this protects the business from unauthorized use.

(Top image modified from Young-Adams AP: *Kinn's the administrative medical assistant,* ed 8, St. Louis, 2014, Saunders.)

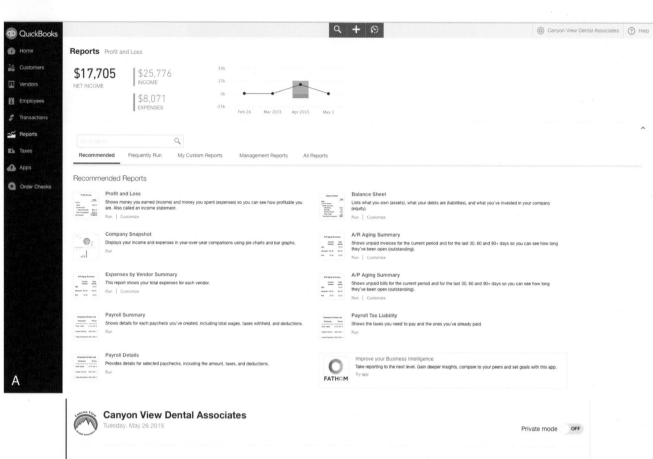

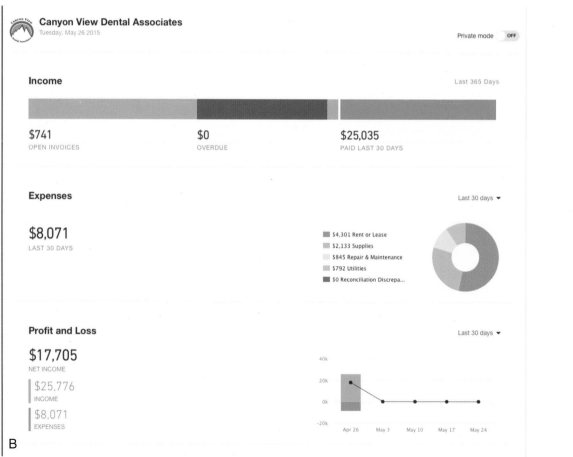

FIGURE 16-1 **A,** A variety of reports are available to run through an accounting software program such as QuickBooks®. **B,** An example of a QuickBooks® report. (Screen capture © Intuit, Inc. All rights reserved.)

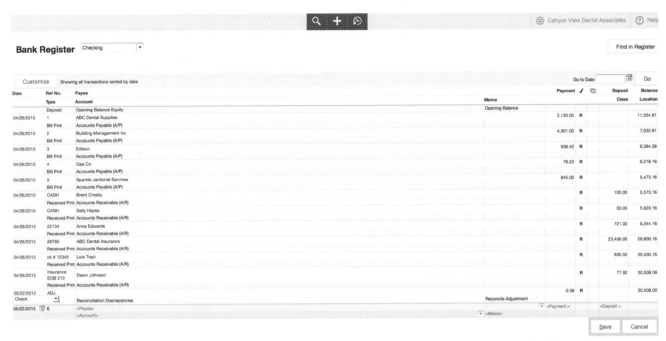

FIGURE 16-2 Example of a computer-generated check register using QuickBooks®. (Screen captures © Intuit, Inc. All rights reserved.)

PROCEDURES

Steps in Writing a Check

Manual Check Writing

1. Use ink that cannot be changed or altered (ink pen, typewriter, or computer). Technology makes it easy to counterfeit checks. The use of special paper and embossing instruments helps to eliminate the possibility that a check can be counterfeited or altered.
2. Write neatly, legibly, and accurately.
3. Correctly enter the name of the payee (person or company receiving the check). Write company names as they appear on their statements (check the statement for this information under the heading "Make checks payable to"). When issuing a check to an individual, you need not use titles (e.g., Mr., Mrs.).
4. Clearly write the amount of the check. The amount is written in two different ways, alpha and numeric:
   - $346.75
   - Three hundred forty-six and 75/100 dollars
5. Transfer information to the check register: check number, payee, and amount. Fill in all spaces on the check so that the amount or the payee cannot be altered.
6. After checks are written or printed, have them signed by an authorized person. Usually the dentist or the business manager will sign all checks. Sound accounting practices are very clear that the same person who writes the checks must not be the person who signs the checks. This protects both the business and the employee from improperly transferred funds.
7. If an error is made in the writing of a check, the check is voided and a new check issued. It is important to keep the voided check for documentation. When voiding a check, write *void* across the face of the check. Other methods include tearing the check in half and then taping it back together, writing *void* in the check signature area, or tearing the signature area from the check.
8. Checks will not be paid if there are insufficient funds in the account. Before mailing checks or processing electronic transfers, balance the account and verify that sufficient funds are available to cover the payments.

Computer-Generated Check Writing

1. Print checks using special paper stock designed for checks. The paper may contain specialized markings and other characteristics that will protect from unauthorized reproduction.
2. Use a font style and size that is easy to read.
3. Correctly enter the information into the software program. Check to make sure the name of the company is spelled correctly and you have included the correct billing information, such as address and account number.
4. Double-check that you have entered the correct dollar amount. The software program will correctly enter the alpha and numeric information.
5. Check and verify that the information has been entered correctly.
6. A check can be voided in the program and will appear on the check register as voided. If your checks are preprinted with the check number, the check will need to be destroyed using the same method as the manual system.

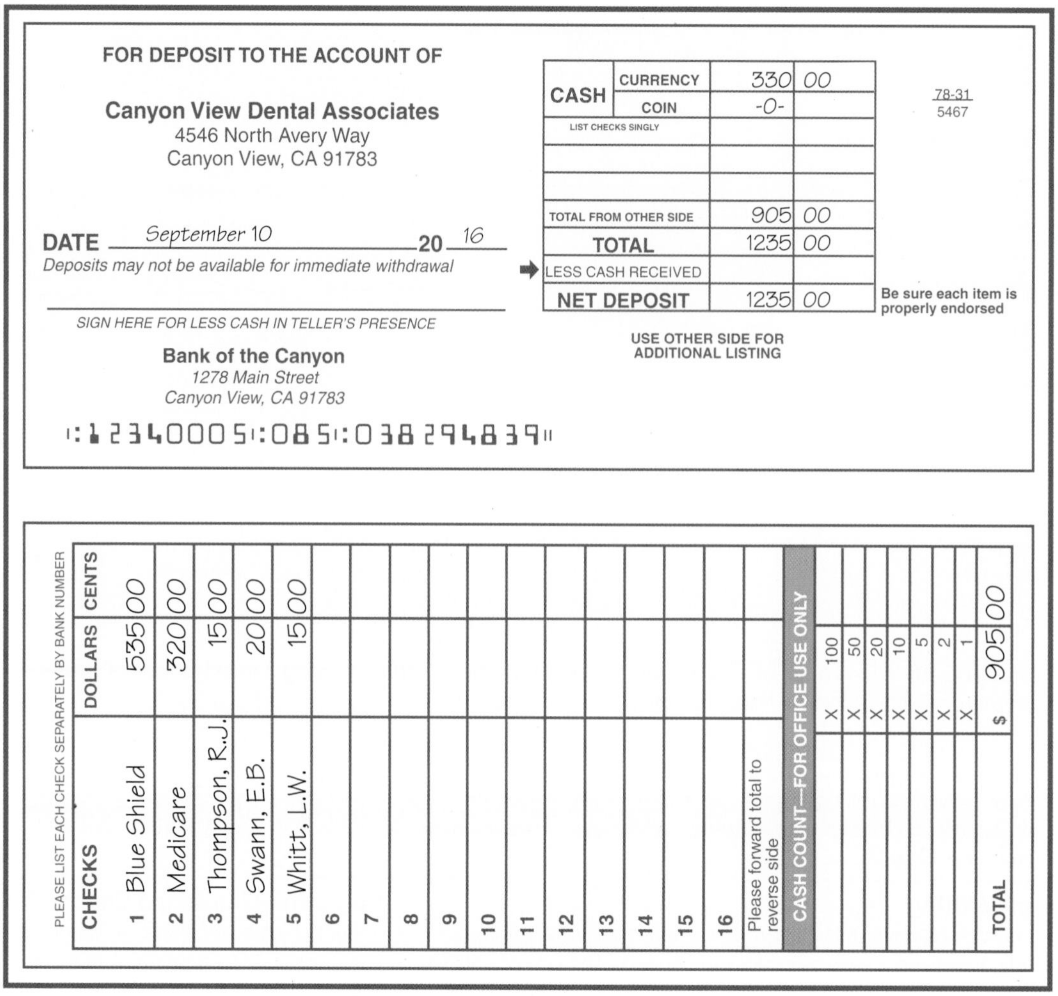

FOR DEPOSIT TO THE ACCOUNT OF

Canyon View Dental Associates
4546 North Avery Way
Canyon View, CA 91783

DATE _September 10_ 20 _16_
Deposits may not be available for immediate withdrawal

SIGN HERE FOR LESS CASH IN TELLER'S PRESENCE

Bank of the Canyon
1278 Main Street
Canyon View, CA 91783

⑈⑈⑈123400051:085i:038294839⑈

CASH	CURRENCY	330	00
	COIN	-0-	
	LIST CHECKS SINGLY		
TOTAL FROM OTHER SIDE		905	00
TOTAL		1235	00
LESS CASH RECEIVED			
NET DEPOSIT		1235	00

78-31
5467

Be sure each item is properly endorsed

USE OTHER SIDE FOR ADDITIONAL LISTING

CHECKS	DOLLARS	CENTS
1 Blue Shield	535	00
2 Medicare	320	00
3 Thompson, R.J.	15	00
4 Swann, E.B.	20	00
5 Whitt, L.W.	15	00
6		
7		
8		
9		
10		
11		
12		
13		
14		
15		
16		
Please forward total to reverse side		
TOTAL	$ 905	00

PLEASE LIST EACH CHECK SEPARATELY BY BANK NUMBER

CASH COUNT—FOR OFFICE USE ONLY
× 100
× 50
× 20
× 10
× 5
× 2
× 1

A

Canyon View Dental Associates
DEPOSIT DETAIL
April 6 - May 26, 2015

DATE	TRANSACTION TYPE	NUM	CLIENT	VENDOR	MEMO/DESCRIPTION	CLR	AMOUNT
Checking							
04/07/2015	Deposit				Opening Balance	R	13,467.81
							13,467.81
04/26/2015	Payment	22134	Anna Edwards			R	721.00
			Anna Edwards				-721.00
04/26/2015	Payment	CASH	Brent Crosby			R	100.00
			Brent Crosby				-100.00
04/26/2015	Payment	Insurance EOB 213	Dawn Johnson			R	77.92
			Dawn Johnson				-77.92
04/26/2015	Payment	ck # 12345	Lois Tract			R	630.00
			Lois Tract				-630.00
04/26/2015	Payment	CASH	Sally Hayes			R	50.00
			Sally Hayes				-50.00
04/26/2015	Payment	28765	ABC Dental Insurance			R	23,456.00
			ABC Dental Insurance				-23,456.00

B

FIGURE 16-3 A, Sample bank deposit slip for a manual accounts payable system. **B,** Electronic deposit summary generated using QuickBooks®. (**A,** Modified from Young-Adams AP: *Kinn's the administrative medical assistant,* ed 8, St. Louis, 2014, Saunders. **B,** Software © Intuit, Inc. All rights reserved.)

RECONCILING A BANK STATEMENT

At the end of each month or banking period, you will receive a bank statement (Figure 16-4). The statement may be delivered in either electronic or paper format. When the bank statement is received, the account should be reconciled. This ensures that your records and the bank records are in agreement.

Information Listed on a Bank Statement

• Date and amount of each deposit. Deposits are identified by type. For example, direct deposits may have been

0821-402054

#821

IIIuuuluIIuIuuIuIuIIImuIIIIuIIuuIuIuIuuIuII

N
2

CALL (888) 555-2932
24 HOURS/DAY, 7 DAYS/WEEK
FOR ASSISTANCE WITH
YOUR ACCOUNT.

PAGE 1 OF 2   THIS STATEMENT COVERS: 6/22/16 THROUGH 7/22/16

INTEREST CHECKING
0821-402054

SUMMARY

PREVIOUS BALANCE	252.10		MINIMUM BALANCE	142.55
DEPOSITS	68.74 +		AVERAGE BALANCE	220.00
INTEREST EARNED	.18 +		ANNUAL PERCENTAGE	
WITHDRAWALS	109.55 −		YIELD EARNED	.96 %
CUSTOMER SERVICE CALLS	.00 −			
INTERLINK/PURCHASE FEE	.00 −		INTEREST EARNED 1994	2.23
MONTHLY CHECKING FEE				
AND OTHER CHARGES	.00 −			

▶ **NEW BALANCE**   **211.47**

USE YOUR EXPRESS CARD TO MAKE UNLIMITED PURCHASES AT RETAILERS DISPLAYING
THE INTERLINK SYMBOL. (A $1 MONTHLY FEE MAY APPLY.)

TRY IT TODAY AT ARCO . . . MOBIL . . . LUCKY . . . RALPHS . . . SAFEWAY & MORE!

CHECKS AND WITHDRAWALS	CHECK 202	DATE PAID 7/05	AMOUNT 15.05	CHECK 203	DATE PAID 7/15	AMOUNT 94.50

DEPOSITS				DATE POSTED	AMOUNT
	CUSTOMER DEPOSIT			7/22	68.74
	INTEREST PAYMENT THIS PERIOD			7/22	.18

BALANCE INFORMATION	DATE 6/22	BALANCE 252.10	DATE 7/05	BALANCE 237.05	DATE 7/15	BALANCE 142.55
					7/22	211.47

24 HOUR CUSTOMER SERVICE	EACH ACCOUNT COMES WITH 3 COMPLIMENTARY CALLS PER STATEMENT PERIOD.
	CALLS TO 24 HOUR CUSTOMER SERVICE THIS STATEMENT PERIOD: 0

INTEREST INFORMATION

FROM	THROUGH	INTEREST RATE	ANNUAL PERCENTAGE YIELD (APY)
6/22	7/22	1.00%	1.01%

INTEREST RATE/APY AS OF 7/22/02 IF YOUR BALANCE IS

$ 0 - 4,999 . . . . .1.00%		1.01%
$ 5,000 - 9,999 . . . . .1.00%		1.01%
$ 10,000 AND OVER 1.00%		1.01%

CALL 1-800-555-2932 IN CALIFORNIA ANYTIME FOR CURRENT RATES.

MEMBER FDIC

STATEMENT

FIGURE 16-4 Sample bank statement for a standard checking account. (Modified from Young-Adams AP: *Kinn's the administrative medical assistant,* ed 8, St. Louis, 2014, Saunders.)

received from insurance companies or credit card companies. In addition to direct deposits, deposits that contain both checks and cash have been made from the office.

- Date, check number, and amount of each check processed by the bank.
- Debit items and other amounts that have been deducted from the account (i.e., automatic payments, electronic transfers, bank charges, service charges).
- Daily totals of debits and credits.
- Beginning and ending balances.
- Canceled checks, unless they are kept by the bank, are returned with the bank statement.

Items Needed for Reconciling the Account

- Check register (pegboard, checkbook register, or computerized register)
- Deposit records (documentation of all deposits made by the dental practice)
- Bank statement and all documentation sent from the bank (canceled checks and electronic transfer debit and credit slips)

Steps in Reconciling the Account

Verify Debits

1. Compare each debit document from the bank with the corresponding entry on the check register (these are the items that did not require a paper check: electronic transfer, automatic payment, and returned checks).
2. Mark the item to identify that the item has been verified and processed. Place the mark on the check register, next to the cleared item in the appropriate column (electronic or manual).
3. If a debit item has not been entered on the register, enter the item and recalculate the total.

Verify Deposits

4. Gather all duplicate deposit slips and place them in chronological order.
5. Gather all direct deposit memos and place them in chronological order.
6. Verify deposits with the statement. Record other credits, such as interest earned.

Verify Canceled Checks

7. Arrange the canceled checks in numeric order.
8. Compare the checks with the register.
9. Identify checks that have been cleared by the bank by placing a mark on the register (electronic or manual).
10. Checks may have been received that were included in a previous reconciliation. Go back and find the check number in the register and identify the check as cleared.

Verify the Balance

Manual	Electronic
11. The worksheet (Figure 16-5) (included with each monthly bank statement) contains directions for calculating the balance. This form provides space for inclusion of outstanding items (checks and deposits that have not been processed by the bank). When the form is completed and the totals checked, they should be the same as the totals on the checkbook register.	11. In the software program, begin the reconcile process. You will need information from the monthly bank statement such as statement ending date, opening balance, and ending balance. The program will also ask you to identify service charges and interest earned. Once the dialogue box (Figure 16-6) has been completed, the program will bring up a screen with a list of deposits and other credits and checks and payments (Figure 16-7). Follow the instructions and complete the process.

12. If the totals are not the same, the error must be located. If the bank has made the error, the bank must be notified. If the error is found in calculations on the checkbook register, corrections must be made there and the totals recalculated. The error could also be made in the calculations on the worksheet; double-check all calculations.

Making Corrections to the Register

Manual	Electronic
13. Make all necessary adjustments to the account and clearly identify the source of these adjustments.	13. Record adjustments in the software program.
14. Recalculate the totals of all columns on the register (if changes or additions have been made). Corrections are made by drawing a line through the figure and entering the correct figure. Never totally cover an entry by crossing it out or using correction fluid.	14. The software program will make the adjustment. The program keeps a log of all transactions and will identify the date, time, and person who made the adjustment.

15. You are finished when the adjusted balance in the check register matches the ending balance on the monthly bank statement worksheet. The bank statement and worksheet can be filed or print a copy of the reconciliation report for the accountant (Figure 16-8).

THIS WORKSHEET IS PROVIDED TO HELP YOU BALANCE YOUR ACCOUNT

1. Go through your register and mark each check, withdrawal, Express ATM transaction, payment, deposit or other credit listed on this statement. Be sure that your register shows any interest paid into your account, and any service charges, automatic payments, or Express Transfers withdrawn from your account during this statement period.

2. Using the chart below, list any outstanding checks, Express ATM withdrawals, payments or any other withdrawals (including any from previous months) that are listed in your register but are not shown on this statement.

3. Balance your account by filling in the spaces below.

ITEMS OUTSTANDING		
NUMBER	AMOUNT	
TOTAL	$	

ENTER

The NEW BALANCE shown on
this statement _ _ _ _ _ _ _ _ _ _ _ _ _ _ _ _ _ _ $_____

ADD

Any deposits listed in your register $_____
or transfers into your account $_____
which are not shown on this $_____
statement.   +$_____

                                  TOTAL _ _ _ _ _ _ _ +$_____

CALCULATE THE SUBTOTAL _ _ _ _ _ _ _ _ . $_____

SUBTRACT

The total outstanding checks and
withdrawals from the chart at left _ _ _ _ _ _ _ _ −$_____

CALCULATE THE ENDING BALANCE

This amount should be the same
as the current balance shown in
your check register _ _ _ _ _ _ _ _ _ _ _ _ _ _ _ _ $_____

IF YOU SUSPECT ERRORS OR HAVE QUESTIONS ABOUT ELECTRONIC TRANSFERS

If you believe there is an error on your statement or Express ATM receipt, or if you need more information about a transaction listed on this statement or an Express ATM receipt, please contact us immediately. We are available 24 hours a day, seven days a week to assist you. Please call the telephone number printed on the front of this statement. Or, you may write to us at United Trust Company, P.O. Box 327, Anytown, USA.

1) Tell us your name and account number or Express card number.

2) As clearly as you can, describe the error or the transfer you are unsure about, and explain why you believe there is an error or why you need more information.

3) Tell us the dollar amount of the suspected error.

You must report the suspected error to us no later than 60 days after we sent you the first statement on which the problem appeared. We will investigate your question and will correct any error promptly. If our investigation takes longer than 10 business days (or 20 days in the case of electronic purchases), we will temporarily credit your account for the amount you believe is in error, so that you may have use of the money until the investigation is completed.

FIGURE 16-5 Sample worksheet to help with reconciliation of a checking account. (From Young-Adams AP: *Kinn's the administrative medical assistant,* ed 8, St. Louis, 2014, Saunders.)

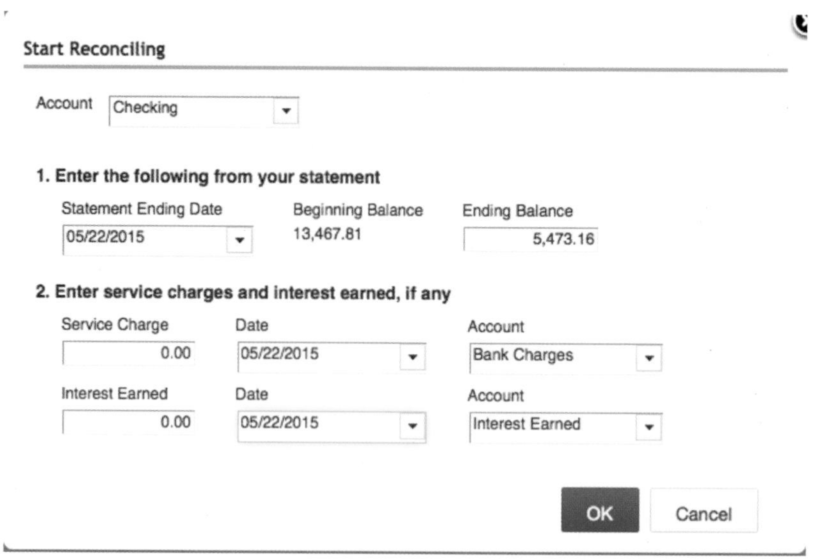

Start Reconciling

Account [Checking ▾]

1. Enter the following from your statement

Statement Ending Date	Beginning Balance	Ending Balance
05/22/2015 ▾	13,467.81	5,473.16

2. Enter service charges and interest earned, if any

Service Charge	Date	Account
0.00	05/22/2015 ▾	Bank Charges ▾

Interest Earned	Date	Account
0.00	05/22/2015 ▾	Interest Earned ▾

[OK]   [Cancel]

FIGURE 16-6 In QuickBooks® this dialogue box prompts the user to enter required information to help reconcile the monthly statement. (Screen capture © Intuit, Inc. All rights reserved.)

Canyon View Dental Associates
CHECK DETAIL
April 1 - May 26, 2015

DATE	TRANSACTION TYPE	NUM	NAME	MEMO/DESCRIPTION	CLR	AMOUNT
Checking						
04/26/2015	Bill Payment (Check)	1	ABC Dental Supplies		R	-2,133.00
						-2,133.00
04/26/2015	Bill Payment (Check)	2	Building Management Inc		R	-4,301.00
						-4,301.00
04/26/2015	Bill Payment (Check)	3	Edison		R	-639.42
						-639.42
04/26/2015	Bill Payment (Check)	4	Gas Co		R	-76.23
						-76.23
04/26/2015	Bill Payment (Check)	5	Sparkle Janitorial Services		R	-845.00
						-845.00
05/22/2015	Check	ADJ		Reconcile Adjustment	R	-0.08
						0.08

FIGURE 16-7 Electronic checking account reconciliation worksheet using QuickBooks®. (Screen capture © Intuit, Inc. All rights reserved.)

Steps to Take When the Account Does Not Balance

1. Check to see that all checks were properly entered on the check register (the same totals are listed on the check and recorded on the bank statement).
2. Check to see whether all totals on the deposits are the same as those listed on the bank statement.
3. Make sure that all checks are accounted for: Either verify that they have been cleared by the bank or list them on the worksheet as outstanding checks. Do not forget to check previous statements for outstanding checks.
4. Make sure all electronic debits and credits are accounted for. Have they been entered on the check register?
5. Make sure all service charges are accounted for. Have they been entered on the check register?
6. Check to see that worksheet calculations are correct.
7. Double-check all addition and subtraction entries in the checkbook. Are they listed in the correct column? Were the debits (service charges, electronic payments, canceled checks, returned checks, corrections in deposits) subtracted

Canyon View Dental Associates
Reconciliation Report
Checking, Period Ending 05/22/2015
Reconciled on: 05/22/2015 (any changes to transactions after this date aren't reflected on this report)
Reconciled by: Linda Gaylor

Summary

Statement Beginning Balance	5,473.16
Checks and Payments cleared	0.00
Deposits and Other Credits cleared	+25,034.92
Adjustment	-0.08
Statement Ending Balance	30,508.00
Register Balance as of 05/22/2015	30,508.00

Details

Deposits and Other Credits cleared

Date	Type	Num	Name	Amount
04/26/2015	Payment	22134	Anna Edwards	721.00
04/26/2015	Payment	CASH	Brent Crosby	100.00
04/26/2015	Payment	Insurance EOB 213	Dawn Johnson	77.92
04/26/2015	Payment	ck # 12345	Lois Tract	630.00
04/26/2015	Payment	CASH	Sally Hayes	50.00
04/26/2015	Payment	28765	ABC Dental Insurance	23,456.00
Total				25,034.92

FIGURE 16-8 Completed electronic reconciliation report generated via QuickBooks®. (Software © Intuit, Inc. All rights reserved.)

from the balance? Were the credits (deposits, direct deposits, interest) added to the balance?

8. If the checkbook still does not balance, you may wish to request help from a co-worker, bank worker, or accountant.

PAYROLL

Creating and maintaining payroll records, calculating payroll, producing payroll reports, and depositing payroll taxes may be duties assigned to the administrative dental assistant. The Internal Revenue Service (IRS) Publication 15, Circular E, *Employer's Tax Guide,* outlines important information on this topic. This circular is updated annually and can be obtained from the IRS or from the Internet (www.irs.gov/pub/irs-pdf/p15.pdf).

Creating the Payroll Record

Each employee must have a separate payroll record with proper documentation. New employees must complete the Immigration and Naturalization Service (INS) Form I-9, Employment Eligibility Verification (Figure 16-9). You can obtain this form from the INS. After the form has been completed, it is the responsibility of the employer to check approved documentation (see the Lists of Accepted Documents in Figure 16-9).

The Social Security Number (SSN) must be recorded with the employee's name and address. If an employee does not have an SSN, he or she must contact the Social Security Administration (SSA) and apply for a card. If the name on the card is different from the name provided by the employee (because of marriage or divorce), instruct the employee to contact the SSA and request a name change. For government

reporting, the name as it appears on the card should be used until an official change has been documented. All employees must have a card because the SSN is needed for tax reports and W-2 forms (reports of wages earned). A copy of the card can be kept in the employee's payroll record.

Employees must also complete a W-4 form (Figure 16-10), Employee's Withholding Allowance Certificate (Internal Revenue Service). The withholding allowance and filing status are used to calculate the amount of income tax that should be withheld from the employee's wages. Employees must complete a new W-4 when a change has occurred in filing status, number of deductions, or name. When employees file for an exempt withholding allowance, they must complete the form annually (see the IRS calendar for the correct dates).

Form W-5 is used for those who qualify for an advance earned income credit (EIC). To obtain these payments, the employee must complete and sign the form (contact the IRS for additional help).

> **! REMEMBER**
>
> It is your responsibility to follow the guidelines. Read the publications offered by the Internal Revenue Service (IRS) and seek the advice of the dental practice accountant.

Payroll Records

Each employee must have a separate payroll record. This record can be a form that is filled in by the payroll clerk, it can be an electronic record, or it can be a payroll card that is used in a one-write system. Each record must include the same type of information (see Anatomy of a Payroll Record).

PUBLICATION 15, CIRCULAR E, *EMPLOYER'S TAX GUIDE*

Department of the Treasury
Internal Revenue Service

Publication 15
Cat. No. 10000W

(Circular E), Employer's Tax Guide

For use in **2015**

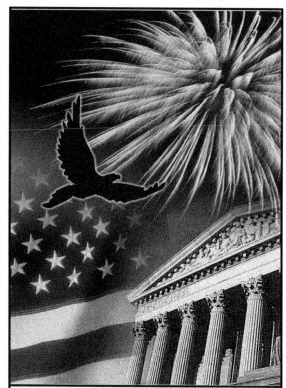

Get forms and other information faster and easier at:
- *IRS.gov* (English)
- *IRS.gov/Spanish* (Español)
- *IRS.gov/Chinese* (中文)
- *IRS.gov/Korean* (한국어)
- *IRS.gov/Russian* (Русский)
- *IRS.gov/Vietnamese* (TiếngViệt)

Dec 22, 2014

Contents

What's New 1

Reminders 2

Calendar 8

Introduction 9

1. Employer Identification Number (EIN) 10

2. Who Are Employees? 11

3. Family Employees 12

4. Employee's Social Security Number (SSN) ... 13

5. Wages and Other Compensation 14

6. Tips 17

7. Supplemental Wages 18

8. Payroll Period 20

9. Withholding From Employees' Wages 20

10. Required Notice to Employees About the
    Earned Income Credit (EIC) 24

11. Depositing Taxes 25

12. Filing Form 941 or Form 944 30

13. Reporting Adjustments to Form 941 or
    Form 944 32

14. Federal Unemployment (FUTA) Tax 35

15. Special Rules for Various Types of
    Services and Payments 37

16. Third Party Payer Arrangements 42

17. How To Use the Income Tax Withholding
    Tables 43

How To Get Tax Help 67

Index 69

Future Developments

For the latest information about developments related to Publication 15 (Circular E), such as legislation enacted after it was published, go to *www.irs.gov/pub15*.

What's New

COBRA premium assistance credit. Effective for tax periods beginning after December 31, 2013, the credit for COBRA premium assistance payments cannot be claimed on Form 941, Employer's QUARTERLY Federal Tax Return (or Form 944, Employer's ANNUAL Federal Tax Return). Instead, after filing your Form 941 (or Form

(From Internal Revenue Service, Department of the Treasury, Washington, DC.)

Instructions for Employment Eligibility Verification

Department of Homeland Security
U.S. Citizenship and Immigration Services

USCIS
Form I-9
OMB No. 1615-0047
Expires 03/31/2016

Read all instructions carefully before completing this form.

Anti-Discrimination Notice. It is illegal to discriminate against any work-authorized individual in hiring, discharge, recruitment or referral for a fee, or in the employment eligibility verification (Form I-9 and E-Verify) process based on that individual's citizenship status, immigration status or national origin. Employers **CANNOT** specify which document(s) they will accept from an employee. The refusal to hire an individual because the documentation presented has a future expiration date may also constitute illegal discrimination. For more information, call the Office of Special Counsel for Immigration-Related Unfair Employment Practices (OSC) at 1-800-255-7688 (employees), 1-800-255-8155 (employers), or 1-800-237-2515 (TDD), or visit **www.justice.gov/crt/about/osc**.

What Is the Purpose of This Form?

Employers must complete Form I-9 to document employee (both citizen and noncitizen) hired aft of the Northern Mariana Islands (CNMI), emplo employment authorization of each new employe should have used Form I-9 CNMI between Nov

General Instructions

Employers are responsible for completing and r "employer" means all employers, including thos agricultural employers, or farm labor contractor

Form I-9 is made up of three sections. Employe retaining completed forms. Do not mail comple Immigration and Customs Enforcement (ICE).

Section 1. Employee Information and A

Newly hired employees must complete and sign Section 1 should never be completed before the

Provide the following information to complete S

Name: Provide your full legal last name, fi surname. If you have two last names or a hy name is your given name. Your middle initi middle name, if any.

Other names used: Provide all other name names, write "N/A."

Address: Provide the address where you cu applicable), City, State, and Zip Code. Do n from Canada or Mexico may use an internat

Date of Birth: Provide your date of birth i written as 01/23/1950.

U.S. Social Security Number: Provide you is voluntary. However, if your employer par

E-mail Address and Telephone Number (number. Department of Homeland Security the information provided and the information "N/A" if you choose not to provide this info

Form I-9 Instructions 03/08/13 N

Employment Eligibility Verification

Department of Homeland Security
U.S. Citizenship and Immigration Services

USCIS
Form I-9
OMB No. 1615-0047
Expires 03/31/2016

▶**START HERE.** Read instructions carefully before completing this form. The instructions must be available during completion of this form. **ANTI-DISCRIMINATION NOTICE:** It is illegal to discriminate against work-authorized individuals. Employers **CANNOT** specify which document(s) they will accept from an employee. The refusal to hire an individual because the documentation presented has a future expiration date may also constitute illegal discrimination.

Section 1. Employee Information and Attestation (Employees must complete and sign Section 1 of Form I-9 no later than the **first day of employment**, but not before accepting a job offer.)

| Last Name (Family Name) | First Name (Given Name) | Middle Initial | Other Names Used (if any) |

| Address (Street Number and Name) | Apt. Number | City or Town | State | Zip Code |

| Date of Birth (mm/dd/yyyy) | U.S. Social Security Number |

I am aware that federal law provides for imprison connection with the completion of this form.

I attest, under penalty of perjury, that I am (check

☐ A citizen of the United States
☐ A noncitizen national of the United States (See i
☐ A lawful permanent resident (Alien Registration N
☐ An alien authorized to work until (expiration date, if ap (See instructions)

For aliens authorized to work, provide your Alien

1. Alien Registration Number/USCIS Number:_____

OR

2. Form I-94 Admission Number:_____

If you obtained your admission number from C States, include the following:

Foreign Passport Number:_____

Country of Issuance:_____

Some aliens may write "N/A" on the Foreign P

Signature of Employee:

Preparer and/or Translator Certification (To
employee.)

I attest, under penalty of perjury, that I have assi
information is true and correct.

Signature of Preparer or Translator

Last Name (Family Name)

Address (Street Number and Name)

Form I-9 03/08/13 N

LISTS OF ACCEPTABLE DOCUMENTS
All documents must be UNEXPIRED

Employees may present one selection from List A
or a combination of one selection from List B and one selection from List C.

LIST A	LIST B	LIST C
Documents that Establish Both Identity and Employment Authorization	**Documents that Establish Identity**	**Documents that Establish Employment Authorization**
OR	AND	
1. U.S. Passport or U.S. Passport Card	1. Driver's license or ID card issued by a State or outlying possession of the United States provided it contains a photograph or information such as name, date of birth, gender, height, eye color, and address	1. A Social Security Account Number card, unless the card includes one of the following restrictions: (1) NOT VALID FOR EMPLOYMENT (2) VALID FOR WORK ONLY WITH INS AUTHORIZATION (3) VALID FOR WORK ONLY WITH DHS AUTHORIZATION
2. Permanent Resident Card or Alien Registration Receipt Card (Form I-551)	2. ID card issued by federal, state or local government agencies or entities, provided it contains a photograph or information such as name, date of birth, gender, height, eye color, and address	2. Certification of Birth Abroad issued by the Department of State (Form FS-545)
3. Foreign passport that contains a temporary I-551 stamp or temporary I-551 printed notation on a machine-readable immigrant visa	3. School ID card with a photograph	3. Certification of Report of Birth issued by the Department of State (Form DS-1350)
4. Employment Authorization Document that contains a photograph (Form I-766)	4. Voter's registration card	4. Original or certified copy of birth certificate issued by a State, county, municipal authority, or territory of the United States bearing an official seal
5. For a nonimmigrant alien authorized to work for a specific employer because of his or her status: a. Foreign passport; and b. Form I-94 or Form I-94A that has the following: (1) The same name as the passport; and (2) An endorsement of the alien's nonimmigrant status as long as that period of endorsement has not yet expired and the proposed employment is not in conflict with any restrictions or limitations identified on the form.	5. U.S. Military card or draft record	5. Native American tribal document
	6. Military dependent's ID card	6. U.S. Citizen ID Card (Form I-197)
	7. U.S. Coast Guard Merchant Mariner Card	7. Identification Card for Use of Resident Citizen in the United States (Form I-179)
	8. Native American tribal document	8. Employment authorization document issued by the Department of Homeland Security
	9. Driver's license issued by a Canadian government authority	
6. Passport from the Federated States of Micronesia (FSM) or the Republic of the Marshall Islands (RMI) with Form I-94 or Form I-94A indicating nonimmigrant admission under the Compact of Free Association Between the United States and the FSM or RMI	**For persons under age 18 who are unable to present a document listed above:** 10. School record or report card 11. Clinic, doctor, or hospital record 12. Day-care or nursery school record	

Illustrations of many of these documents appear in Part 8 of the Handbook for Employers (M-274).

Refer to Section 2 of the instructions, titled "Employer or Authorized Representative Review and Verification," for more information about acceptable receipts.

Form I-9 03/08/13 N

Page 9 of 9

FIGURE 16-9 U.S. Citizenship and Immigration Services Employment Eligibility Verification form, along with Lists of Acceptable Documents and instructions. (From U.S. Citizenship and Immigration Services, Department of Homeland Security, Washington, DC.)

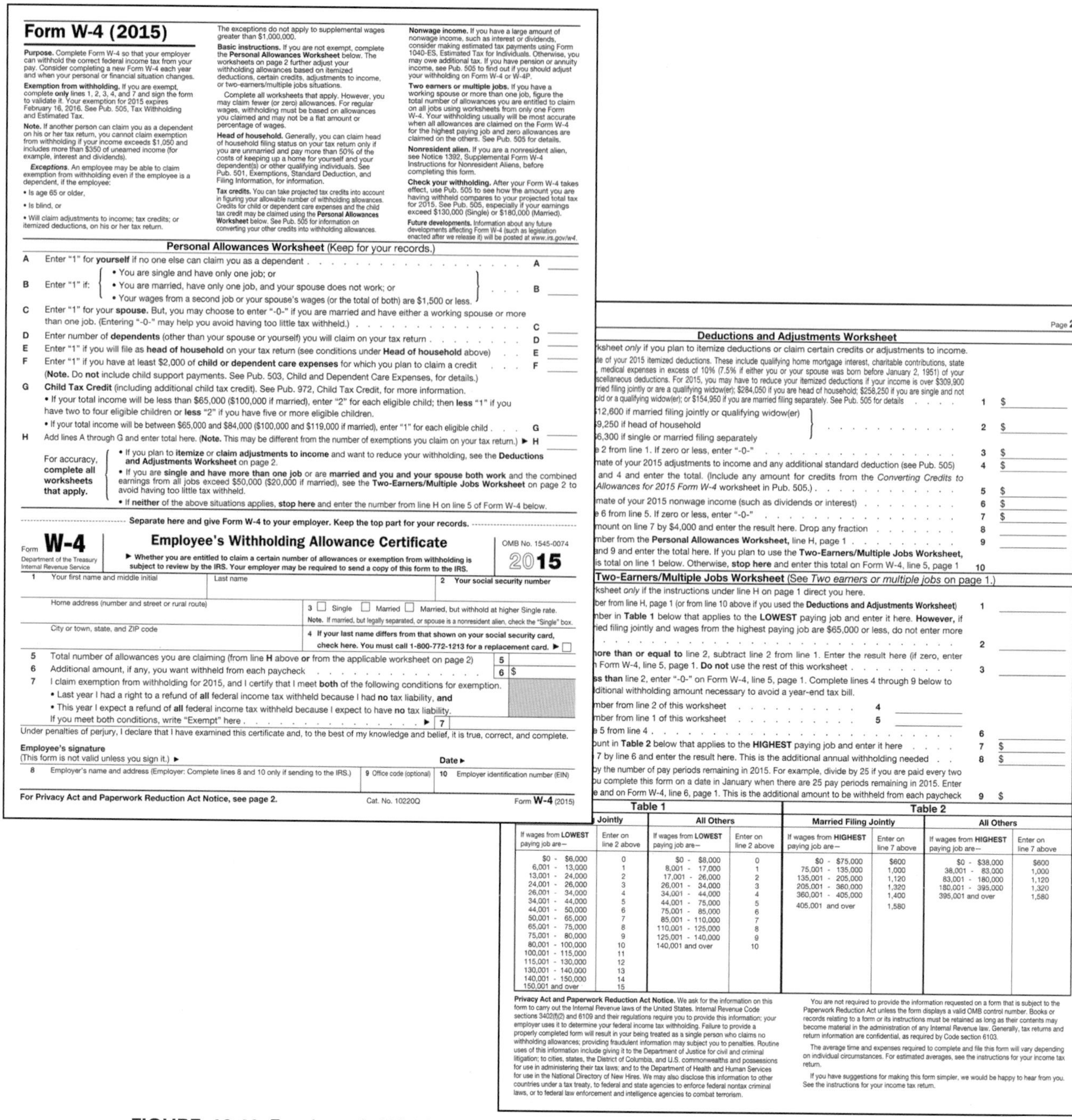

Form W-4 (2015)

Personal Allowances Worksheet (Keep for your records.)

A Enter "1" for **yourself** if no one else can claim you as a dependent . . . A ____

B Enter "1" if: • You are single and have only one job; or • You are married, have only one job, and your spouse does not work; or • Your wages from a second job or your spouse's wages (or the total of both) are $1,500 or less. . . . B ____

C Enter "1" for your **spouse**. But, you may choose to enter "-0-" if you are married and have either a working spouse or more than one job. (Entering "-0-" may help you avoid having too little tax withheld.) . . . C ____

D Enter number of **dependents** (other than your spouse or yourself) you will claim on your tax return . . . D ____

E Enter "1" if you will file as **head of household** on your tax return (see conditions under **Head of household** above) . . E ____

F Enter "1" if you have at least $2,000 of **child or dependent care expenses** for which you plan to claim a credit . . . F ____
(**Note.** Do **not** include child support payments. See Pub. 503, Child and Dependent Care Expenses, for details.)

G **Child Tax Credit** (including additional child tax credit). See Pub. 972, Child Tax Credit, for more information.
• If your total income will be less than $65,000 ($100,000 if married), enter "2" for each eligible child; then **less** "1" if you have two to four eligible children or **less** "2" if you have five or more eligible children.
• If your total income will be between $65,000 and $84,000 ($100,000 and $119,000 if married), enter "1" for each eligible child . . . G ____

H Add lines A through G and enter total here. (**Note.** This may be different from the number of exemptions you claim on your tax return.) ► H ____

For accuracy, complete all worksheets that apply.
• If you plan to **itemize or claim adjustments to income** and want to reduce your withholding, see the **Deductions and Adjustments Worksheet** on page 2.
• If you are **single and have more than one job** or are **married and you and your spouse both work** and the combined earnings from all jobs exceed $50,000 ($20,000 if married), see the **Two-Earners/Multiple Jobs Worksheet** on page 2 to avoid having too little tax withheld.
• If **neither** of the above situations applies, **stop here** and enter the number from line H on line 5 of Form W-4 below.

Separate here and give Form W-4 to your employer. Keep the top part for your records.

Form **W-4** Department of the Treasury Internal Revenue Service

Employee's Withholding Allowance Certificate

► Whether you are entitled to claim a certain number of allowances or exemption from withholding is subject to review by the IRS. Your employer may be required to send a copy of this form to the IRS.

OMB No. 1545-0074 **2015**

1 Your first name and middle initial | Last name | 2 Your social security number

Home address (number and street or rural route) | 3 ☐ Single ☐ Married ☐ Married, but withhold at higher Single rate.

City or town, state, and ZIP code | 4 If your last name differs from that shown on your social security card, check here. You must call 1-800-772-1213 for a replacement card. ► ☐

5 Total number of allowances you are claiming (from line **H** above **or** from the applicable worksheet on page 2) 5

6 Additional amount, if any, you want withheld from each paycheck . . . 6 $

7 I claim exemption from withholding for 2015, and I certify that I meet **both** of the following conditions for exemption.
• Last year I had a right to a refund of **all** federal income tax withheld because I had **no** tax liability, **and**
• This year I expect a refund of **all** federal income tax withheld because I expect to have **no** tax liability.
If you meet both conditions, write "Exempt" here . . . ► 7

Under penalties of perjury, I declare that I have examined this certificate and, to the best of my knowledge and belief, it is true, correct, and complete.

Employee's signature
(This form is not valid unless you sign it.) ► Date ►

8 Employer's name and address (Employer: Complete lines 8 and 10 only if sending to the IRS.) | 9 Office code (optional) | 10 Employer identification number (EIN)

For Privacy Act and Paperwork Reduction Act Notice, see page 2. Cat. No. 10220Q Form **W-4** (2015)

Page **2**

Deductions and Adjustments Worksheet

Two-Earners/Multiple Jobs Worksheet (See *Two earners or multiple jobs* on page 1.)

Table 1 | Table 2

FIGURE 16-10 Employee's Withholding Allowance Certificate (Form W-4). (From Internal Revenue Service, Department of the Treasury, Washington, DC.)

> **! REMEMBER**
>
> Payroll records are important documents that must be kept for a period of 4 years (check current government regulations). Personnel records are different from payroll records. Personnel records contain information regarding performance reviews and contracts. These are confidential and must be kept separate from payroll records.

Computerized Payroll

Computer programs are available that calculate and record all payroll information. These programs use the information kept in a payroll record (Figure 16-11). After the account has been established, payroll information is entered and the program determines the amount of tax and other deductions. A paper check can be printed or the funds direct deposited into

ANATOMY OF A PAYROLL RECORD

| | Marital status __④_____ |
| | Number of Exp _____④_____ |

EMPLOYEE'S PAYROLL RECORD

Name: _①_____ Social Security Number _③_____

Address ___①_____ City _____ Zip code _____

Telephone _____ Date of Birth _②_____

Occupation: _____ Date of employment _②_____

Pay rate: _⑤_____

	Date	Check number	Gross salary	Fed W/H	FICA	M/C	State W/H	Other	Net check
	1/ / ⑥		⑦	⑧	⑧	⑧	⑧	⑧	⑨
	1/ /								
	1/ /								
	1/ /								
	JAN TOTAL		⑩	⑩	⑩	⑩	⑩	⑩	⑩
	2/ /								
	2/ /								
	2/ /								
	2/ /								
	FEB TOTAL								
	3/ /								
	3/ /								
	3/ /								
	MAR TOTAL								
	FIRST QT. TOTALS		⑪	⑪	⑪	⑪	⑪	⑪	⑪

① NAME AND ADDRESS OF EMPLOYEE

② PERSONAL DATA

Date of birth, date of employment, and home telephone number.

③ SOCIAL SECURITY NUMBER

Mandated by law.

④ NUMBER OF DEDUCTIONS AND FILING STATUS

Information taken from W-4.

⑤ PAY RATE

How much the employee is being paid, and how it is calculated (hourly, weekly, monthly).

⑥ DATE CHECK IS ISSUED

⑦ GROSS PAY

The total amount earned before deductions.

⑧ DEDUCTIONS

These are amounts that are subtracted from the gross pay. They include income tax withholdings (federal and state if applicable), FICA (Federal Insurance Contributions Act [social security]), and Medicare. In some states, other taxes may be withheld. In addition to taxes, deductions may include insurance, pension fund contributions, and savings deposits.

⑨ NET SALARY

The amount remaining after all deductions have been subtracted.

⑩ MONTHLY TOTALS

The total gross salary, total deductions for each category, and total net salary.

⑪ QUARTERLY TOTALS

These are the totals of the three monthly totals. This information is used by the accountant when completing the quarterly government payroll reports. At the end of the year, these totals are added up to make the "Year End Total," which is then used to complete the year end reports for government agencies. Each employee is given a copy of this report (W-2 form). This information is used by the employees when calculating their tax liability for the year and must be attached to their tax form.

Edit employee details

First name*   M.I.   Last name*

Clifford   P   Usher

1   **What are Clifford's withholdings?**

   Single, with no allowances

2   **How often do you pay Clifford?**

   Every Friday ▼   starting 05/01/2015

3   **How much do you pay Clifford?**

   Salary ▼ $ 5,000.00   per month ▼

   ☐ Clifford works part-time

   Add additional pay types

4   **Does Clifford have any deductions? (Examples: retirement, health care)**

   No (most common)

5   **How do you want to pay Clifford?**

   Paper check

Sample check (Based on the pay schedule and rate you enter)

Canyon View Dental Associates
4546 North Avery Way
Alta Loma, CA 91701

PAY TO   Clifford P. Usher $801.19

SAMPLE CHECK

GROSS PAY	
Regular	$1,153.85

TAXES WITHHELD	
Federal Income Tax	$196.52
Social Security	$71.54
Medicare	$16.73
CA Income Tax	$57.49
CA State Disability Ins	$10.38

SUMMARY	
Total pay	$1,153.85
Taxes	$352.66
Net pay this check	**$801.19**

FIGURE 16-11 A sample electronic payroll record generated through QuickBooks®. (Software © Intuit, Inc. All rights reserved.)

the employees bank account. Reports are generated on the basis of information stored in the employee database.

Payroll Services

Banks and third party vendors who calculate payroll provide payroll services. Such services maintain records, generate payroll checks, provide reports, and complete government forms. In addition, they arrange for direct deposit of payroll into employees' personal accounts, thereby eliminating the need for paper checks. The IRS provides a list of companies who have passed the IRS Assurance Testing System (ATS) and/or Business Acceptance Testing (BAT) requirements for software developers, reporting agents, and transmitters of electronic business returns to the IRS.

Calculating Payroll

Before payroll checks can be written, the amount due must be calculated through determination of taxes and other deductions. In a manual system this may be the duty of an

administrative assistant. Gross salary is the amount of pay given before any deductions have been taken out. Deductions are subtracted from the gross salary to calculate the net salary or "take home" salary (the amount for which the check is written).

Employment Tax Rates

Federal tax deductions include withholding taxes, Social Security tax (FICA), and Medicare taxes. Federal unemployment (FUTA) taxes are paid by the employer on behalf of an employee. In addition to federal taxes, individual state taxes may be collected. Other deductions include contributions to a pension fund, a health insurance plan, a life and disability insurance program, and a savings program.

Employment tax rates and wage bases in 2015. Social Security tax

- Tax rate: 6.2% for each employer and employee
- Wage base: $118,500

EXAMPLES OF PAYROLL CALCULATIONS

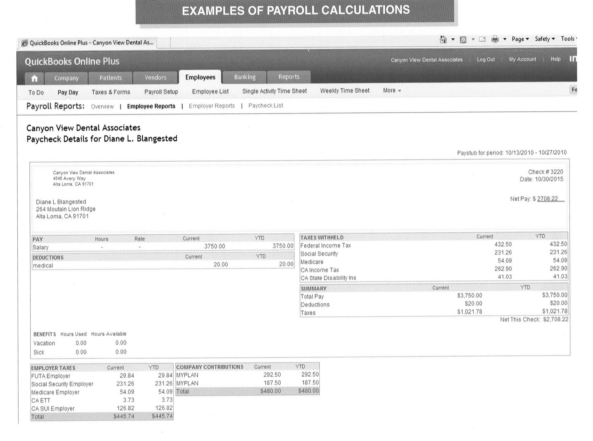

Scenario #1.

Diana Blangested is the office manager. Her monthly salary is $7,500.00 (gross salary). She is paid semi-monthly on the 1st and 15th of each month. This information was entered into the payroll program during the initial employee setup. Each payday the administrative assistant makes a request for a payroll check, and the deductions are automatically calculated.

Percentage Method Tables for Income Tax Withholding
(For Wages Paid in 2015)

TABLE 1—WEEKLY Payroll Period

(a) SINGLE person (including head of household)—

If the amount of wages (after subtracting withholding allowances) is:
Not over $44 . . . . $0

Over—	But not over—	The amount of income tax to withhold is:	of excess over—
$44	—$222	$0.00 plus 10%	—$44
$222	—$764	$17.80 plus 15%	—$222
$764	—$1,789	$99.10 plus 25%	—$764
$1,789	—$3,685	$355.35 plus 28%	—$1,789
$3,685	—$7,958	$886.23 plus 33%	—$3,685
$7,958	—$7,990	$2,296.32 plus 35%	—$7,958
$7,990		$2,307.52 plus 39.6%	—$7,990

(b) MARRIED person—

If the amount of wages (after subtracting withholding allowances) is:
Not over $165 . . . . $0

Over—	But not over—	The amount of income tax to withhold is:	of excess over—
$165	—$520	$0.00 plus 10%	—$165
$520	—$1,606	$35.50 plus 15%	—$520
$1,606	—$3,073	$198.40 plus 25%	—$1,606
$3,073	—$4,597	$565.15 plus 28%	—$3,073
$4,597	—$8,079		
$8,079	—$9,105		
$9,105			

TABLE 2—BIWEEKLY Payroll Period

(a) SINGLE person (including head of household)—

If the amount of wages (after subtracting withholding allowances) is:
Not over $88 . . . . $0

Over—	But not over—	The amount of income tax to withhold is:	of excess over—
$88	—$443	$0.00 plus 10%	—$88
$443	—$1,529	$35.50 plus 15%	—$443
$1,529	—$3,579	$198.40 plus 25%	—$1,529
$3,579	—$7,369	$710.90 plus 28%	—$3,579
$7,369	—$15,915	$1,772.10 plus 33%	—$7,369
$15,915	—$15,981	$4,592.28 plus 35%	—$15,915
$15,981		$4,615.38 plus 39.6%	—$15,981

(b) MARRIED person—

If the amount of wages (after subtracting withholding allowances) is:
Not over $331 . . . .

Over—	But not over—
$331	—$1,040
$1,040	—$3,212
$3,212	—$6,146
$6,146	—$9,194
$9,194	—$16,158
$16,158	—$18,210
$18,210	

TABLE 3—SEMIMONTHLY Payroll Period

(a) SINGLE person (including head of household)—

If the amount of wages (after subtracting withholding allowances) is:
Not over $96 . . . . $0

Over—	But not over—	The amount of income tax to withhold is:	of excess over—
$96	—$480	$0.00 plus 10%	—$96
$480	—$1,656	$38.40 plus 15%	—$480
$1,656	—$3,877	$214.80 plus 25%	—$1,656
$3,877	—$7,983	$770.05 plus 28%	—$3,877
$7,983	—$17,242	$1,919.73 plus 33%	—$7,983
$17,242	—$17,313	$4,975.20 plus 35%	—$17,242
$17,313		$5,000.05 plus 39.6%	—$17,313

(b) MARRIED person—

If the amount of wages (after subtracting withholding allowances) is
Not over $358 . . . . $0

Over—	But not over—
$358	—$1,127
$1,127	—$3,479
$3,479	—$6,658
$6,658	—$9,960
$9,960	—$17,504
$17,504	—$19,727
$19,727	

TABLE 4—MONTHLY Payroll Period

(a) SINGLE person (including head of household)—

If the amount of wages (after subtracting withholding allowances) is:
Not over $192 . . . . $0

Over—	But not over—	The amount of income tax to withhold is:	of excess over—
$192	—$960	$0.00 plus 10%	—$192
$960	—$3,313	$76.80 plus 15%	—$960
$3,313	—$7,754	$429.75 plus 25%	—$3,313
$7,754	—$15,967	$1,540.00 plus 28%	—$7,754
$15,967	—$34,483	$3,839.64 plus 33%	—$15,967
$34,483	—$34,625	$9,949.92 plus 35%	—$34,483
$34,625		$9,999.62 plus 39.6%	—$34,625

(b) MARRIED person—

If the amount of wages (after subtracting withholding allowances) is
Not over $717 . . . .

Over—	But not over—
$717	—$2,254
$2,254	—$6,958
$6,958	—$13,317
$13,317	—$19,921
$19,921	—$35,008
$35,008	—$39,454
$39,454	

Publication 15 (2015)

Page 45

Scenario #2.

Deanna Rogers is a part-time hourly employee. She has worked a total of 32.5 hours for this pay period. Her hourly wage is $15.00. She has a filing status of single and is claiming 0 deductions.

EMPLOYEE'S PAYROLL RECORD

Marital status *S*
Number of Exp *O*

Name: *Deanna Rogers*   Social Security Number: *123-45-6778*
Address: *42 S. Eagle Nest*   City *Canyon View*   Zip code *91711*
Telephone: *626-555-4664*   Date of Birth *11/24/80*
Occupation: *Part time chairside asst.*   Date of employment *9/12/98*
Pay rate: *$15.00 per hour*

Date	Check number	Gross salary	Fed W/H	FICA	M/C	State W/H	Other	Net check
1/2/11	2683	487.50	42.23	30.23	7.07	—	—	$407.97
1/ /								
1/ /								
1/ /								
JAN TOTAL								
2/ /								
2/ /								
2/ /								
2/ /								
FEB TOTAL								
3/ /								
3/ /								
3/ /								
MAR TOTAL								
FIRST QT. TOTALS								

Steps to determine her semimonthly take home salary

1. Determine semimonthly salary.......$15.00 × 32.5 = $487.50
2. Determine federal withholding
   using Percentage Method of $487.50 − $442.00 = $45.50 (see table 3 on the left)
   Withholding...................................$45.50 × 0.15 (15%) = $6.83
                                              $6.83 + 35.40 = $42.23
3. Determine FICA............................$487.50 × .062 (6.2%) = $30.23
4. Determine Medicare.....................$487.50 × .0145 (1.45%) = $7.07

Medicare tax
- Tax rate: 1.45% for each employer and employee
- All wages are subject to Medicare tax

Federal unemployment tax
- Tax rate: 6% before state credits (employers only)
- Wage base: $7000

Calculating Net Salary

With the help of tax tables and percentage calculation guides, the administrative dental assistant must calculate the various taxes that are deducted from each employee's pay. Several steps are followed in determining the net salary of each employee.

Salary can be calculated in various ways. Hourly employees are paid according to the number of hours worked during a pay period. Salaried employees have a set amount they are paid each month, regardless of the number of hours worked. Contract employees may be paid according to the amount of work they produce or the amount of money they collect, or by a daily rate. Some employees may be paid a base salary with incentives added on the basis of different conditions, such as amount of money collected or the level of treatment produced. It is important to understand the different pay levels and how the salaries should be calculated.

Withholding tax is determined by the filing status (married or single) and the number of deductions stated on the employee's W-4 form. Withholding tax can be calculated in two ways. The first is with the use of a tax table (Figure 16-12). These tables are provided in IRS Publication 15. Locate the table that describes the pay period: daily, weekly, biweekly, semimonthly, or monthly. Then select the table for the correct filing status (single or married) and locate the gross salary and number of deductions.

A Percentage Method of Withholding formula can be used to calculate the amount of withholding tax. The correct table is identified by the payroll period and filing status (Figure 16-13).

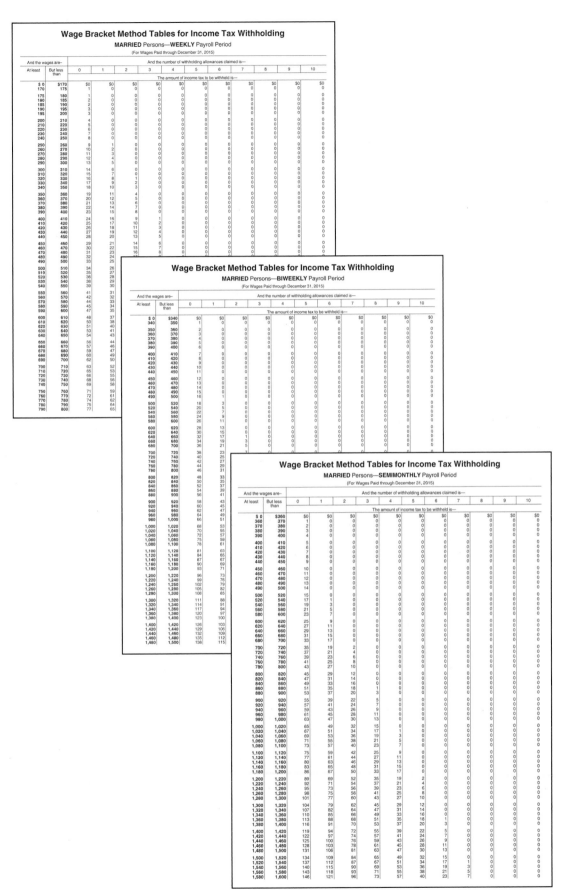

FIGURE 16-12 Example of employer tax tables from Publication 15. (From Internal Revenue Service, Department of the Treasury, Washington, DC.)

Percentage Method Tables for Income Tax Withholding

(For Wages Paid in 2015)

TABLE 1—WEEKLY Payroll Period

(a) SINGLE person (including head of household)—
If the amount of wages (after subtracting withholding allowances) is: Not over $44 . . . . The amount of income tax to withhold is: $0

Over—	But not over—	The amount of income tax to withhold is:	of excess over—
$44	—$222	$0.00 plus 10%	—$44
$222	—$764	$17.80 plus 15%	—$222
$764	—$1,789	$99.10 plus 25%	—$764
$1,789	—$3,685	$355.35 plus 28%	—$1,789
$3,685	—$7,958	$886.23 plus 33%	—$3,685
$7,958	—$7,990	$2,296.32 plus 35%	—$7,958
$7,990		$2,307.52 plus 39.6%	—$7,990

(b) MARRIED person—
If the amount of wages (after subtracting withholding allowances) is: Not over $165 . . . . The amount of income tax to withhold is: $0

Over—	But not over—	The amount of income tax to withhold is:	of excess over—
$165	—$520	$0.00 plus 10%	—$165
$520	—$1,606	$35.50 plus 15%	—$520
$1,606	—$3,073	$198.40 plus 25%	—$1,606
$3,073	—$4,597	$565.15 plus 28%	—$3,073
$4,597	—$8,079	$991.87 plus 33%	—$4,597
$8,079	—$9,105	$2,140.93 plus 35%	—$8,079
$9,105		$2,500.03 plus 39.6%	—$9,105

TABLE 2—BIWEEKLY Payroll Period

(a) SINGLE person (including head of household)—
If the amount of wages (after subtracting withholding allowances) is: Not over $88 . . . . The amount of income tax to withhold is: $0

Over—	But not over—	The amount of income tax to withhold is:	of excess over—
$88	—$443	$0.00 plus 10%	—$88
$443	—$1,529	$35.50 plus 15%	—$443
$1,529	—$3,579	$198.40 plus 25%	—$1,529
$3,579	—$7,369	$710.90 plus 28%	—$3,579
$7,369	—$15,915	$1,772.10 plus 33%	—$7,369
$15,915	—$15,981	$4,592.28 plus 35%	—$15,915
$15,981		$4,615.38 plus 39.6%	—$15,981

(b) MARRIED person—
If the amount of wages (after subtracting withholding allowances) is: Not over $331 . . . . The amount of income tax to withhold is: $0

Over—	But not over—	The amount of income tax to withhold is:	of excess over—
$331	—$1,040	$0.00 plus 10%	—$331
$1,040	—$3,212	$70.90 plus 15%	—$1,040
$3,212	—$6,146	$396.70 plus 25%	—$3,212
$6,146	—$9,194	$1,130.20 plus 28%	—$6,146
$9,194	—$16,158	$1,983.64 plus 33%	—$9,194
$16,158	—$18,210	$4,281.76 plus 35%	—$16,158
$18,210		$4,999.96 plus 39.6%	—$18,210

TABLE 3—SEMIMONTHLY Payroll Period

(a) SINGLE person (including head of household)—
If the amount of wages (after subtracting withholding allowances) is: Not over $96 . . . . The amount of income tax to withhold is: $0

Over—	But not over—	The amount of income tax to withhold is:	of excess over—
$96	—$480	$0.00 plus 10%	—$96
$480	—$1,656	$38.40 plus 15%	—$480
$1,656	—$3,877	$214.80 plus 25%	—$1,656
$3,877	—$7,983	$770.05 plus 28%	—$3,877
$7,983	—$17,242	$1,919.73 plus 33%	—$7,983
$17,242	—$17,313	$4,975.20 plus 35%	—$17,242
$17,313		$5,000.05 plus 39.6%	—$17,313

(b) MARRIED person—
If the amount of wages (after subtracting withholding allowances) is: Not over $358 . . . . The amount of income tax to withhold is: $0

Over—	But not over—	The amount of income tax to withhold is:	of excess over—
$358	—$1,127	$0.00 plus 10%	—$358
$1,127	—$3,479	$76.90 plus 15%	—$1,127
$3,479	—$6,658	$429.70 plus 25%	—$3,479
$6,658	—$9,960	$1,224.45 plus 28%	—$6,658
$9,960	—$17,504	$2,149.01 plus 33%	—$9,960
$17,504	—$19,727	$4,638.53 plus 35%	—$17,504
$19,727		$5,416.58 plus 39.6%	—$19,727

TABLE 4—MONTHLY Payroll Period

(a) SINGLE person (including head of household)—
If the amount of wages (after subtracting withholding allowances) is: Not over $192 . . . . The amount of income tax to withhold is: $0

Over—	But not over—	The amount of income tax to withhold is:	of excess over—
$192	—$960	$0.00 plus 10%	—$192
$960	—$3,313	$76.80 plus 15%	—$960
$3,313	—$7,754	$429.75 plus 25%	—$3,313
$7,754	—$15,967	$1,540.00 plus 28%	—$7,754
$15,967	—$34,483	$3,839.64 plus 33%	—$15,967
$34,483	—$34,625	$9,949.92 plus 35%	—$34,483
$34,625		$9,999.62 plus 39.6%	—$34,625

(b) MARRIED person—
If the amount of wages (after subtracting withholding allowances) is: Not over $717 . . . . The amount of income tax to withhold is: $0

Over—	But not over—	The amount of income tax to withhold is:	of excess over—
$717	—$2,254	$0.00 plus 10%	—$717
$2,254	—$6,958	$153.70 plus 15%	—$2,254
$6,958	—$13,317	$859.30 plus 25%	—$6,958
$13,317	—$19,921	$2,449.05 plus 28%	—$13,317
$19,921	—$35,008	$4,298.17 plus 33%	—$19,921
$35,008	—$39,454	$9,276.88 plus 35%	—$35,008
$39,454		$10,832.98 plus 39.6%	—$39,454

FIGURE 16-13 Example of percentage withholding tables from Publication 15. (From Internal Revenue Service, Department of the Treasury, Washington, DC.)

Payroll Taxes: Reports and Deposits

After taxes have been calculated, they are reported to the IRS and deposited. Taxes to be reported include Federal Income, Social Security, and Medicare taxes. In addition to these taxes, the employer must pay FUTA taxes.

Federal Income, Social Security, and Medicare taxes are reported on Form 941, Employer's Quarterly Federal Tax Return (Figure 16-14). This form, which is filed with the IRS on a quarterly basis (every 3 months beginning in January), is completed by the bookkeeper, accountant, or payroll service with the use of information documented in the payroll records.

The employer's FUTA tax is calculated quarterly. The type of tax being deposited, the amount of the deposit, and reporting requirements determine deposit schedules. These schedules are outlined in the IRS Publication 15 (Circular E) for the current year. If it is your responsibility to file the tax reports and make the deposits, you will need to know the dates and make the deposits as scheduled. If deposits are not received by the due date, a penalty will be assessed.

The IRS requires that all tax deposits be made using Electronic Fund Transfer (EFT) technology. This can be done through your bank or you can make the deposit directly to the Treasury Department using the Electronic Federal Tax Payment System (EFTPS).

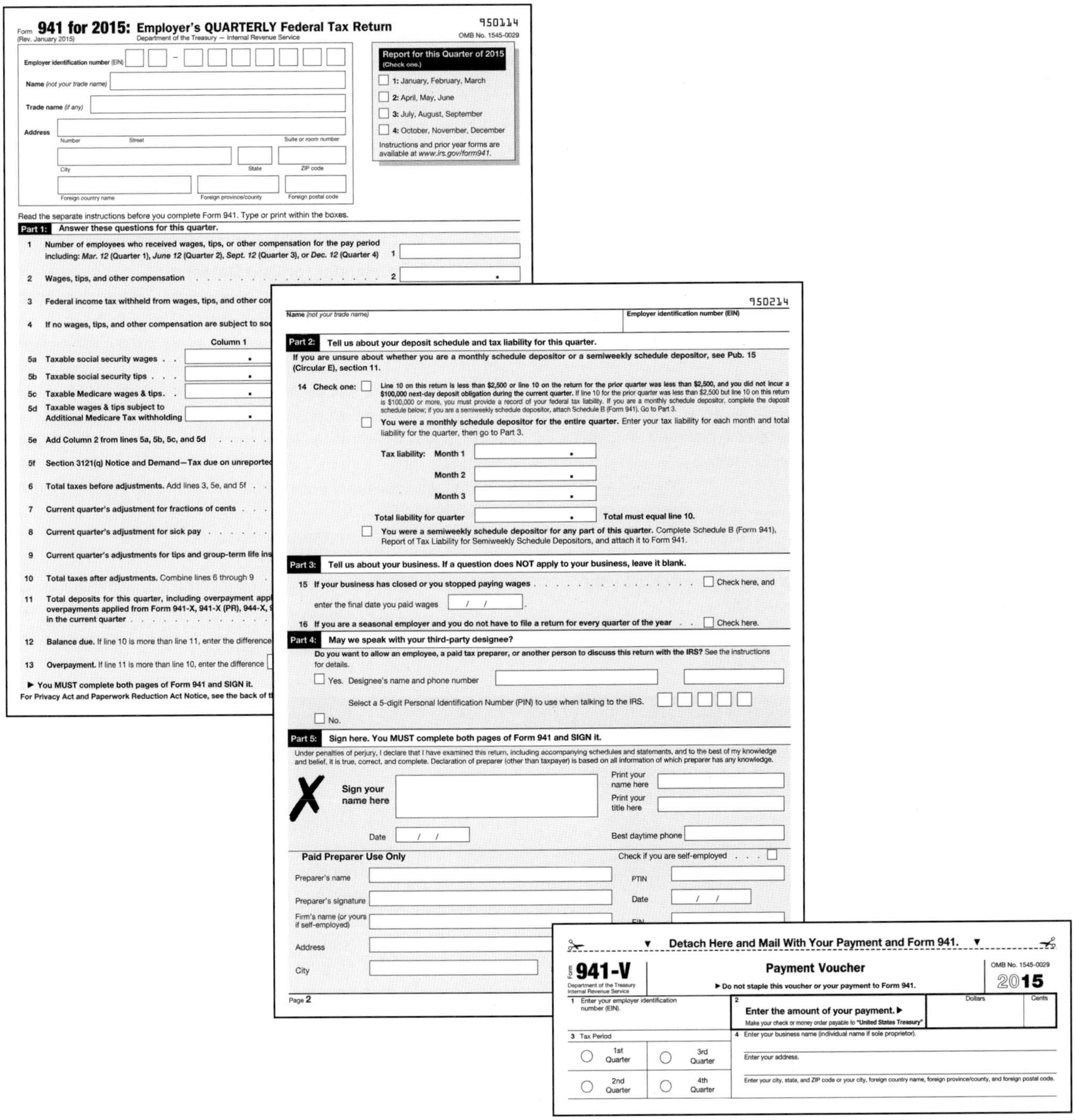

Form **941 for 2015: Employer's QUARTERLY Federal Tax Return** 950114
(Rev. January 2015) Department of the Treasury — Internal Revenue Service OMB No. 1545-0029

Employer identification number (EIN)
Name (not your trade name)
Trade name (if any)
Address Number Street Suite or room number
City State ZIP code
Foreign country name Foreign province/county Foreign postal code

Report for this Quarter of 2015 (Check one.)
- 1: January, February, March
- 2: April, May, June
- 3: July, August, September
- 4: October, November, December

Instructions and prior year forms are available at *www.irs.gov/form941*.

Read the separate instructions before you complete Form 941. Type or print within the boxes.

Part 1: Answer these questions for this quarter.

1 Number of employees who received wages, tips, or other compensation for the pay period including: *Mar. 12* (Quarter 1), *June 12* (Quarter 2), *Sept. 12* (Quarter 3), or *Dec. 12* (Quarter 4) 1

2 Wages, tips, and other compensation 2

3 Federal income tax withheld from wages, tips, and other co

4 If no wages, tips, and other compensation are subject to so

Column 1

5a Taxable social security wages

5b Taxable social security tips

5c Taxable Medicare wages & tips.

5d Taxable wages & tips subject to Additional Medicare Tax withholding

5e Add Column 2 from lines 5a, 5b, 5c, and 5d

5f Section 3121(q) Notice and Demand—Tax due on unreporte

6 Total taxes before adjustments. Add lines 3, 5e, and 5f

7 Current quarter's adjustment for fractions of cents

8 Current quarter's adjustment for sick pay

9 Current quarter's adjustments for tips and group-term life ins

10 Total taxes after adjustments. Combine lines 6 through 9

11 Total deposits for this quarter, including overpayment appl overpayments applied from Form 941-X, 941-X (PR), 944-X, in the current quarter

12 Balance due. If line 10 is more than line 11, enter the difference

13 Overpayment. If line 11 is more than line 10, enter the difference

▶ You MUST complete both pages of Form 941 and SIGN it.

For Privacy Act and Paperwork Reduction Act Notice, see the back of t

---

950214

Name (not your trade name) | Employer identification number (EIN)

Part 2: Tell us about your deposit schedule and tax liability for this quarter.

If you are unsure about whether you are a monthly schedule depositor or a semiweekly schedule depositor, see Pub. 15 (Circular E), section 11.

14 Check one: ☐ Line 10 on this return is less than $2,500 or line 10 on the return for the prior quarter was less than $2,500, and you did not incur a $100,000 next-day deposit obligation during the current quarter. If line 10 for the prior quarter was less than $2,500 but line 10 on this return is $100,000 or more, you must provide a record of your federal tax liability. If you are a monthly schedule depositor, complete the deposit schedule below; if you are a semiweekly schedule depositor, attach Schedule B (Form 941). Go to Part 3.

☐ You were a monthly schedule depositor for the entire quarter. Enter your tax liability for each month and total liability for the quarter, then go to Part 3.

Tax liability: Month 1
Month 2
Month 3
Total liability for quarter — Total must equal line 10.

☐ You were a semiweekly schedule depositor for any part of this quarter. Complete Schedule B (Form 941), Report of Tax Liability for Semiweekly Schedule Depositors, and attach it to Form 941.

Part 3: Tell us about your business. If a question does NOT apply to your business, leave it blank.

15 If your business has closed or you stopped paying wages ☐ Check here, and enter the final date you paid wages / /

16 If you are a seasonal employer and you do not have to file a return for every quarter of the year ☐ Check here.

Part 4: May we speak with your third-party designee?

Do you want to allow an employee, a paid tax preparer, or another person to discuss this return with the IRS? See the instructions for details.

☐ Yes. Designee's name and phone number

Select a 5-digit Personal Identification Number (PIN) to use when talking to the IRS.

☐ No.

Part 5: Sign here. You MUST complete both pages of Form 941 and SIGN it.

Under penalties of perjury, I declare that I have examined this return, including accompanying schedules and statements, and to the best of my knowledge and belief, it is true, correct, and complete. Declaration of preparer (other than taxpayer) is based on all information of which preparer has any knowledge.

Sign your name here — Print your name here — Print your title here

Date / / — Best daytime phone

Paid Preparer Use Only — Check if you are self-employed ☐

Preparer's name — PTIN
Preparer's signature — Date / /
Firm's name (or yours if self-employed) — EIN
Address
City

Page 2

▼ Detach Here and Mail With Your Payment and Form 941. ▼

Form **941-V** Department of the Treasury Internal Revenue Service — **Payment Voucher** ▶ Do not staple this voucher or your payment to Form 941. — OMB No. 1545-0029 **2015**

1 Enter your employer identification number (EIN).

2 **Enter the amount of your payment.** ▶ Make your check or money order payable to "United States Treasury" — Dollars — Cents

3 Tax Period: ○ 1st Quarter ○ 2nd Quarter ○ 3rd Quarter ○ 4th Quarter

4 Enter your business name (individual name if sole proprietor).
Enter your address.
Enter your city, state, and ZIP code or your city, foreign country name, foreign province/county, and foreign postal code.

FIGURE 16-14 Employer's Quarterly Federal Tax Return form (Form 941) and Payment Voucher (Form 941-V). (From Internal Revenue Service, Department of the Treasury, Washington, DC.)

EMPLOYER RESPONSIBILITIES

The following list provides a brief summary of your basic responsibilities. Because the individual circumstances for each employer can vary greatly, their responsibilities for withholding, depositing, and reporting employment taxes can differ.

New Employees

- Verify work eligibility of employees
- Record employees' names and Social Security Numbers (SSNs) from social security cards
- Ask employees for Form W-4

Each Payday

- Withhold federal income tax based on each employee's Form W-4
- Withhold employee's share of Social Security and Medicare taxes
- Include advanced earned income credit payment in paycheck if employee requested it on Form W-5
- Deposit:
  - Withheld income tax
  - Withheld and employer Social Security taxes
  - Withheld and employee Medicare taxes

NOTE: The due date of the deposit generally depends on your deposit schedule (monthly or semiweekly).

Annually (By January 31)

- File Form 944 (pay tax with return if not required to deposit)

Quarterly (by April 30, July 31, October 31, and January 31)

- Deposit FUTA tax in an authorized financial institution if undeposited amount is more than $500
- File Form 941 (pay tax with return if not required to deposit)

Annually (See Calendar for Due Dates)

- Remind employees to submit a new Form W-4 if they need to change their withholding
- Ask for a new Form W-4 from employees claiming exemption from income tax withholding
- Reconcile Forms 941 with Forms W-2 and W-3
- Furnish each employee with a Form W-2
- File Copy A of Forms W-2 and the transmittal Form W-3 with the SSA
- Furnish each payee a Form 1099 (for example, Forms 1099-R and 1099-MISC)
- File Forms 1099 and the transmittal Form 1096
- File Form 940 or Form 940-EZ
- File Form 945 for any nonpayroll income tax withholding

Modified from Publication 15 (Circular E), Employer's Tax Guide (December 2014). Courtesy Internal Revenue Service.

RECORD KEEPING

A record of all employment taxes must be kept for at least 4 years. These records must be available for Internal Revenue Service (IRS) review and must contain the following information:

- Employer identification number (EIN)
- Amounts and dates of all wage, annuity, and pension payments
- Amount of tips reported
- Fair market value of in-kind wages paid
- Names, addresses, Social Security Numbers (SSNs), and occupations of employees and recipients

- Employee copies of Form W-2 that were returned as undeliverable
- Dates of employment
- Periods for which employees and recipients were paid while absent because of sickness or injury and the amount and weekly rate of payments you or third-party payers made to them
- Copies of employees' and recipients' income tax withholding allowance certificates (Forms W-4, W4P, W-S, and W-4V)
- Dates and amounts of tax deposits made
- Copies of returns filed
- Records of fringe benefits provided, including substantiation

Employer Identification Number

All employers who report employment taxes or provide tax statements to employees will need an Employer identification number (EIN). The EIN is a nine-digit number that is issued by the IRS. Digits are arranged as follows: 00-0000000. The EIN is used to identify the tax accounts of employers. The EIN must be placed on all items sent to the IRS or the SSA.

KEY POINTS

- Accounts payable is a system by which all dental practice expenditures are organized, verified, and categorized. Organization of these accounts is necessary to ensure that timely payments are made.
- Check writing has been expanded to include paper instruments, electronic transfers, and the use of credit and debit cards. Checks can be generated with the use of computers, one-write systems, and outside services. Accountants use information from the check register to categorize expenditures and create reports.

- A bank statement must be reconciled to ensure that all records are in agreement. Steps in reconciling include verifying debits, deposits, and canceled checks and comparing balances.
- Payroll functions include calculating payroll, deducting taxes, writing checks, and filing tax reports. These functions can be performed manually, with the use of a computer software package, or by an outside agency.

CAREER-READY PRACTICES

Career-Ready Practices activities are designed to provide students with experiences that can be "practiced" in preparation for skills needed on the job. In each of the following exercises, a variety of approaches may be used to address the problem, rather than "right" or "wrong" answers. Below each exercise, next to the compass icon, is a listing of suggested Career-Ready Practice numbers that correspond to the listing of 12 practices in the front of the text (see p. viii-ix); these practices provide suggestions for approaches to complete the exercise.

1. You have been tasked with writing a detailed job description for an accounts payable clerk in the dental office. Outline the tasks that will be required and explain how these tasks (manually or with a computer) will be performed. Include a timeline for specific tasks, list the reports that will need to be generated and describe the safeguards that should be in place to protect the employer and the employee from unauthorized use of funds. Use information given in this chapter as well as outside resources to support your plan.

Career-Ready Practices

2 *Apply appropriate academic and technical skills.*

4 *Communicate clearly, effectively, and with reason.*

5 *Consider the environmental, social, and economic impacts of decisions.*

8 *Utilize critical thinking to make sense of problems and persevere in solving them.*

17

Bookkeeping Procedures: Accounts Receivable

LEARNING OBJECTIVES

1. Explain the role of the administrative dental assistant in the management of patient financial transactions.
2. Identify the components of financial records organization.
3. Perform the steps in the daily routine for managing patient transactions.
4. List and explain the types of financial reports used in a dental office.

INTRODUCTION

Dentistry, like any business, is mandated by federal and state regulations to maintain a system that documents the collection of monies. Smart business practice also requires that a financial system be maintained, with both accounts receivable and accounts payable. Accounts receivable is the system that records all financial transactions between a patient and the dental practice. This system calculates the amount of money owed to the dental practice by accounting for charges and payments. Accounts payable is the system that records all monies the dental practice owes others. It is the responsibility of the administrative dental assistant to maintain accurate records in the management of accounts receivable and accounts payable.

Two separate procedures are required in the maintenance of financial records and reports. The administrative dental assistant is responsible for bookkeeping. Bookkeeping is the method of recording all financial transactions. The second procedure is accounting. Accounting is the method used to verify and classify all transactions (accounts payable and accounts receivable) and is usually the duty of an accountant. An accountant may be employed by large dental practices. Smaller dental practices usually seek the outside services of an accountant who will audit bookkeeping procedures, calculate taxes, and write financial reports.

COMPONENTS OF FINANCIAL RECORDS ORGANIZATION

Patient information
- Identifies person responsible for payment of the account
- Identifies insurance coverage

Method of recording transactions
- Computerized
- Manual bookkeeping, "pegboard," or "one-write" system

Billing
- Patient
- Insurance company

Patient Information

The first step is to determine who is financially responsible for the account. Information can be obtained from the financial information section of a patient registration form (Figure 17-1, A). Insurance information, both primary (first coverage) and secondary (second coverage), is listed on the same form. This information can also be found in the database of a practice management software system (Figure 17-1, B).

Methods of Recording Transactions
Computerized Bookkeeping Systems

A computerized bookkeeping system uses a program (function) to organize, track, and calculate the accounts receivable. This function is usually a main component in a full management system of the type used in most dental practices (discussed in Chapter 7). The advantage of using a comprehensive practice management system is that the information has been recorded in an electronic clinical record creating a database that is shared with other components of the system. The database can be used for a variety of different financial tasks, including tracking treatment, billing insurance, billing patients, preparing deposit slips, formulating accounting reports, and forecasting the financial health of the dental practice. The software program has the capability to seamlessly perform many of the daily tasks typically performed by the administrative dental assistant in managing patient transactions.

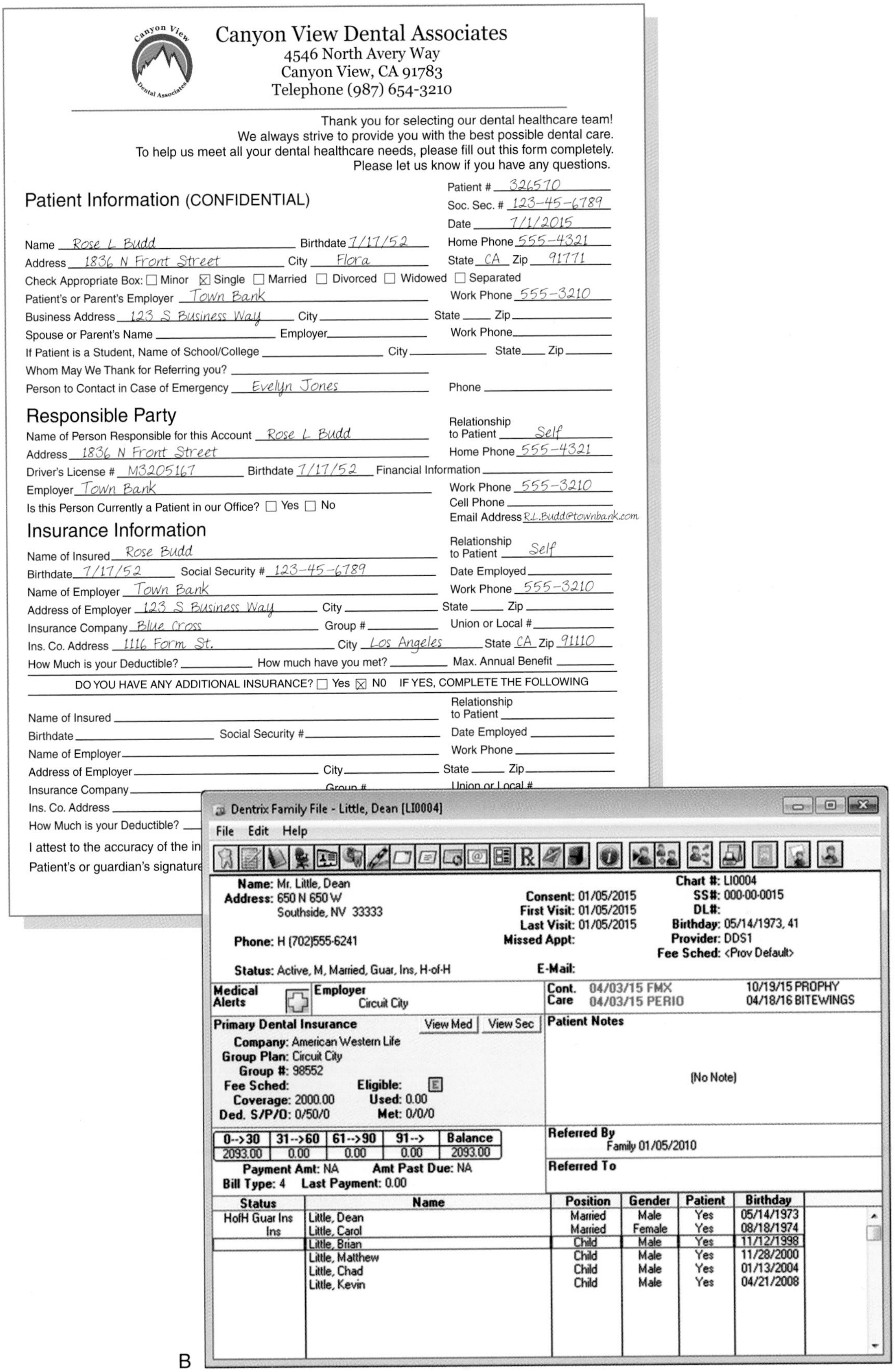

Canyon View Dental Associates
4546 North Avery Way
Canyon View, CA 91783
Telephone (987) 654-3210

Thank you for selecting our dental healthcare team!
We always strive to provide you with the best possible dental care.
To help us meet all your dental healthcare needs, please fill out this form completely.
Please let us know if you have any questions.

Patient Information (CONFIDENTIAL)

Patient # 326570
Soc. Sec. # 123-45-6789
Date 7/1/2015

Name Rose L Budd Birthdate 7/17/52 Home Phone 555-4321
Address 1836 N Front Street City Flora State CA Zip 91771
Check Appropriate Box: ☐ Minor ☒ Single ☐ Married ☐ Divorced ☐ Widowed ☐ Separated
Patient's or Parent's Employer Town Bank Work Phone 555-3210
Business Address 123 S Business Way City State Zip
Spouse or Parent's Name Employer Work Phone
If Patient is a Student, Name of School/College City State Zip
Whom May We Thank for Referring you?
Person to Contact in Case of Emergency Evelyn Jones Phone

Responsible Party

Name of Person Responsible for this Account Rose L Budd Relationship to Patient Self
Address 1836 N Front Street Home Phone 555-4321
Driver's License # M3205167 Birthdate 7/17/52 Financial Information
Employer Town Bank Work Phone 555-3210
Is this Person Currently a Patient in our Office? ☐ Yes ☐ No Cell Phone
Email Address R.L.Budd@townbank.com

Insurance Information

Name of Insured Rose Budd Relationship to Patient Self
Birthdate 7/17/52 Social Security # 123-45-6789 Date Employed
Name of Employer Town Bank Work Phone 555-3210
Address of Employer 123 S Business Way City State Zip
Insurance Company Blue Cross Group # Union or Local #
Ins. Co. Address 1116 Form St. City Los Angeles State CA Zip 91110
How Much is your Deductible? How much have you met? Max. Annual Benefit

DO YOU HAVE ANY ADDITIONAL INSURANCE? ☐ Yes ☒ NO IF YES, COMPLETE THE FOLLOWING

Name of Insured Relationship to Patient
Birthdate Social Security # Date Employed
Name of Employer Work Phone
Address of Employer City State Zip
Insurance Company Group # Union or Local #
Ins. Co. Address
How Much is your Deductible?
I attest to the accuracy of the in
Patient's or guardian's signature

A

Dentrix Family File - Little, Dean [LI0004]
File Edit Help

Name: Mr. Little, Dean
Address: 650 N 650 W
Southside, NV 33333
Phone: H (702)555-6241
Status: Active, M, Married, Guar, Ins, H-of-H
Consent: 01/05/2015
First Visit: 01/05/2015
Last Visit: 01/05/2015
Missed Appt:
E-Mail:
Chart #: LI0004
SS#: 000-00-0015
DL#:
Birthday: 05/14/1973, 41
Provider: DDS1
Fee Sched: <Prov Default>

Medical Alerts
Employer Circuit City
Cont. Care 04/03/15 FMX 04/03/15 PERIO 10/19/15 PROPHY 04/18/16 BITEWINGS

Primary Dental Insurance View Med View Sec
Company: American Western Life
Group Plan: Circuit City
Group #: 98552
Fee Sched: Eligible: E
Coverage: 2000.00 Used: 0.00
Ded. S/P/O: 0/50/0 Met: 0/0/0

Patient Notes
[No Note]

0-->30	31-->60	61-->90	91-->	Balance
2093.00	0.00	0.00	0.00	2093.00

Payment Amt: NA Amt Past Due: NA
Bill Type: 4 Last Payment: 0.00

Referred By
Family 01/05/2010
Referred To

Status	Name	Position	Gender	Patient	Birthday
HofH Guar Ins	Little, Dean	Married	Male	Yes	05/14/1973
Ins	Little, Carol	Married	Female	Yes	08/18/1974
	Little, Brian	Child	Male	Yes	11/12/1998
	Little, Matthew	Child	Male	Yes	11/28/2000
	Little, Chad	Child	Male	Yes	01/13/2004
	Little, Kevin	Child	Male	Yes	04/21/2008

B

FIGURE 17-1 A, Completed patient registration form, including financial and insurance information. **B,** The same registration information is also found in the patient database of the practice management software system. (**B,** Dentrix screen capture courtesy Henry Schein Practice Solutions, American Fork, Utah.)

Manual Bookkeeping Systems

The most common manual (paper and pencil) bookkeeping system used in a dental practice is the pegboard system. This system uses a variety of forms designed to be placed one on top of another for the purpose of entering the information one time (also referred to as a "one-write system"). Once the information is entered (handwritten), it is the responsibility of the administrative dental assistant to calculate totals and balance the spreadsheets (Figure 17-2, A).

Use of a pegboard system requires that the administrative dental assistant be familiar with each step and know how to make entries properly, use receipts and superbills, produce monthly statements, and use a 10-key adding machine or calculator (preferably with a tape for verification of entries).

BILLING

Billing is the procedure that notifies a responsible party (individual or insurance carrier) regarding the current status of an account. Insurance carriers are sent the attending dentist's statements (claim forms) and patients are sent statements. A statement indicates the date of service, identifies the patient, and lists all transactions (treatment and payment). The purposes of the statement are to inform the patient and to request payment for the balance due. It is important that statements are easy for patients to read and understand. Traditional paper statements are printed and sent via the postal service (Figure 17-3, A). Electronic patient statements are generated by the practice management software and sent directly to the patient via e-mail or through a third-party billing service (Figure 17-3, B).

No matter what method of billing is used it is important to remember that patient billing is an organized procedure that should be performed at the same time each month. A key to successful billing is to be consistent each month. Patients usually pay bills around their paydays. The most common pay periods are the 1st and 15th of each month. Therefore if you want the bills to be paid around those dates, schedule your billing period so that patients receive their statements around the 10th or 23rd of each month. Not all statements need to be sent on the same day. If you are working in a very large office, statements can be divided and sent weekly or bimonthly.

Insurance companies are billed with the attending dentist's statements or encounter forms, as discussed in Chapter 15. In addition to billing the insurance company directly, superbills can be given to patients; it then becomes the responsibility of the patient to bill the insurance company. Superbills can be computer generated or may be completed using a pegboard system.

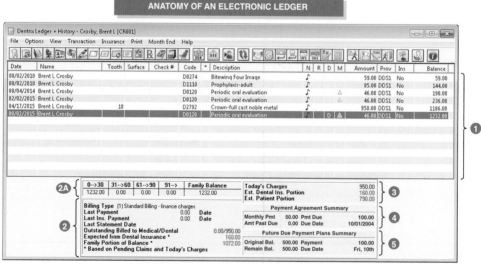

ANATOMY OF AN ELECTRONIC LEDGER

1. The Transaction Log lists all transactions posted to the patient/family's account. For each transaction, the Ledger lists the date, patient or guarantor name, tooth number (when applicable), procedure code or type, a description, amount of the transaction, and the transaction provider. It also indicates whether insurance has been billed or not. Several symbols can appear in the Description column to provide additional information about the transaction.

2. Account Information includes the Billing Type, the amount and date of the last guarantor payment, and the amount and date of the last insurance payment. The Last Statement Date is the last time a Billing Statement was printed for the account. Outstanding Billed to Insurance is the estimated amount that insurance will pay on all outstanding dental claims. Family Portion of Balance is the estimated amount the patient will owe after insurance has paid.

2A. The account balance is shown in the appropriate aging bracket(s). The total account balance is shown under Family Balance.

3. Today's Charges is the total of all transactions with today's date. Est. Dental Ins. Portion is the estimated amount that dental insurance will pay according to the coverage setup in the Family File. Est. Patient Portion is the estimated amount the Patient owes according to the coverage setup in the Family File.

4. If a Payment Agreement exists for the account, the current status of the agreement is shown here.

5. If a Future Due Payment Plan exists for the account, the current status of the payment plan is shown here.

(Dentrix screen capture courtesy Henry Schein Practice Solutions, American Fork, Utah.)

DAILY LOG OF CHARGES AND RECEIPTS

DATE 1/31/15 SHEET NUMBER _____ A   B1   B2   C   D

DATE	FAMILY MEMBER	PROFESSIONAL SERVICES	CHARGE	PYMTS.	ADJ.	NEW BALANCE	PREVIOUS BALANCE	NAME
1/31	Rose	ins. pmt./adj.		98 00	12 00	80 00	190 00	Rose Budd
1/31	Frank	NSF	80 00	—	—	80 00	-0-	Frank Williams
1/31	Jodi	payment	—	62 00	—	<22 00>	40 00	Jodi Coulson
1/31	Dawn	Restorative	230 00	-0-	—	240 00	10 00	Dawn Johnson
1/31	Maria	prophy/c.pmt.	62 00	62 00	—	-0-	-0-	Marie Gonzales
1/31	Angela	FMX		62 00	—	80 00	62 00	Angela Brown
1/31	Mark	Composite	246 00	—	24 00	221 40	-0-	Mark Vail
1/31	Lois	ins. pmt.	—	630 00	20 00	171 00	821 00	Lois Tract

TOTALS

COL. D TOTAL
PLUS COL. A
SUB TOTAL
LESS COLS. B
MUST EQUAL

A

DAY SHEET (CHRONOLOGICAL)
Dentrix Dental Practice
04/17/2015

Date: 04/17/2015   Page: 1

ENTRY DATE	PROCEDURE DATE	PATIENT NAME	TH	CODE	DESCRIPTION	CHARGES	PAYMENTS	BT	PROV	PHONE #
04/17/2015	04/17/2015	Little, Dean		D1110	Prophylaxis-adult	85.00		4	DDS1	(702)555-6241
04/17/2015	04/17/2015	Little, Dean		D0274	Bitewing Four Image	59.00		4	DDS1	(702)555-6241
04/17/2015	04/17/2015	Little, Dean		D0180	Comprehensive perio evaluati	89.00		4	DDS1	(702)555-6241
04/17/2015	04/17/2015	Edwards, Anna	18	D2150	ML Amalgam-2 surf. prim/perm	161.00		4	ENDO	(702)555-7101
04/17/2015	04/17/2015	Hayes, Sally		D1110	Prophylaxis-adult	85.00		10	DDS1	( )
04/17/2015	04/17/2015	Davis, Karen		D1110	Prophylaxis-adult	85.00		1	DDS1	(702)555-1530
04/17/2015	04/17/2015	Brown, Mary		D1110	Prophylaxis-adult	85.00		1	DDS2	(702)555-4509
04/17/2015	04/17/2015	Brown, Mary		D0120	Periodic oral evaluation	46.00		1	DDS2	(702)555-4509

GRAND TOTALS:	CURRENT	MONTH-TO-DATE	YEAR-TO-DATE	PREVIOUS MONTH
CHARGES:	695.00	5717.00	5717.00	0.00
PAYMENTS:	0.00	0.00	0.00	0.00
CREDIT ADJUSTMENTS:	0.00	0.00	0.00	0.00
CHARGE ADJUSTMENTS:	0.00	0.00	0.00	0.00
FINANCE CHARGES:	0.00	0.00	0.00	0.00
LATE CHARGES:	0.00	0.00	0.00	0.00
CHARGES BILLED TO INSURANCE:	0.00	0.00	0.00	0.00
NEW PATIENTS SEEN:	0	1	1	0
PATIENTS SEEN:	5			
AVG PROD PER PATIENT:	139.00			
AVG CHG PER PROCEDURE:	86.87			
PREVIOUS BALANCE	5022.00			
BALANCE AS OF 04/17/2015	5717.00			
NET CHANGE	695.00			

SMITH, DENNIS - DDS1 TOTALS:				
CHARGES:	403.00	4845.00	4845.00	0.00
PAYMENTS:	0.00	0.00	0.00	0.00
CREDIT ADJUSTMENTS:	0.00	0.00	0.00	0.00
CHARGE ADJUSTMENTS:	0.00	0.00	0.00	0.00
FINANCE CHARGES:	0.00	0.00	0.00	0.00
LATE CHARGES:	0.00	0.00	0.00	0.00
CHARGES BILLED TO INSURANCE:	0.00	0.00	0.00	0.00
NEW PATIENTS SEEN:	0	1	1	0
PATIENTS SEEN:	3			
AVG PROD PER PATIENT:	134.33			
AVG CHG PER PROCEDURE:	80.60			
PREVIOUS BALANCE	4442.00			
BALANCE AS OF 04/17/2015	4845.00			
NET CHANGE	403.00			

B

FIGURE 17-2 A, Manual pegboard daysheet. **B,** The practice management program also organizes, tracks, and calculates accounts receivable and can quickly generate a daysheet. (**B,** Dentrix form courtesy Henry Schein Practice Solutions, American Fork, Utah.)

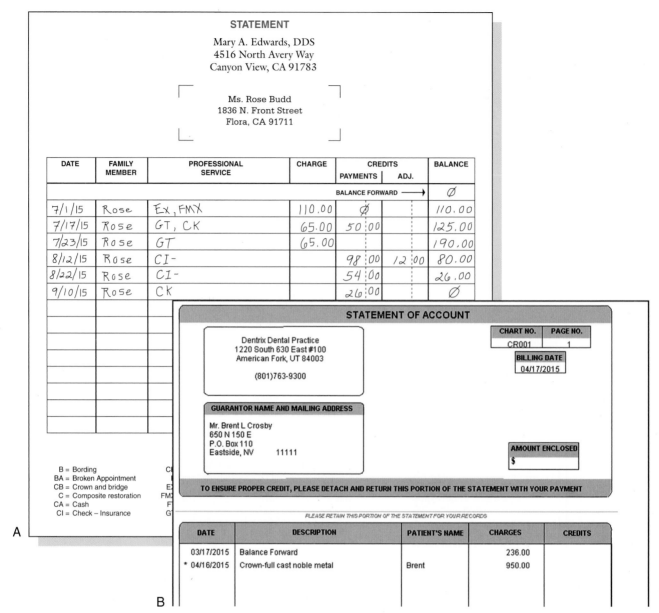

FIGURE 17-3 A, Pegboard statement (copy of ledger card). **B,** Computer-generated statement. (**B,** Dentrix form courtesy Henry Schein Practice Solutions, American Fork, Utah.)

Electronic Financial Record

An **electronic ledger** stores all of the necessary financial information for a patient. From the ledger you can generate an insurance claim, create a pretreatment estimate, post payments, and make adjustments. From the ledger you will be able to see a summary of the day's transaction (by family or individual patient), a history of charges and payments, insurance status, the financial plan, the age of the account, and a total family balance.

Pegboard System

Components of the pegboard system include NCR (no carbon required) paper with carbon strips placed on the backs of receipts. This system allows the administrative dental assistant to write the information one time. When all forms are aligned correctly, the information is transferred to the corresponding column on the receipt, ledger card, and **daily journal.** In addition, an NCR-treated deposit slip can be attached to the appropriate section of the daily journal, providing for a "one-write" deposit slip.

DAILY ROUTINE FOR MANAGING PATIENT TRANSACTIONS

PROCEDURES

Steps in Managing Patient Transactions

1. Identify patients.
2. Produce routing slips.
3. Post financial transactions.
4. Document patient treatments.
5. Document payments.
6. Complete end-of-day procedures.

! REMEMBER

All of the following tasks can be performed using a manual system, computerized system, or combination of both systems. Although techniques will differ in the completion of tasks, all systems will contain the same types of tasks: identifying patients, producing routing slips, posting transactions, and completing end-of-day procedures.

Identify Patients

Identify patients who are going to be seen during the day. The day before treatment, review the patients' clinical records, confirm appointments, prepare the daily schedule, and check pending treatments. Members of the dental healthcare team can review the charts before patients arrive. This process allows the team to become acquainted with the schedule, check for adverse medical conditions, determine what type of anesthetic will be used, acquire information that can be used to personalize a conversation with a patient, check whether laboratory work has been returned, and mentally prepare for the day. It is at this point that the team can have a short meeting to discuss the patients and cases for the day.

Produce Routing Slips

Routing slips are used to communicate treatment information between the treatment area and the business office and establish a check and balance system to ensure that all transactions are posted (Figure 17-4). Computerized routing slips may contain information about the patient, such as treatment plan, date of last visit, and list of other family members who are patients. Financial information includes previous balance, payment plan, financial arrangements, and

insurance balance. Routing slips can be complex, computer-generated forms or simple charge slips. Superbills and encounter forms are frequently used as routing slips.

HIPAA

Privacy Rule

Routing slips contain protected health information (PHI) and must be kept out of the sight of all nonauthorized personnel.

At the end of the day, it is the responsibility of the administrative dental assistant to account for all patients seen during the day. If there is not a system in place to account for the patients such as routing slips or other reports, the administrative dental assistant will not be able to certify that all transactions have been posted correctly. This is extremely important to the financial health of the dental practice. There are many different techniques that can be used to ensure that all patient transactions have been posted, such as numbering the routing slips, comparing the routing slips with the appointment book, or using a system linked to an electronic scheduler that identifies missing transactions. If a patient's transactions cannot be accounted for, the missing information must be identified and posted before the audit of daily transactions is completed.

Post Transactions

Entering or transferring treatment information and associated fees to an accounting system accomplishes posting transactions. When a computerized system is used, the information is stored in the patient's database and used to generate the patient's ledger, billing statement, and insurance claim. If a one-write system is used, the treatment information is recorded on the daysheet and the patient's financial ledger.

Several methods can be used to organize the daily posting routine. All methods, although they vary, include the same elements: identify each patient seen during the day, communicate treatment information from the clinical area to the business office, post all transactions (charges, payment, and adjustments), and verify the daysheet report at the end of the day to ensure accounting accuracy, and prepare an audit report to ensure that all transactions have been posted (Figure 17-2, *B*). Missing one or two chargeable transactions daily can cost the dental practice hundreds of dollars.

PATIENT ROUTE SLIP

Friday - April 17, 2015 at 8:00am — For Ms. Mary Brown (Ms. Brown)

PATIENT INFORMATION

PATIENT NAME:
Ms. Mary Brown (Ms. Brown)
760 N 750 W
Apt. 304
Eastside, NV 11111
HOME: (702)555-4509   **WORK:** (702)555-2000

☐ **PATIENT CLAIMS PENDING**
(Patient has Medical Ins.)

EMPLOYER: Allied Plumbing
SOC SEC NUMBER: 000-00-0004   **CHART NUMBER:** BR0001
MEDICAL ALERTS: Allergy - Hay Fever

PRIMARY PROVIDER: DDS2   **SECONDARY PROVIDER:**
FIRST VISIT DATE: 01/04/2010   **YEARS AS A PATIENT:** 5
LAST VISIT DATE: 04/17/2015   **CCDATES:** 10/29/2013 FMX
LAST PROPHYLAXIS: 04/17/2015   04/02/2014 BITEWINGS
MISSED APPT NUM: 4   **LAST MISSED APPT:** 08/02/2010
LAST REFERRED BY: Phone Survey, 01/04/2010
LAST REFERRED TO: Dr. Clark, Robert S (Oral and Maxillofacial Surgery),
 # REFERRALS: 0   **LAST REFERRAL:**
LAST GRATUITY:

Patient Notes:

ACCOUNT INFORMATION

GUARANTOR NAME:
Ms. Mary Brown
760 N 750 W
Apt. 304
Eastside, NV 11111
HOME: (702)555-4509   **WORK:** (702)555-2000
EMPLOYER: Allied Plumbing
SOC SEC NUMBER: 000-00-0004
BILLING TYPE: 1
LAST PAYMENT: **LAST STATEMENT:**
NEXT PAYMENT: NA   **LAST PMT AMT:** 0.00
   PAYMENT DUE: NA

☐ **FAMILY CLAIMS PENDING**

0==>30	31==>60	61==>90	91==>	INS EST	BALANCE
711.00	0.00	0.00	0.00	81.00	711.00

INSURANCE INFORMATION

PRIMARY CARRIER: Ameritas
SUBSCRIBER: Mary Brown (Self)
EMPLOYER: Allied Plumbing
GROUP NUMBER: 11220   **MAXIMUM BENEFITS:** 2000.00
BENEFITS USED: 0.00   Jan   **BENEFITS REMAINING:** 2000.00
DED OWED S/P/O: PAT-0/50/0, FAM-0/0/0

PREV: 100%	BASIC: 80%	MAJOR: 50%	ORTHO: 50%

SECONDARY CARRIER:
SUBSCRIBER:
EMPLOYER:
GROUP NUMBER: **MAXIMUM BENEFITS:**
BENEFITS USED: **BENEFITS REMAINING:**
DED OWED S/P/O:

PREV:	BASIC:	MAJOR:	ORTHO:

NAME (1 of 1)	POSITION	GEN	BIRTHDAY	AGE	LAST VISIT	LAST PROPHY	CCDATE	NEXT APPT	TP
*Ms. Mary Brown	Single	F	05/15/1984	30	04/17/2015	04/17/2015	10/29/2013(+)		U

APPOINTMENT INFORMATION

APPT DATE: 04/17/2015   **TIME:** 8:00am   **SCHEDULED TIME:** 60 Minutes   **APPT AMOUNT:** 131.00
OPERATORY: OP-1   **PROVIDER:** DDS2   **ADD'L PROVIDER:**   **APPT STATUS:**

NOTES:

DATE	ORDER	TOOTH	CODE	PROCEDURE	AMOUNT
04/17/2015	?		D0120	Periodic oral evaluation	46.00
04/17/2015	?		D1110	Prophylaxis-adult	85.00
	1	18	D3330	Endodontic therapy - molar	930.00
	2		D0470	Diagnostic casts	100.00
	3	18	D2750	Crown-porc fuse high noble mtl	995.00
	?	1	D7140	Extract,erupted th/exposed rt	0.00
	?	16	D7140	Extract,erupted th/exposed rt	0.00
	?	17	D7140	Extract,erupted th/exposed rt	0.00
	?	32	D7140	Extract,erupted th/exposed rt	0.00

TX TOTAL: 2156.00

DATE	TIME	PROVIDER	REASON

FIGURE 17-4 Sample routing slip generated from the practice management program. Routing slips communicate information from the treatment room to the business office. (Dentrix form courtesy Henry Schein Practice Solutions, American Fork, Utah.)

PROCEDURES

Steps in Managing Patient Transactions Using a Computerized System

1. Checking the patient in
   - Ask the patient to update his or her health history, insurance information, and billing address. This can be completed electronically (using a computer kiosk [Figure 17-5] or a digital tablet such as an iPad). It can also be accomplished by handing the patient a clipboard with the necessary forms.

   - Change the status of the patient in the electronic scheduler to "in the office." By changing the status you alert other members of the dental healthcare team that the patient has arrived (typically the status change is noted by changing the color in the scheduler [Figure 17-6]). Changing the status in the scheduler also prompts the program

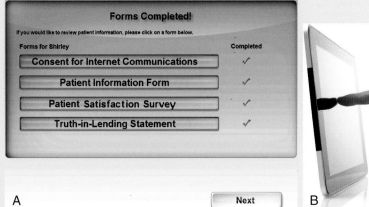
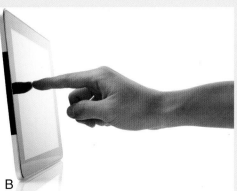

FIGURE 17-5 The in-office computer kiosk or digital tablet can be a convenient way for patients to update their own information electronically. A. (Dentrix screen capture courtesy Henry Schein Practice Solutions, American Fork, Utah.) B. (Copyright © 2012 blackred, iStock.com. All rights reserved.)

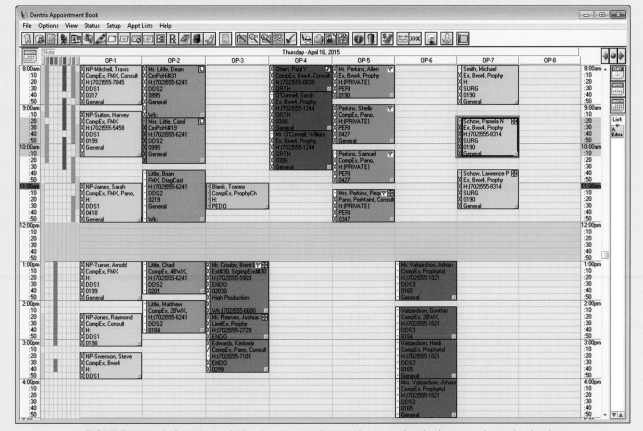

FIGURE 17-6 A function within the electronic appointment book changes the color in the space directly to the left of the patient name (in the box with the letter *X*) to indicate that a patient is in the office. In the Dentrix program, this is indicated by changing this area to blue. (Dentrix screen capture courtesy Henry Schein Practice Solutions, American Fork, Utah.)

PROCEDURES

Steps in Managing Patient Transactions Using a Computerized System—cont'd

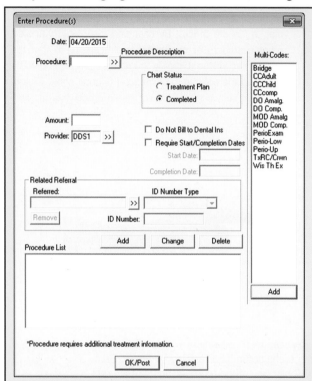

FIGURE 17-7 The Enter Procedure(s) screen allows the user to record each treatment procedure performed. (Dentrix screen capture courtesy Henry Schein Practice Solutions, American Fork, Utah.)

to open other features that will expedite checking the patient out at the end of the appointment.

2. Recording treatment
   - Clinical staff (dentist, assistant, or hygienist) records the patient's treatment for the day in the electronic record (Figure 17-7).
   - Clinical staff may also schedule the patient's next appointment.

3. Checking the patient out
   - Administrative dental assistant checks the patient's clinical record and, if necessary, records treatment. Once the patient's treatment has been entered with all of the necessary information, such as tooth number, surface, and type of procedure, the computer program automatically posts the information to the patient's electronic ledger (Figure 17-8).
   - Collect and post payment for services (Figure 17-9).
   - Cue the system to process the insurance claim.
   - Schedule the next appointment (if not completed by the clinical staff [Figure 17-10]).
   - Print a walkout statement for the patient (Figure 17-11).
   - Provide post-treatment care instructions, if necessary.

4. End-of-day procedure
   The following can be done anytime during the day as time permits:
   - Post mail payments, insurance payments, or electronic transfer payments to the patient's account (see Figure 17-9).

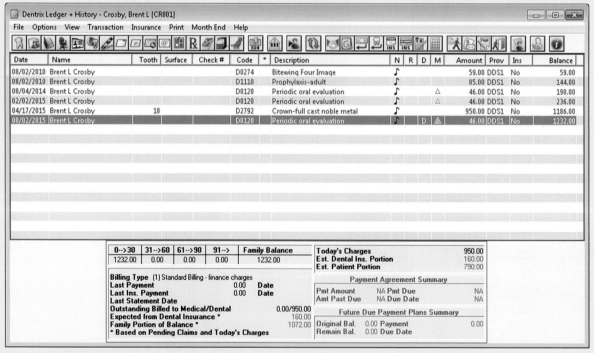

FIGURE 17-8 Treatment information is automatically posted to the patient's ledger. (Dentrix screen capture courtesy Henry Schein Practice Solutions, American Fork, Utah.)

Continued

PROCEDURES

Steps in Managing Patient Transactions Using a Computerized System—cont'd

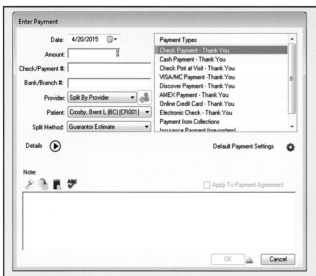

FIGURE 17-9 The administrative dental assistant can easily record and post payments within the electronic system. (Dentrix screen capture courtesy Henry Schein Practice Solutions, American Fork, Utah.)

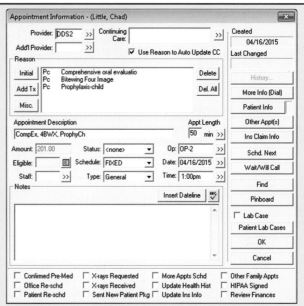

FIGURE 17-10 During checkout, the administrative dental assistant can quickly and easily schedule the patient's next appointment if the clinical staff has not already done so. (Dentrix screen capture courtesy Henry Schein Practice Solutions, American Fork, Utah.)

- Print the routing slips for the next day.
  - Check notes for allergies, needed laboratory work, or other information and follow up to ensure that there are no surprises on the day of the appointment (see Figure 17-4).
- Confirm the next day's appointments.
  The following should be performed after all of the transactions for the day have been posted to the system.
- Generate the daysheet report (check the report for completeness [see Figure 17-2, *A*]).
- Print any reports that are normally run on a daily or weekly basis, such as reports by provider, procedure, insurance, recall, etc.
- Complete banking procedures: print deposit slip, prepare deposit, and deliver to the bank.

PROCEDURES

Steps in Managing Patient Transactions Using a Computerized System—cont'd

STATEMENT OF SERVICES RENDERED

Dentrix Dental Practice
1220 South 630 East #100
American Fork, UT 84003

(801)763-9300

CHART NO.	PAGE NO.
CR001	1

BILLING DATE
04/20/2015

GUARANTOR NAME AND MAILING ADDRESS

Mr. Brent L Crosby
650 N 150 E
Eastside, NV 11111

PATIENT	TOOTH	SURF	DESCRIPTION	CHARGE	CREDIT
Brent			Comprehensive oral evaluation	80.00	

PRIOR BALANCE	CURRENT CREDITS	CURRENT CHARGES	NEW BALANCE	DENTAL INS. EST.	PLEASE PAY
1232.00	0.00	80.00	1312.00	80.00	1232.00

PATIENT	DATE	TIME	REASON

FIGURE 17-11 The practice management software allows the user to easily print a walkout statement during patient checkout. (Dentrix form courtesy Henry Schein Practice Solutions, American Fork, Utah.)

Posting Payments

In addition to receiving payments at the time of service, the practice will receive payments in a variety of forms such as daily mail, electronic transfer, and automatic payment via a third party. Checks from patients and insurance companies are posted to accounts receivable in the same manner as daily transactions (see Figure 17-9).

Most insurance companies do not pay 100% of the amount billed. The balance is therefore billed to the patient as the patient portion. Some contracts with insurance carriers stipulate that a patient cannot be charged a fee higher than the fee allowable by the contract. If a higher fee is charged, the disallowed amount (clearly stated on the explanation of benefits [EOB] form) must be adjusted. The amount is entered in the adjustment dialog box and subtracted from the patient portion.

Posting Credit Card Payments

Payment may be made by credit card. In addition to traditional credit cards, there are debit cards and third-party dental payment plan cards. All cards are processed in the same manner. The card is swiped through an electronic credit card terminal. The terminal electronically sends data to a card center for approval. The credit card terminal also serves as a printer and produces a transaction receipt for the patient and the office (Figure 17-12). Money is directly deposited into the specified account from the card center. The transaction is posted to the patient's ledger (electronically or handwritten) in the same way that a cash or check payment is recorded and coded accordingly.

Adjustments

Adjustments are made to an account for a variety of reasons. Disallowed insurance charges, professional courtesies, senior discounts, credit card and payment plan fees, and uncollectible fees are all examples of adjustments that reduce the patient's balance (Figure 17-13).

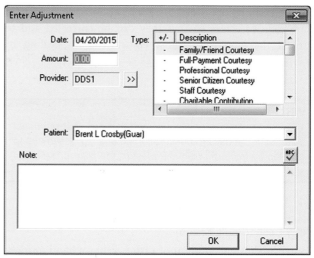

FIGURE 17-13 Adjustments are made to an account for a variety of reasons. (Dentrix screen capture courtesy Henry Schein Practice Solutions, American Fork, Utah.)

When a credit card, debit card, or third-party dental payment plan is used there will be a transaction fee. The fee will be reflected in the deposit to the bank account, which will cause your totals for money collected and the bank deposit to be out of balance. In a computer system this function will vary depending on the software system used. It is important to remember that the daily fees collected will need to match the bank deposit totals. Also remember you cannot charge the patient the fee charged by the credit card company.

One adjustment that raises a patient's balance is a returned check. NSF (nonsufficient funds) checks are checks that are not honored by the bank. Stop payment checks are another form of returned item from the bank. The amount of the check has already been deducted from the patient's account balance; therefore it is necessary to recharge the patient. In addition, most banks add a service charge for returned items, which can be passed on to the patient.

Credit balances are created when there has been a payment that is larger than the balance due. This may occur when a patient pays in advance of treatment. When a credit balance remains at the conclusion of treatment, a refund will be made to the patient.

It may be necessary to give overdue accounts to an outside agency for collection. This is done after a reasonable attempt has been made to collect payment. The agency charges a commission to collect the amount and the commission will be adjusted from the patient's balance.

Completing the Audit Report

The purpose of an audit report is to track all daily transactions and verify that all transactions were posted correctly. This is an important step and should not be skipped. At the end of the day the report is run and any missing transactions or questions in the report need to be addressed in order to complete the end-of-day procedure.

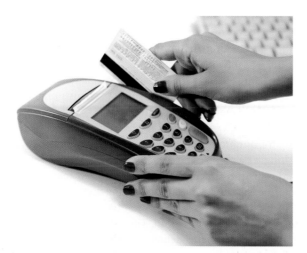

FIGURE 17-12 The credit card terminal is a necessity in the modern dental office to ensure that patients who wish to pay via this method can do so. (Copyright © 2012 photobac, iStock.com. All rights reserved.)

The audit report is necessary for two reasons: to identify omissions or errors so that they can be corrected and to protect the employer against embezzlement (stealing by an employee).

WHAT WOULD YOU DO?

The business manager is concerned that not all of the transactions for the day are being recorded and has asked you to develop a structured plan and present the plan to the office staff at their next meeting.

Petty Cash (Change Fund)

Sometimes a small amount of cash is kept on hand to make change and to purchase small items. The amount of money placed in the fund varies but must be tracked. When an item is purchased with petty cash, the receipt is placed in the petty cash file and the amount is recorded in the petty cash journal. If the doctor or another staff member requests cash from petty cash, a voucher must be filled out with the amount and date and signed by the person taking the money. When money is replenished, a check is drawn and cashed at the bank and the new amount is entered into the journal. A check is used for the purpose of tracking the transaction. Cash should not be taken from a deposit because it will change the amount of the deposit so that the deposit total will not match the amount of money collected for the day.

Routine for Managing Financial Transactions
Day Before
- Review the patient's charts.
- Confirm appointments.
- Prepare a daily schedule and make copies for each treatment room and other areas (electronic and paper).
- Check on laboratory work that is due.
- Fill the schedule, if needed, from the call list.

Day of Appointment
- Produce routing slips.
- Check schedule.
- Review charts with office staff (mini staff meeting).
- When a patient arrives, update financial, medical, and insurance information.
- When treatment is completed, proceed with patient checkout, post transactions, and schedule next appointment.
- Process payments.

End of Day
- Complete posting of daily transactions.
- Prepare bank deposit.
- Generate a daysheet report.
- Complete audit report and account for all transactions.
- Complete insurance processing.

REPORTS

Reports are used to summarize and outline various conditions. Reports that are often used in a dental practice identify patients who are due for recall appointments, patients who have not completed treatment plans, and outstanding insurance claims. In addition to the many reports that identify what needs to be done, some reports illustrate the financial status of the dental practice. Reports enable the dental healthcare team to identify strong and weak areas of the practice and to make necessary corrections. Reports are used by accountants and bookkeepers for the purpose of reporting financial information to government agencies and are considered legal documents.

Reports are written with information that is tabulated and collected. Without a computer to organize and store information, report writing can be long and laborious. Reports can be generated in different formats and according to different criteria. Information for financial reports is obtained from check registers, deposit records, and bank statements. Style and criteria are determined by the nature of the report and the needs of the dentist or accountant.

The administrative dental assistant is responsible for collecting and maintaining financial data to help the accountant generate financial reports. Organizing and maintaining financial records that are inaccurate *is not* an option. This information is used to produce legal documents and must be maintained and protected with the utmost care and accuracy.

Types of Reports

Financial reports are used to determine the financial health of a dental practice. Accountants use them to report business, income, and payroll taxes.

Profit and loss statements are used to identify overhead (the cost it takes to operate a business). They also show whether the dental practice is making or losing money.

Accounts receivable reports categorize the monies patients and insurance companies owe the dental practice. When money is slow in being paid to the dental practice, all members of the team are affected. In addition to the amount of money that is owed, the length of time the money is owed is important. **Aging** the accounts receivable reports shows how much of the money that is owed is 30, 60, 90, or 120 days past due. Most dental practices do not charge interest on money owed; therefore each day money remains unpaid, the value of the money depreciates (loses value). Accounts receivable reports draw attention to the overdue accounts by identifying the amount of money owed, by whom it is owed, and how long it has been since the last payment. With this report, the administrative dental assistant is able to take action in expediting the collection of outstanding accounts.

Production reports identify what type of procedures have been performed and by whom. These reports can be used to determine whether the dental team is productive. Offices with associate dentists and hygienists whose salaries are based on production use these reports to calculate compensation.

Additional Reports

Insurance Reports

- Outstanding insurance claims
- Amount of money owed by insurance companies
- Aging of insurance claims
- Incomplete dental treatment
- Work completed but not submitted for payment
- Preauthorized dental treatment

Accounts Payable Reports

- Money owed to others (bills)
- Account balances
- Categories of expenditures (used in financial reports)

Bank Account Reports

- Account balances
- Average daily balance
- Interest
- Credits and debits

Payroll

- Employee accounting (salary, deductions, taxes paid)
- Payment of payroll tax (by the dentist)
- Payment of workers' compensation insurance
- Payment to pension and employee benefits funds

KEY POINTS

- Accounts receivable is the system by which all financial transactions between the patient and the dental practice are recorded. Accounts payable is the system by which money owed by the dental practice to others is recorded. It is the responsibility of the administrative dental assistant to keep accurate records in the management of accounts receivable and accounts payable.
- Patient financial information is recorded in a computer system or a manual bookkeeping ledger. The computerized system uses an electronic ledger and the manual system most often uses a pegboard system.

- Managing financial transactions, either computerized or manual, includes:
  - Posting transactions
  - Completing audit reports (ensuring that all transactions have been posted)
  - Billing patients and insurance carriers
- **Reports** are used to illustrate different financial and patient trends. Financial reports are used by accountants and members of the dental healthcare team to determine the fiscal health of the dental practice. These reports are also used for mandated documentation and account reporting to government agencies.

CAREER-READY PRACTICES

Career-Ready Practices activities are designed to provide students with experiences that can be "practiced" in preparation for skills needed on the job. In each of the following exercises, a variety of approaches may be used to address the problem, rather than "right" or "wrong" answers. Below each exercise, next to the compass icon, is a listing of suggested Career-Ready Practice numbers that correspond to the listing of 12 practices in the front of the text (see p. viii-ix); these practices provide suggestions for approaches to complete the exercise.

1. Your dental office has just converted to a new computerized practice management system and there is a computer terminal in each of the treatment areas. The business manager feels it will be more efficient if the clinical assistant enters the treatment and makes appointments directly from the treatment area, bypassing the administrative dental assistant. How do you think the division of duties will affect you, the administrative dental assistant? What will be the positive and negative consequences?

 Career-Ready Practices
  1 Act as a responsible and contributing citizen and employee.
  5 Consider the environmental, social and economic impacts of decisions.
  2 Apply appropriate academic and technical skills.

2. In small groups, compare the value of having patient treatment entered by the clinical assistant or the administrative dental assistant. How will the tasks required for managing patient transactions be divided?

 Career-Ready Practices
  8 Utilize critical thinking to make sense of problems and persevere in solving them.
  5 Consider the environmental, social and economic impacts of decisions.
  12 Work productively in teams while using cultural/global competence.

3. In your group, explain the task each staff member will be responsible for and write procedures and policies that will ensure that there is a check and balance in managing patient transactions.

 Career-Ready Practices
  9 Model integrity, ethical leadership and effective management.
  11 Use technology to enhance productivity.
  12 Work productively in teams while using cultural/global competence.
  6 Demonstrate creativity and innovation.

PART V

Managing Your Career

18 Employment Strategies, 273

Employment Strategies

1. List career opportunities for administrative dental assistants.
2. Identify and explain the steps to be followed in developing an employment strategy. Discuss the function of each step, including:
   - Construct a high-quality resume and cover letter.

- Identify the avenues of where to look for employment.
- Explain the function of a personal career portfolio and discuss its advantages.
- Identify and respond to common interview questions.
- Explain the proper way to accept and leave a job.

INTRODUCTION

Hundreds of jobs are waiting for the right person to fill them. The hiring decision is based on the ability of the prospective employee to successfully present himself or herself. Convincing the employer that you are the best person for the job is not easy. The process begins with a self-study and ends with a personal interview. Along the way, you will identify career options, answer questions about yourself, research possible employment opportunities, produce a quality resume, construct a letter of introduction, complete an application, and prepare mentally and physically for an interview.

CAREER OPPORTUNITIES FOR ADMINISTRATIVE DENTAL ASSISTANTS

While completing your training as an administrative dental assistant, you have learned about available career options in dentistry. During your on-the-job training, you may have had the opportunity to experience different avenues of dental assisting in different settings.

Private Practice

Private practice offers the administrative dental assistant a variety of job opportunities, depending on the size and specialty of the practice.

Small Practice

A small practice with one or two dentists and a hygienist can offer an assistant the opportunity to use multiple skills. For example, administrative dental assistants may be responsible for most of the business office tasks. In addition, they may be cross-trained in clinical assisting to help in the clinical area when needed.

Benefits of working in a small dental practice

- The assistant may have the opportunity to be cross-trained in business office skills and clinical area skills. This becomes necessary when few people are available to perform many tasks.
- A family atmosphere develops because all members of the dental healthcare team work closely together on a daily basis. Patients are familiar with all team members because they see the same members at each visit. This relationship can also extend into the community when patients and team members meet at the supermarket, work together on other projects, and attend social functions.
- Loyalty toward the dental practice seems to be stronger because of the close relationship between team members.

Large Practice

Larger dental practices, or corporate practices with several locations, need assistants who have specialized skills. For example, in a large practice the administrative dental assistant may be responsible only for insurance billing. This type of setting provides the assistant with the opportunity to become specialized or an expert in a single area of the business office.

Benefits of working in a large dental practice

- The administrative dental assistant will have the opportunity to become specialized in a single area.
- Professional interaction is greater because of the ability to draw from several different types of professional experiences.
- Advancement opportunities are greater.
- Employee benefits packages will have a greater number of choices.
- Networking within a large organization is possible.

Insurance Companies

Insurance companies use trained administrative dental assistants for a variety of jobs. Insurance processing trainers hold workshops on how to complete insurance claim forms correctly. Assistants familiar with dental terminology and procedures are assigned to claims processing. The environment of an insurance company provides an opportunity for administrative dental assistants to expand their business and administrative skills.

Management and Consulting Firms

Administrative dental assistants who gain experience and develop management skills may consider a position with a management and consulting firm. These firms specialize in consulting and training for individual and group dental practices. They make recommendations based on the needs of the dental practice. Dental practices may use consultants to improve patient relations, enhance productivity, develop efficient computer systems, or build a professional healthcare team. In addition to large firms that specialize in these services, individuals and small groups may provide management services.

Teaching

Working as a dental assisting educator is a rewarding career choice because it enables you to share with others the knowledge and experience you have acquired in the dental profession. Settings in which dental assisting educators are used include high school programs, community colleges, adult education programs, and proprietary schools.

Qualifications and credentials vary according to educational system and state requirements. Typically, a school requires an applicant to have acquired a set number of years of work experience, to have completed teaching methodology coursework (or to be working toward completion), and to have earned dental assisting certification (CDA [certified dental assistant]) or appropriate state licensure. Additional requirements may include a bachelor's degree and graduation from an accredited dental assisting program.

Future Career Opportunities

As computers become more advanced, additional career opportunities will be created. Within a dental practice, computer skills will be applied to a greater number of functions and well-trained staff will be required. Distributors of software packages will need the skills of experienced administrative dental assistants for their sales force and training staffs.

Technology will also open doors to new avenues for administrative and clinical dental assistants. The ability of the dental assistant to acquire new skills and perform increasingly challenging tasks will result in the creation of a dental healthcare team of lifelong learners.

STEPS FOR DEVELOPING EMPLOYMENT STRATEGIES

You have already taken the first step toward exploring dental career opportunities by enrolling in a dental assisting program. As you prepare for completion of this course, you may be given the opportunity to train in a dental practice setting. This experience will give you the opportunity to acquire work experience in a dental practice, ask questions, and work side by side with a dental professional. Additional career exploration opportunities may include job shadowing, career research, networking, and career fairs.

As you go through the job search process, you will proceed through a series of steps:
- Assessing yourself and your career options
- Gathering information
- Composing a resume
- Writing cover letters
- Looking for a job
- Going on an interview
- Accepting a job offer

Assessing Yourself and Your Career Options

The first step is to assess yourself and identify what you are looking for in a job. What are the things that are important to you? Formulate a list. Consider the number of hours per week that you can or want to work. What is the distance you are willing to travel? Do you prefer to work in a large or a small dental practice? What position do you want (administrative or clinical assistant)? Identify your personal philosophy and describe the type of dentist you would like to work for. Complete a budget and decide how much salary you need to make to survive. Rate your findings. Finally, are you willing to compromise?

Gathering Information

To fill out an application, compose a resume, prepare for an interview, and complete an employment record, you will need to gather specific pieces of information. These include the following:
- **Social Security card.** You must enter your Social Security number on an application and a copy of your Social Security card will be required when you are hired.
- **Driver's license, resident card, or picture identification card.** These documents are required when you are hired.
- **Diplomas, certificates, and licenses.** These documents are used to verify education, certification, and licensure.
- **Master application information.** A master application is a form that organizes information that will be used to complete applications and employment records. Not all of this information will be used on every document but by gathering this information and recording it on a master form, you will be able to complete applications and answer questions quickly and efficiently.
  - Name, address, telephone number
  - Date and place of birth, U.S. citizenship, resident card number, passport or visa
  - Details of any conviction for a crime and whether you are bondable
  - *Emergency information:* Name and address of a physician who should be contacted in case of an emergency; insurance information; list of disabilities, medications, or allergies

- *Education:* Names, dates, and locations of schools attended and your grade point averages
- *Additional information:* Special training received, skills attained, machines or equipment you can operate, extracurricular activities in which you participate, hobbies or outside interests, professional organizations to which you belong, and honors or awards received
- *Availability:* Date available to start, days and times of day (shift) that you are available to work
- Salary requirements
- *U.S. military service:* Branch of service in which you worked, date entered, date discharged, rank, special training, and duties
- *Employment records (paid and nonpaid):* Company name, address, telephone number, dates of employment, rate of pay, name of supervisor, duties of the job, reason for leaving
- *References:* Name, address, telephone number, occupation, number of years acquainted (References are people who know you personally and are willing to verify your abilities, skills, and attitudes. References should be former employers, teachers, counselors, coaches, neighbors, or clergy. Before using a person as a reference, you should first ask his or her permission.)

Composing a Resume

The most important tool of the job search process is the resume. Resumes are personal marketing tools created with one goal—to get a job interview. A strong resume will give you a competitive advantage, help you to organize your thoughts, and help you to make a good impression.

Applicants and employers use resumes in various ways. Resumes may be used to reach a large number of prospective employers in a mass mailing (paper and digital) or to contact a dentist individually in person. The objective is to gain the attention of a prospective employer and be granted an interview. Employers use resumes as the first step in the screening process. They review resumes and select for an interview those persons who seem to meet the qualifications required for the job.

Organizing Information

Before you start writing your resume, take some time to organize your information and to complete a few simple worksheets. You will need your master application information and five pieces of paper with the following headings: Objective, Education, Work Experience, Skills and Abilities, and Miscellaneous (for professional affiliations, certifications, and so forth).

Objective The objective is an important component of your resume. It identifies the position for which you are applying and is supported by information listed in the body of your resume. The objective is written to meet the employer's needs, outline the job you are seeking, and identify the skills you have to offer the employer. This is accomplished in a brief statement of one or two sentences. The following list of questions and answers will help you to formulate the job objective:

- *What job do you want?* Identify the job for which you are applying—for example, dental assistant, administrative dental assistant, office manager, business manager, insurance clerk, or chairside dental assistant. Try to be specific and use actual job titles. With the use of a computer, it is easy to change a few key words in a resume to customize it for a specific job title.
- *For whom do you prefer to work?* Identify the setting for the job you would like to have. If you are using a generic job title like business manager, insurance clerk, or office manager, add for whom you would like to work—for example, business manager in a progressive dental practice or insurance clerk for a large dental practice.
- *Where would you like to work?* Identify the setting in which you would like to work—for example, corporate dental practice, solo dental practice, management firm, insurance company, or school.
- *What level of responsibility do you prefer to assume?* Identify your level of training or certification—for example, entry level, Certified Dental Assistant, or Registered Dental Assistant.
- *What skills or abilities do you have?* Brainstorm and think of all of the duties you perform during the day and the skills and abilities they require. Make a long list and then select three or four of the most important skills and abilities.

After you have completed your worksheets, review your answers and formulate your objective. It may not be necessary to list all information as long as the objective is clear and concise and can be supported by information you list in the body of the resume. Be careful not to be too general; give specific information that focuses on the needs of the dental practice as well as your own. Examples of well-worded objectives follow:

- Seeking a position with a group dental practice that would provide an opportunity to demonstrate my experience as a Certified Dental Assistant. Skilled in patient communications, computer applications, and team building.
- Seeking a position with a dental practice as an entry level administrative dental assistant. Offering excellent skills in telephone techniques, computer applications, and filing. Cheerful outlook and a positive attitude.
- Offering dental management, communication, and insurance processing skills. Seeking to apply these skills as an administrative assistant in a dental insurance company.

Identification of an objective followed by a bulleted list of highlights (under the heading Highlights of Qualifications) is an effective format that you may wish to use. This method provides a very short, concise objective supported by qualifications. The highlights of qualifications are written with action verbs (see box titled Resume Action Verbs) that describe your relevant skills, experiences (duties), credentials, and accomplishments. For example:

- Collaborated in the successful design of a computerized recall system that increased the hygiene production by 20%.

ANATOMY OF A RESUME

Ima Graduate ①

1234 Valley Boulevard
Canyon View, CA 12345
① Cell phone (123) 555-7890
imagraduate@comcast.com

Objective ② Interested in obtaining a position as an administrative dental assistant. Offering excellent skills in patient communication, appointment scheduling, and computer applications. Enjoy working as a member of a professional healthcare team.

Education ③ 2014–2015　Canyon View Junior College　Canyon View, CA
Administrative Dental Assistant
Certification of Completion

2010-2014　Canyon View High School　Canyon View, CA
Diploma

Work Experience ④ January–September 2015　Canyon View Dentistry
Canyon View, CA
Administrative Dental Assistant
• Patient scheduling
• Computer data entry and management
• Patient relations

Skills and Abilities ⑤ • Computer skills
• Telephone procedures
• Patient communications
• Enthusiastic team member
• Organized
• Able to work unsupervised

Professional Affiliations and Certification ⑥ • ADAA, American Dental Assistants Association
• CDPMA, Certified Dental Practice Management Assistant
• American Heart Association, CPR–Healthcare Provider
• Radiology Certification

References ⑦ Available upon request

④ **WORK HISTORY**

This section can also come under the heading **Work Experience, Employment History, Professional Experience,** or **Experience.** In this section you will list the name and location of each company or organization, starting and ending dates, and a brief description of your duties. You can also list volunteer work experience, especially if it demonstrates skills and abilities that will enhance your job qualifications (non-paid training can also be listed). List the experience in chronological order.

⑤ **SKILLS AND ABILITIES**

Use this section to highlight skills, abilities, and strengths that are pertinent to the job you are applying for. Statements should be action-oriented, begin with verbs, and be concise.

⑥ **MISCELLANEOUS**

Headings and information include such items as extracurricular activities, clubs, memberships in professional organizations, certification, volunteer activities, awards, and achievements.

⑦ **REFERENCES**

You can include two professional references or state: References furnished upon request. The use of references is optional. When listing references state the name, title or occupation, address, and telephone number.

ORDER OF INFORMATION
Prime space is the top one-third of the page, so list the most important sections first.

MECHANICS
Typed on one page, easy to read, with correct spelling, grammar, and punctuation. Eliminate unessential words or phrases.

MARGINS
The finished resume should appear balanced, centered from top to bottom and left to right.

PAPER
Use heavy stock standard size (8.5" x 11") resume paper of good quality (white, cream, or light gray). Print on high-quality setting or have professionally printed. Pages should be free of streaks, fading, or correction fluid.

A resume is a summary of your skills, abilities, education, and work experience. The completed resume serves as an introduction; depending on your resume, you may or may not obtain an interview.

① **HEADING**

The heading will include full name, address, cell phone number, and e-mail address. For security reasons if the resume is posted online, omit your address.

② **JOB OBJECTIVE**

A job objective focuses on the type of job you are seeking and what you can offer the prospective employer. The statements made should be specific and concise. Information listed in the objective will be supported in the body of the resume.

The objective is considered one of the most important sections of the resume.

③ **EDUCATION**

Information included in your education statement: dates attended, diplomas, degrees, awards and certificates earned. Workshops and seminars that contribute to your qualifications should also be included in this section. List the information in chronological order (start with the most recent date and work back in time).

- Developed a system for tracking and monitoring electronically submitted dental claims.
- Managed a dental office for 3 years. Supervised four administrative and clinical assistants, planned and conducted monthly staff meetings, and prepared payroll.
- Skilled in the use of computer applications (add a list of specific applications).

- Able to work in a dental practice with professionalism and confidence.
- Responsible for the scheduling of three dentists and five hygienists in a high-volume multispecialty practice. Duties included reviewing and entering new patient data, setting up electronic clinical records, maintaining the electronic appointment book, and scheduling staff.

RESUME ACTION VERBS

Management Skills
- Administered
- Analyzed
- Assigned
- Attained
- Chaired
- Consolidated
- Contracted
- Coordinated
- Delegated
- Developed
- Directed
- Evaluated
- Executed
- Improved
- Increased
- Organized
- Oversaw
- Planned
- Prioritized
- Produced
- Recommended
- Reviewed
- Scheduled
- Straightened
- Supervised

Communication Skills
- Addressed
- Arbitrated
- Arranged
- Authored
- Collaborated
- Convinced
- Corresponded
- Developed
- Directed
- Drafted
- Edited
- Enlisted
- Formulated
- Influenced
- Interpreted
- Lectured
- Mediated
- Moderated
- Negotiated
- Persuaded
- Promoted

- Publicized
- Reconciled
- Recruited
- Spoke
- Translated
- Wrote

Research Skills
- Clarified
- Collected
- Critiqued
- Diagnosed
- Evaluated
- Interpreted
- Interviewed
- Investigated
- Organized
- Reviewed
- Summarized
- Surveyed
- Systematized

Technical Skills
- Assembled
- Built
- Calculated
- Computed
- Designed
- Devised
- Engineered
- Fabricated
- Maintained
- Operated
- Overhauled
- Programmed
- Remodeled
- Repaired
- Solved
- Upgraded

Teaching Skills
- Adapted
- Advised
- Clarified
- Coached
- Communicated
- Coordinated
- Developed
- Enabled

Continued

RESUME ACTION VERBS—cont'd

- Encouraged
- Evaluated
- Explained
- Facilitated
- Guided
- Informed
- Instructed
- Persuaded
- Set goals
- Stimulated
- Trained

Financial Skills
- Administered
- Allocated
- Analyzed
- Appraised
- Audited
- Balanced
- Budgeted
- Calculated
- Computed
- Developed
- Forecasted
- Managed
- Marketed
- Planned
- Projected
- Researched

Creative Skills
- Acted
- Conceptualized
- Created
- Customized
- Designed
- Developed
- Directed
- Established
- Fashioned
- Founded
- Illustrated
- Initiated
- Instituted
- Integrated
- Introduced
- Invented
- Originated
- Performed
- Planned
- Revitalized
- Shaped

Helping Skills
- Assessed
- Assisted
- Clarified
- Coached
- Counseled
- Demonstrated

- Diagnosed
- Educated
- Expedited
- Facilitated
- Familiarized
- Guided
- Motivated
- Referred
- Rehabilitated
- Represented

Clerical or Detail Skills
- Approved
- Arranged
- Catalogued
- Classified
- Collected
- Compiled
- Dispatched
- Executed
- Generated
- Implemented
- Inspected
- Monitored
- Operated
- Organized
- Prepared
- Processed
- Purchased
- Recorded
- Retrieved
- Screened
- Specified
- Systematized
- Tabulated
- Validated

Accomplishments
- Achieved
- Attained
- Convinced
- Expanded
- Expedited
- Founded
- Improved
- Increased
- Initiated
- Introduced
- Invented
- Originated
- Overhauled
- Pioneered
- Reduced
- Resolved
- Restored
- Revitalized
- Spearheaded
- Strengthened
- Transformed
- Upgraded

DESCRIPTIVE RESUME PHRASES

- Strong sense of responsibility
- Flexible and willing to take on a variety of tasks
- Neat, efficient, thorough
- Strong managerial skills
- Able to prioritize a heavy workload
- Cheerful outlook, positive attitude
- Strong motivation and dedication to the job
- Extensive artistic background
- Able to make important decisions on my own
- Take pride in a job well done
- Committed to completing a job
- Attentive to time schedules
- Self-motivated
- Goal-oriented
- Dedicated to the highest quality of work
- Resourceful problem solver

- Good organizational skills
- Willing to do extra work to gain valuable experience
- Ability to learn quickly
- Open-minded and imaginative
- Reliable and prompt
- Get along well with others
- Excellent communication skills
- Accurate in spelling and grammar
- Able to work well under pressure
- Able to work well unsupervised
- Outstanding leadership skills
- Good with numbers
- Enjoy a challenge
- Well organized
- Able to meet deadlines
- Enthusiastic team member

Education Using the information you listed on your master application sheet, list the schools you attended; the dates you attended; relevant courses you have taken; and the diplomas, certificates, and degrees you have earned.

Work experience List paid and unpaid job positions, start and end dates, and employers and their locations. It is important to include all work experience that relates to the job for which you are applying (if you have had several jobs that do not apply to the new position, they will be listed on your application).

Skills and abilities Be sure to list unpaid or volunteer positions that demonstrate responsibility, specific job skills, and work habits. Employers are looking for not only *hard skills* (skills and experience that are specific to a task or job) but also **soft skills.** Soft skills (a component of Career Ready Practices) are a set of personal qualities, habits, attitudes, and social skills that are needed for successful job performance. Examples of *soft skills* are:

- *Strong work ethic:* You are motivated to do your best to get the job done, no matter what. You are on time and ready to work. You are honest.
- *Time management:* You are able to prioritize tasks. You are able to anticipate what needs to be done next. You are able to work on more than one project or task at a time. You use your time efficiently.
- *Positive attitude:* You look for the best in a situation. You are energetic and upbeat. You smile.
- *Communication skills:* You can make your case and express your needs in a way that builds bridges with customers, colleagues, and vendors. You articulate verbally and are a good listener.
- *Problem solver:* You are able to see a problem, assess the needs, and creatively develop a solution. You work well with others to help solve problems. You are part of the solution, not the problem.
- *Team player:* You work well with others. You are cooperative. You are able to assume the role of a leader when appropriate.

- *Ability to accept and learn from criticism:* You are able to accept criticism. You are coachable and open to learning. You want to grow as a person and as a professional.
- *Self-confident:* You truly believe you can do the job. You project a sense of calm and inspire confidence in others. You have the courage to ask questions that need to be asked and to freely contribute your ideas.
- *Flexibility/adaptability:* You easily adapt to change and new ideas. You enjoy challenges.
- *Work well under pressure:* You are able to handle the stress that comes with deadlines and crisis. You can be counted on to come through in a pinch.

! REMEMBER

The combination of your technical skills and soft skills is what sets you apart from the crowd!

Miscellaneous List all activities that you have been involved in, including clubs, memberships in professional organizations, and volunteer activities. Keep a list of all of your certificates, licenses, and awards.

Constructing the Resume

After you have gathered all of the information and completed the worksheets, organize the information and put it into a resume format. Resumes are individual works that represent the writer. Be creative and gain the attention of the reader. It has been noted that the most important part of the resume is the top one third of the page. Information that you want noticed should go in this area. Resumes can be prepared using three basic formats: chronological, functional, and hybrid.

- **Chronological resumes** arrange information in order of occurrence, with the most recent information presented first. The objective is presented, followed by work experience, education background (order can be reversed depending on the importance), skills and abilities acquired, and miscellaneous information.

- **Functional resumes** place skills and abilities first, according to importance, regardless of the time of occurrence. After objective statements are listed, skills and abilities are highlighted, followed by information on work experiences, educational background, and miscellaneous information.
- **Hybrid resumes** combine the best features of chronological and functional resumes; information is rearranged and the focus is only on information that is relevant to the current job objective. The hybrid resume begins with a job objective that is followed by highlights of qualifications, relevant skills and experiences, chronological work history, and a listing of relevant education and training.

Online resumes are posted on websites for prospective employers to review. Before posting your resume, you *must* take precautions to protect yourself and preserve your personal identity. To better understand how posting your resume works, you first must understand the "business" side of the process. A job placement website will not charge you a fee to post your resume; they generate revenue by selling employers access to their resume database. The database is typically sold to anyone who is willing to pay the fee; this means that they do not filter who will receive your information. Because of the lack of security involved in posting a resume, it is recommended that you follow some simple precautions before you do so.

1. Remove your standard contact information.
   - Name
   - Address
   - Phone numbers
   - Business e-mail
   - Personal e-mail
   - Add a new personal e-mail address that is located on a large web-based service—for example, Yahoo, Gmail, or Hotmail. When you select your new e-mail address, use a name that is general in nature and reflects the "professional" you. Cute e-mail addresses are fine for your friends but they will not impress a prospective employer.
2. Do not use names of companies in your work history. You can change the wording to say the same thing but leave out who you worked for. For example, instead of stating that you worked for Dr. Mary Edwards, DDS, you could say, "Worked in single doctor dental office; my duties included…"
3. Review privacy statements of the website.

Resume Services

Some businesses and organizations write resumes. They charge a fee and use information given to them by the applicant. Such a service may be expensive but these companies do create resumes of professional quality.

Electronic resumes are resumes that are available through the Internet. Resume services will scan your resume or transfer it to a digitized copy. Prospective employers contact the service and request copies of resumes. The service does not charge the employee for this service. The prospective employer pays for a copy of your resume. Cover letters and resumes can be directed to prospective employers by way of e-mail (without use of a service). This method is relatively new to the dental profession. This may eventually become the way that all cover letters and resumes are submitted.

Cover letters and resumes can also be faxed to prospective employers. Unfortunately, you will lose the ability to place your resume on quality paper. If this method is used, care should be taken to create a resume that will transfer easily and maintain a professional appearance.

Writing Cover Letters

The purpose of a **cover letter** (letter of introduction or application) is to introduce yourself to a prospective employer. Cover letters should accompany all resumes sent by mail (including those sent via electronic transfer and fax). They can also be used as an introduction during an informational interview. Cover letters are personalized and addressed to a specific individual. They express an interest in working with a specific employer or company. They should convey enthusiasm and commitment. Cover letters balance professionalism with personal warmth and friendship and outline specifically what you are seeking and offering.

Looking for a Job

With proper marketing tools (resume and cover letter), you are ready to begin seriously looking for employment. The first question may be, "Where do I look?" You can start the process by identifying various avenues that may lead to employment: social media, professional networking, professional dental organizations, newspaper advertisements, employment agencies, temporary agencies, school placement, yellow pages, co-workers, family, and friends.

Social media are popular among many employers and job seekers. Although they are not for everyone (employer or job seeker), they are key players in the job search process. Sites like Facebook, Twitter, LinkedIn, and Google+ allow employers to get a look at who you are outside of your resume, cover letter, or interview. Therefore it is very important that the person they see on social media is the one they would like to hire. Employers check to see if the information you share on your resume is consistent, how you spend your time outside of work, if you have good communication skills, and how you speak of former employers and jobs. Job seekers can also learn about perspective employers using social media. Social networking allows you to connect with current and former employees, hear about job openings instantaneously, and gain insight on your career choice.

Professional networking, including social networking, is a means of contacting other dental professionals and letting them know that you are seeking employment. This is an informal job placement service and is one of the most effective means of seeking employment. The informal nature benefits the job seeker because people share more information about

ANATOMY OF A COVER LETTER

1234 Valley Boulevard
Canyon View, CA 12345
Phone (123) 555-7890

April 12, 2015

1 Family Dental Center
3841 Oak Drive
Canyon View, CA 91786

Dear Dr. Lamoure:

2 I am interested in working as an administrative dental assistant for your organization. I am a knowledgeable administrative assistant with a year of experience to offer you. I enclose my resume as a first step in exploring the possibilities of employment with Family Dental Centers.

3 My most recent experience was scheduling coordinator for Canyon View Dentistry. I was responsible for patient scheduling. I also coordinated revision of the practice policies and procedures manual. In addition, I initiated the conversion of patient scheduling from manual to computer.

As an administrative dental assistant with your organization, I would bring a focus on quality and enthusiasm to your dental team. Furthermore, I work well with others, and I am experienced in patient relations.

4 I would appreciate your keeping this inquiry confidential. I will call you in a few days to arrange an interview at a convenient time for you. Thank you for your consideration.

Sincerely,

Ima Graduate

Ima Graduate

1 **INSIDE ADDRESS AND SALUTATION**
Target the letter to a specific employer. Address the letter to a specific person, by name if possible.

2 **PARAGRAPH ONE**
Tell why you are contacting the employer and identify the position in which you are interested.

3 **PARAGRAPHS TWO AND THREE**
Express interest in the position and the dental practice or company. If applicable, tell how you became attracted to the particular dental practice (answering your ad in the Sunday paper, referred by John Evatt of the ABC Company). This demonstrates that you have done some research. Mention skills or qualifications that you possess that would be of particular interest to the dental practice. Identify at least one thing about you that is unique (must be relevant to the position).

4 **PARAGRAPH FOUR**
Summarize specifically what you are asking and offering. Describe just what you will do to follow through.

- Your letter should be well organized, grammatically correct, and typed. If the letter accompanies a resume, use the same type of high-quality paper.

- Have someone proofread the letter before it is sent.

- Keep a copy in your personal career portfolio.

the job, personalities of the dental healthcare team, working conditions, benefits, advantages, and disadvantages. Benefits to the employer are basically the same; they can let other professionals know that they have an open position and let them recommend possible applicants and get the word out. Professional networking includes:

- Attending local dental assistant society meetings, participating in study clubs, and volunteering at local dental clinics
- Connecting with current dental professionals, hearing about job openings instantaneously, and gaining insight on your career choice
- Talking to supply house representatives who visit several dental offices in a local area (they may know when there is an open position and who may be looking for a position)

Professional organizations, such as local chapters of the American Dental Association (ADA) and the American Dental Assistants Association (ADAA), may offer placement services for their members. A dental assistant can register with the local chapter by completing an informational survey. This survey will identify special skills, quantity of experience acquired, and type of employment sought and will ask for your telephone number. Member dentists who have an opening can request a list of all applicants and will contact those who meet their qualifications. Other professional dental organizations also may offer an employment placement service.

Newspaper advertisements are placed by employers and are an advertisement describing the position available and inviting applicants to call for an appointment or send their resumes.

An **employment agency** offers placement services. It can be state run or may be a private business. State agencies usually provide their services free of charge whereas private employment agencies charge the applicant or the employer. When you use a private agency, make sure you understand your liability and responsibilities.

Temporary agencies place applicants in positions for a specified length of time. The agency charges a fee to the employer. The applicant works in a temporary position and is paid by the agency. When you work for a temporary agency, make sure you understand the details of your contract.

Educational institutes often provide career placement services for their students. Depending on the institution, services can range from posting job opportunities to actually placing graduates in dental practices.

Other job search resources include the yellow pages (for a list of dentists; you may wish to send a cover letter and resume to attempt to schedule an interview). Former co-workers and employers may notify you when they learn of a job opening. Family and friends are also often willing to help you make a professional contact.

Organizing the Job Search

After you have identified sources and decided which direction you wish to pursue, take time to do some research on prospective employers. The primary reason for research is to help you gain information about a dental practice, including the type of practice—specialty, corporate, large group, or small solo practice. You can identify the type of dental insurance, if any, that they accept, the types of financial plans they offer, whether they use an active recall system, and whether they are members of a professional organization. This information can be gathered during informal networking or by checking the web page of the organization. Such information will:

- Prepare you for the interview
- Demonstrate your initiative and ability to organize
- Help you feel more confident about your ability to respond to questions
- Assist you in deciding whether the dental practice meets your standards for employment

Job Search Log

The purpose of the **job search log** is to help you organize, plan, and follow through with employment leads. It tracks submitted applications and resumes and identifies the company name and telephone numbers of contact persons. Additionally, the log provides space in which you can keep track of important information for interviews and follow-up questions, such as directions, parking, date, time, name of interviewer, date of planned follow-up, and comments.

Personal Career Portfolios

A collection of documents that support your professional career is called a **personal career portfolio.** Such portfolios are used as a source of information and a means of illustrating your skills, abilities, and strengths. Information contained in a portfolio is collected over time and is constantly changed and updated. Because they are personal collections, portfolios vary from person to person in content and appearance. They provide information for your use as you prepare applications and resumes and can serve as a study guide when you are preparing for a job interview. The portfolio is also a marketing tool; it presents your accomplishments, highlights your professional activities, and demonstrates to prospective employers your organizational abilities.

Components of a personal career portfolio

- Resume
- Completed application
- Personal information

    Write one or two paragraphs about yourself to be included in this section. To help you write a statement, see the box titled Adjectives Describing Personal Qualities for a list of adjectives that describe personal qualities. Complete the following statement: I am (select an adjective from the box). I have demonstrated this quality by _____. This quality is important in this field because _____.

ADJECTIVES DESCRIBING PERSONAL QUALITIES

- Accurate
- Ambitious
- Articulate
- Assertive
- Careful
- Committed
- Confident
- Conscientious
- Considerate
- Consistent
- Creative
- Decisive
- Dedicated
- Dependable
- Diligent
- Disciplined
- Efficient
- Energetic
- Enterprising
- Enthusiastic
- Flexible
- Friendly
- Goal-oriented

- Honest
- Humorous
- Independent
- Insightful
- Knowledgeable
- Leader
- Loyal
- Motivated
- Neat
- Open-minded
- Organized
- Outgoing
- Patient
- Positive
- Productive
- Professional
- Quick
- Responsible
- Skillful
- Strong
- Thorough
- Tolerant

Include a list of personal qualities that make you an excellent candidate for employment, personal references, volunteer experiences, areas of personal interest, and information on former employers along with salary history.

Have photocopies of report cards and transcripts, Social Security card, driver's license or picture ID, resident card (if not a U.S. citizen), and passport.

Achievements are a good marketing tool. Keep a high-quality copy of certificates you have earned and write a brief description that explains how you earned the award. Items that may be placed in this section of your portfolio include the following:

- Records of certificates earned
- Records of awards, honors, and leadership shown
- Records of volunteer and extracurricular activities
- Records of published articles

Personal letters help you to follow up on current leads and serve as models for future letters. These include:

- Cover letters
- Research letters
- Information interview letters
- Career information request letters

Reference letters are written by people who know you personally and are willing to speak on your behalf. Reference letters verify your abilities, skills, and positive attitude. Keep a quality letter in your portfolio, along with additional copies to give prospective employers when requested.

- **Thank-you cards and letters** are letters that you have received from others.

- **Performance documentation** may include recent performance reviews, positively written comments regarding the quality of your work, and evidence of volunteer and non-paid activities.
- **Work samples** may include actual completed works (samples of professional letters you have written) or pictures of completed work with a written statement that tells about the sample.

Going on an Interview

The purpose of the job interview is to share information; interviewers want to get to know the applicant better and the applicant wants to tell why he or she is the best person for the job. During the interview, the interviewer asks questions designed to reveal information about the skills, abilities, and attitude of the applicant. The ways in which applicants respond to these questions help the prospective employer to determine whether to offer the applicant the job. Sometimes the person who is offered the job is not the best qualified but is the one who made the best impression.

Preparing for Interview Questions

During the interview, you will be asked several questions. These may range from "Tell me about yourself" to "Do you have any questions for me?" See the box titled Sample Interview Questions and Answers for a list of commonly asked questions. Take some time to answer each one of these questions. Write down your responses and keep them in your personal career portfolio. Before you go on an interview, review these questions and your responses to them.

SAMPLE INTERVIEW QUESTIONS AND ANSWERS

- *Please tell me about yourself.* This question is designed to reveal your level of self-confidence and your ability to handle yourself under pressure. The interviewer should be familiar with the information you listed on the job application and your resume. Mention things that are easy for you to talk about but keep them job related. For example, discuss your skills, abilities, personal qualities, work experience, or career technical training. Keep your response short.

- *What are your strengths and weaknesses?* Always answer this question in a positive tone. Be prepared to talk about your strengths. When asked to identify weaknesses, use this as an opportunity to list a weakness that may be a positive for the job for which you are applying. Becoming bored with simple tasks may be seen as positive in a job that requires complex tasks. When talking about a negative, give a positive solution: I have a tendency to procrastinate but I work well under pressure.

- *Why do you want to work here?* On the basis of your research information, state reasons why you would like to work in this particular dental practice instead of another dental practice. Everyone wants to feel special and this is a chance to show that you have done your homework and have considered other options.

- *How do you spend your spare time?* This question is designed to see if you spend your time constructively. Answer in a positive tone and do not mention things that will appear negative or boring.

- *Where do you see yourself in 3 to 5 years?* This question is meant to reveal your goals. Be prepared to state your career goals. Goals can be stated in broad, generic terms: "I see myself working in a profession that will provide room for growth and advancement."

- *Why should I hire you? How are you qualified for this job?* This question allows the interviewer to see whether your skills, abilities, and personal qualities match the job description. You can answer the question by listing the qualifications of the job and explaining how your qualifications match them.

- *What did you like or dislike about your last job or class?* Reference a similarity between your last job and the one you are applying for and explain why you liked it. Use personal traits: "I enjoyed helping patients. I like to make them feel comfortable when they come to the dental office." It is wise not to say negative things about a previous job because the interviewer may know your previous employer.

- *Do you have any questions for me?* The final question of the interview normally gives the applicant a chance to ask questions. Remember, you are also interviewing the prospective employer. Be prepared to ask one or two questions. Questions may relate to the future growth or expansion of the practice, a job description, or examples of a typical day, specific procedures, or opportunities for team development. Questions may also seek information on when the position will be filled and on whether you can answer any other questions about your qualifications.

During the interview, be prepared to think! Questions are designed to highlight your strengths and to assess your ability to respond when under pressure. These questions may identify personal work habits and philosophy; for example:

- Accomplishments that make you feel proud
- Who has had a positive influence on your life and why
- What rewards, other than money, motivate you
- Why you chose this career
- What you have learned from participation in extracurricular activities
- How a former employer or teacher would describe you
- A major problem you have encountered and how you dealt with it

For an interview to be successful, you must be prepared, make a good impression, and complete the interview process. Suggestions that will result in a successful interview follow.

Before the interview

- Research the company, salary range, and job qualifications.
- Prepare for questions by writing answers to questions that might be asked.
- Prepare questions for the interviewer.
- Review your resume and have a copy available.
- Organize your personal career portfolio to take with you.
- Review material in your portfolio and use it as a study guide.
- Prepare your thank-you letters.
- Locate the interview site, determine travel time, and check available parking.
- Practice good grooming and hygiene. Appropriate clothing for women includes suit, skirt and blouse, or dress with a jacket; medium-heeled shoes with closed toes and heels; and flesh-colored hosiery. Hair should be neatly groomed and jewelry kept to a minimum. Clothing for men includes suit or sport jacket, dress shirt, slacks, tie, belt, and dress shoes and dark socks. Hair should be neatly groomed and cut and facial hair shaved and trimmed. Jewelry on men should be limited to a watch and a ring. Color plays an important role, so choose solid colors or muted stripes for suits. The best colors are thought to be blue (believable) and gray (authoritative).
- Go alone and prepare to arrive at least 15 minutes early.

> **! REMEMBER**
>
> Dress conservatively. Clothing and accessories should not be trendy. Do not wear bright colors or extreme or excessive makeup and jewelry. This applies to both men and women.

During the interview

- Introduce yourself to the receptionist.
- Do not chew gum or smoke (before or during the interview).
- Introduce yourself to the interviewer, shake hands firmly (if the interviewer offers a hand), and be seated when directed.
- Maintain eye contact with the interviewer.

- Be enthusiastic.
- Keep a businesslike attitude.
- Demonstrate good posture and mannerisms.
- Emphasize your qualities and skills.
- Ask questions (do not ask about salary until a position has been offered).

After the interview

- Thank the interviewer for his or her time, smile, and shake hands.
- Thank the receptionist and ask for the interviewer's business card (which will provide information for the thank-you letter).
- Send a thank-you letter within 24 hours of the interview. The thank-you letter can be a personal note or a typed letter.
- If you have not heard from the interviewer after 2 or 3 days, telephone the office but keep the number of calls to a minimum.

Accepting a Job Offer

When a job is offered, you may or may not choose to accept it. Before you accept the position, it is necessary to know the particulars of the job: salary, benefits, vacation schedule, work schedule, and so forth. You should base your decision on conditions that you identified in your self-assessment. Do not feel that you are obligated to accept a position if it does not meet your needs. If a compromise cannot be reached, thank the employer for the offer and politely decline.

If you accept the offer, the employer should present an **employment agreement**. This agreement is an outline of conditions for employment. It may include a job title and description, work schedule, and salary and **benefits** (vacation days, sick days, insurance, and retirement plans). The agreement should clearly state when reviews are conducted and should describe termination procedures. The employer and the employee sign the agreement. A copy is given to the employee and one is kept in the employee's personal employment file.

LEAVING A JOB

There are many reasons for leaving a job. It has been estimated that people have five to eight different careers during their lifetimes. This requires moving from job to job. A job change should be viewed as a chance to improve your employment status and achieve future success.

When it is time to leave a job, this must be done in a positive way and in accordance with the employment agreement. You will need to tell your supervisor that you are leaving. State the reason and give a proposed date of exit (2 weeks' notice is average). Offer to train a new employee and thank your employer for the opportunity to work for the organization.

A formal letter of resignation should be given to your employer when you speak to your supervisor. This letter is addressed to the personnel department. In the letter, state the position from which you are resigning, thank the company, and state the date of your resignation.

When employers initiate your termination, they should follow the procedure outlined in your employment agreement. If they ask you to leave without notice, they may offer severance pay. If you think that your termination is occurring without cause, you have rights under the law. For information concerning employment rights and a grievance process, consult the local labor board in your state.

KEY POINTS

- Career opportunities for administrative dental assistants include working in small and large dental practices, insurance companies, management and consulting firms, and educational institutions.
- Developing an employment strategy will prepare the administrative dental assistant for the job search process. The process includes completing a self-assessment, gathering information to be used in developing a master application form, creating a personal career portfolio, and writing a quality resume and cover letter.

- The interview process consists of three parts: preparing for the interview, responding to questions during the interview, and following up with a thank-you note or letter.
- Before you accept a job offer, you should know what your salary requirements are and compare them with the salary offered by the employer. Employment agreements are outlines that highlight job descriptions, salary, benefits, and termination policy. When a job is terminated, this should be done in a professional and positive manner.

CAREER-READY PRACTICES

Career-Ready Practices activities are designed to provide students with experiences that can be "practiced" in preparation for skills needed on the job. In each of the following exercises, a variety of approaches may be used to address the problem, rather than "right" or "wrong" answers. Below each exercise, next to the compass icon, is a listing of suggested Career-Ready Practice numbers that correspond to the listing of 12 practices in the front of the text (see p. viii-ix); these practices provide suggestions for approaches to complete the exercise.

1. To help prepare yourself for employment, complete a self-assessment based on the questions listed earlier in the chapter under "Assessing Yourself and Your Career Options."

 Career-Ready Practices
   10 *Plan education and career path aligned to personal goals.*
   4 *Communicate clearly, effectively and with reason.*
   5 *Consider the environmental, social and economic impacts of decisions.*
   3 *Attend to personal health and financial well-being.*

2. Prepare for an interview by answering the following questions:
   - Would you tell me about yourself?
   - What are your strengths and weaknesses?

- Why would you like to work here?
- How do you spend your spare time?
- Where do you see yourself in 3 to 5 years?
- Why should I hire you?
- In what ways are you qualified for this job?
- What rewards, other than money, motivate you?
- How would a former employer or teacher describe you?

 Career-Ready Practices
   4 *Communicate clearly, effectively and with reason.*
   5 *Consider the environmental, social and economic impacts of decisions.*
   9 *Model integrity, ethical leadership and effective management.*

3. Research current trends in job seeking to gain insight on how you can expand your prospects of gaining employment.

 Career-Ready Practices
   7 *Employ valid and reliable research strategies.*
   2 *Apply appropriate a academic and technical skills.*
   6 *Demonstrate creativity and innovation.*

GLOSSARY

Abutment tooth A tooth, a root, or an implant used for the retention of a fixed or removable prosthesis. (Chapter 2)

Account aging report Report that identifies the length of time that has elapsed since a charge was made. (Chapter 14)

Accounting Method used to verify and classify all transactions (accounts payable and receivable); this is usually the duty of an accountant. (Chapter 17)

Accounts payable System that organizes, verifies, and categorizes all dental practice expenditures. (Chapters 9, 16, 17)

Accounts receivable System that records all financial transactions between a patient and the dental practice. (Chapters 9, 17)

Accounts receivable report Report that categorizes the amount of money patients and insurance companies owe the dental practice. (Chapter 17)

Achievements Awards, honors, certificates, and accomplishments that serve as marketing tools in an employment search. (Chapter 18)

Administrative dental assistant Assistant assigned duties that pertain to the business side of dentistry. (Chapter 1)

Administrative Management Society (AMS) (letter writing) Another name for the simplified style of letter writing that includes open punctuation and a subject line but no salutation or complimentary closing. (Chapter 4)

Administrative Simplification Method designed to make the business of healthcare easier by providing standards for transaction code sets, privacy of patient information, security of patient information, and national provider identifiers. (Chapter 1)

Administrator Person or group of persons who represent dental benefits plans for the purpose of negotiating and managing contracts with dental service providers. (Chapter 15)

Advanced (practice management) system Practice management system that integrates the business office with the clinical practice. Dental healthcare team members are responsible for entering the information and accessing the system and treatment room terminals provide for chairside charting and storage of digitized images. (Chapter 7)

Aging Process that identifies how much of the money owed is 30, 60, 90, or 120 days past due. (Chapter 17)

Aging labels File labels that allow for quick and easy visual identification of when a patient was last seen in the dental practice. (Chapter 9)

Allowable charges Maximum amount paid for each procedure by the insurance company. (Chapter 15)

Alphabetic filing System that indexes names for filing purposes. Indexing rules have been standardized by the Association of Records Managers and Administrators (ARMA), which is recognized by the American National Standards Institute (ANSI) as an American National Standard. (Chapter 9)

Amalgam Alloy of various metals, silver in color, used as a dental restorative material. (Chapter 2)

American Dental Assistants Association (ADAA) Professional organization for dental assistants. It performs a variety of functions that promote professional growth, community involvement, and continuing education for its members. (Chapter 1)

Americans with Disabilities Act (ADA) Act signed into law on July 26, 1990, to prohibit discrimination on the basis of disability in employment, programs and services provided by state and local governments, and goods and services provided by private companies and commercial facilities. (Chapter 13)

Amylase Enzyme found in saliva that is a function of the digestive process and serves as a source of minerals (fluorides, calcium, and phosphate) needed in the remineralization of tooth structure. (Chapter 2)

Anatomical chart Type of dental chart that uses an anatomical representation of teeth within the dental arches. (Chapter 2)

Anterior teeth Teeth found toward the front of the mouth; include the central incisors, lateral incisors, and cuspids (canines). (Chapter 2)

Apex Anatomical area at the end of the tooth root. (Chapter 2)

Apical foramen Small opening at the apex of the root, where blood vessels and nerves enter. (Chapter 2)

Application software Software designed for specific tasks, such as word processing, spreadsheet, database, and graphics. (Chapter 13)

Appointment book A tool that, when used efficiently, helps one to organize the daily schedule of the dental practice. It identifies who will be performing the work, on what date, and at what time. (Chapter 10)

Appointment card Written reminder of the patient's next appointment. (Chapter 10)

Appointment scheduler Administrative personnel, within the business office of a dental practice, whose primary functions are to schedule and confirm appointments, maintain the recall system, and track patients who are in need of treatment. (Chapter 1)

Art of scheduling Process that involves working with the dental healthcare team to determine time requirements and develop a process to monitor and adjust scheduling to meet agreed-upon goals. (Chapter 10)

Assignment of benefits Authorization given by the subscriber or patient to a dental benefits plan, directing the company to make payment for dental benefits directly to the providing dentist. (Chapter 15)

Attending dentist statement Form submitted by the dentist to the dental benefits plan that requests payment for services (dental claim form). (Chapter 15)

Attention line (letter writing) Name of the person to whom a particular letter is being sent. (Chapter 4)

Audit Method used by third parties to check the accuracy of dental claim forms by comparing patient clinical records with information submitted on the dental claim form. (Chapter 15)

Automated recall system System involving the use of an electronic database to identify and track recall patients. (Chapter 11)

Avoiding style (conflict resolution) Style of conflict resolution used when an issue is trivial, a cooling-off period is needed, or the benefits do not go beyond the discord that a situation will cause between involved parties. (Chapter 6)

Backorder Items that were ordered but not shipped and will be sent at a later date. (Chapter 12)

Background noise Noise that occurs as the result of activities that are going on outside of the immediate area; it can vary in intensity. Ambient sound level should not be higher than 55 decibels (dB). (Chapter 13)

Balance The amount of funds remaining in the account after all deposits, payments, and outstanding items have been accounted for. (Chapter 16)

Balance billing Billing the patient for the difference between the amount paid by the dental benefits plan and the fee charged by the dentist (according to the specification of the dental benefits plan contract). (Chapter 15)

Bank statements and financial reports Part of financial records that are filed according to subject and then subdivided chronologically. (Chapter 9)

Barcode An optical machine-readable image of symbols and shapes that represents data relating to the object to which it is attached. (Chapter 12)

Basic (practice management) system Method of organizing and creating a database and performing spreadsheet and word processing tasks. (Chapter 7)

Benefit payment Amount paid by the dental benefits plan. (Chapter 15)

Benefit services Services that are paid by the dental benefits plan. (Chapter 15)

Benefits (employee) Vacation days, sick days, insurance, and retirement plan. (Chapter 18)

Billing The procedure that notifies a responsible party (individual or insurance carrier) regarding the current status of an account. (Chapter 17)

Birthday rule Method used to determine which parent is considered the primary provider of a child's dental coverage. This rule establishes that the parent whose birth date comes first during the year is the primary provider. (Chapter 15)

Blocked (letter writing) Letter format in which the margins are the same as those in the full-blocked style with the exception of dateline, complimentary close, company signature, and writer identification, all of which begin at the vertical center of the page. (Chapter 4)

Board of dental examiners Agency that has been assigned the task and authority to issue dental licenses. (Chapter 9)

Body of letter Portion of a letter composed of the introduction, main body, and closing. The purpose of these paragraphs is to relay to the reader concise information that is organized in a logical sequence. (Chapter 4)

Bookkeeper Person who keeps records of the amount of money deposited into checking and savings accounts and uses a check paying system (manual check writing or electronic debt accounts) to pay vendors. (Chapter 1)

Bookkeeping Method of recording all financial transactions. (Chapter 17)

Bookmarks Feature used in appointment books to identify the current week so that it can be turned to quickly. (Chapter 10)

Bridge Fixed prosthetic. (Chapter 2)

Buccal Surface of posterior teeth that faces the cheek. (Chapter 2)

Buccal frena Two buccal structures (right and left) that connect the cheek to the gingiva in the area of the maxillary first molar. (Chapter 2)

Buccal vestibule Junction of the mucous membrane of the cheek and the gingiva. (Chapter 2)

Business manager Person who manages the fiscal operation, develops marketing campaigns, negotiates contracts with managed care providers, and oversees the compliance of insurance, managed care, and government programs. (Chapter 1)

Business office Area where most of the administrative dental assistant's duties are carried out. (Chapter 1)

Business records Business documents that pertain to the operation of the dental practice. They are divided into several different types and require a variety of methods for retrieval and storage. (Chapter 9)

Business reports Reports that focus on the fiscal operation of the dental practice, including profit and loss statements, practice production, and other specified reports that categorize a subject area. They are filed by subject and then subdivided chronologically. (Chapter 9)

C

Call list Organized list that identifies patients who need to be scheduled for dental treatment, who can come in when there is a change in the schedule, or who wish to be notified when an opening in the schedule occurs. (Chapter 10)

Capitation programs Programs in which the dental practice is paid a set amount for each patient who is enrolled in the program. Payment is made for each enrolled patient, regardless of whether he or she receives treatment. (Chapter 15)

Card files (Rolodex) Files designed for quick reference of telephone numbers and addresses and that can be used in a recall system. (Chapter 9)

Cast crown Cast restoration that covers the anatomical crown. (Chapter 2)

Cementum Thin, hard covering of the root surface of a tooth. (Chapter 2)

Central incisors Anterior teeth (toward the front) characterized by thin, sharp incisal edges, which aid in cutting food. (Chapter 2)

Central processing unit (CPU) One of the components of a simple computer system. It is the main operating component of the computer hardware. (Chapter 13)

Certified dental assistant A certification granted by the Dental Assisting National Board, Inc. (DANB). To qualify for this certification, the individual must graduate from a Commission on Dental Accreditation (CODA)–accredited dental assisting program or meet the work experience requirements and pass a written examination. (Chapter 1)

Certified dental practice management assistant (CDPMA) Certification offered to administrative dental assistants who meet specified requirements and pass an examination administered by the National Dental Assisting Board. (Chapter 1)

Cervix Narrow portion of the tooth where the root and the crown meet. (Chapter 2)

Chairside dental assistants Personnel who perform various duties, including scheduling appointments efficiently, communicating with the use of dental terminology, processing dental insurance claims, correctly coding procedures for posting, making entries in patients' clinical records, and doubling as an assistant when additional help is needed in the clinical area. (Chapter 1)

Change Action that can be harmful or beneficial. When not accepted or understood, it places a barrier on communication. For some, it is seen as negative. Good communication provides a means for discussing the need for change and how it will improve the organization. (Chapter 6)

Channel One of the steps in the process of communication. Once the sender has translated his or her idea into a message, it is placed in the appropriate channel. (Chapter 3)

Charting methods Symbolic system used to identify teeth and current dental conditions. (Chapter 3)

Charting symbols Series of symbols, numbers, and colors used to illustrate specific dental conditions. (Chapter 3)

Chronological filing System that allows one to locate documents according to date, month, or year. (Chapter 9)

Chronological resumes Arrangement of information on a resume in the order of occurrence, with the most recent information provided first. The objective is presented, followed by work experience, education (order can be reversed, depending on the importance), skills and abilities, and miscellaneous information. (Chapter 18)

Circulating (roving) assistant Individual who performs a variety of duties, including assisting a dentist or chairside assistant as needed, taking dental x-rays, and maintaining responsibility for sterilization and infection control. (Chapter 1)

Claim (dental) Method used to request payment or authorization for treatment. Each provides necessary information about the patient, the treating dentist, and coded treatment. (Chapter 15)

Claims payment fraud Changing or manipulating information (done by a dental benefits plan) on a claim form that results in payment of a lower benefit to the treating dentist. (Chapter 15)

Claims reporting fraud Changing or manipulating information (done by the dentist) on a claims form that results in payment of a higher benefit by the dental benefits plan. Intentionally falsifying information and services. (Chapter 15)

Clean area Identifiable area of a sterilization center that is used for assembling and storing sterilized instruments and treatment trays. (Chapter 15)

Clinical record (patient chart) Documents used to determine and record patient demographics, medical and dental health history, previous treatment, diagnosed treatment, radiographs, and treatment notes. (Chapter 8)

Closed panel programs Programs that dictate to patients where they can receive their dental treatment. (Chapter 15)

Closing (letter writing) Describes the next step or expected outcomes of the letter. (Chapter 4)

Code on Dental Procedures and Nomenclature (the Code) National standard for codes used to report dental treatment. (Chapters 1, 15)

College degrees (filing) A suffix used as a filing unit. When used, this should be placed in the last filing unit to distinguish between two identical names. (Chapter 9)

Color coding System used in filing that identifies various sections of the alphabet (or numbers) through specific colors or color combinations. Provides visual identification. (Chapter 9)

Columns Divisions of the pages of an appointment book. The functions of these are to organize the schedule and to indicate who is performing the dentistry, who the patient is, why the patient is being seen, and what is going to be done. (Chapter 10)

Combination recall system Method of scheduling appointments according to patient preference. Some patients may be unwilling to schedule an appointment in advance but do not mind if you call them at work to schedule the appointment closer to the actual appointment date. Other patients may be very good at scheduling an appointment as soon as they receive the card in the mail. (Chapter 1)

Commission on Dental Accreditation (CODA) Organization that accredits dental assisting programs. (Chapter 1)

Commissures Corners of the mouth at which the upper and lower lips meet. (Chapter 2)

Communication A two-way process in which information is transferred and shared between a sender and a receiver. (Chapter 3)

Company signature (letter writing) Identifies the company of the person who is sending a letter and is optional. It is used when the sender of the letter is representing the company. (Chapter 4)

Completeness A step in the organizational stage. When checking, make sure you have included all information, facts, and explanations needed by the reader. It is not uncommon to include a phrase that will appeal to the reader's emotions or understanding. (Chapter 4)

Complimentary closing (letter writing) Final message of a letter, such as "sincerely" or "truly yours." (Chapter 4)

Compromising style (conflict resolution) A style that is best used when parties are equally powerful, consensus cannot be reached, integrating or dominating style is not successful, and a temporary solution to a complex problem is needed. (Chapter 6)

Computerized bookkeeping system Uses a program (function) to organize, track, and calculate the accounts receivable. (Chapter 17)

Computerized dental practice management system An integrated system of software or application suites that are seamlessly linked to perform related functions. (Chapter 7)

Concise Term that describes communication that conveys just the right amount of information without overusing words or phrases. (Chapter 4)

Conference calls Several people are present on the telephone line at the same time. (Chapter 3)

Confidential personnel records Information about an employee's employment performance. (Chapter 9)

Confirmation of initial impression stage A process patients go through to confirm or change their initial impression of the dental office. This includes taking into account the office location, outside appearance, signage, appearance of the reception area, greeting, and time spent waiting. (Chapter 5)

Consent form Form used to receive authorization from a patient to continue treatment. (Chapter 8)

Consolidated Omnibus Budget Reconciliation Act (COBRA) Legislation that mandates guaranteed medical and dental overage for a period of 18 months after the loss of group benefits coverage. Individuals are given the option of purchasing their own coverage at a group rate under special contracts. (Chapter 15)

Consultation area Area used for meeting with patients when privacy is needed. (Chapter 15)

Consumable supplies and products Items that are used and that need to be replenished. (Chapter 12)

Contaminated area Identifiable area of the sterilization center where instruments are processed before they are sterilized. (Chapter 12)

Continuing care See *Recall system.* (Chapter 11)

Coordination of benefits (COB) System that coordinates the benefits of two or more insurance policies. The total benefits paid should not be more than 100% of the original service fee. (Chapter 15)

Copayment Portion of the service fee that remains after payment is made by the dental benefits plan. (Chapter 15)

Copy notation (letter writing) The abbreviation "cc" for computer copy or carbon copy, used to notify the reader that the document is being forwarded to another party. (Chapter 15)

Corporate dentistry Type of dental facilities that are owned and operated by companies for the purpose of providing dental care to their employees and dependents. (Chapter 15)

Correspondence log Method used to document various types of correspondence that pertain to the patient. This form is kept in the patient's clinical record. (Chapter 8)

Cover letter (letter of introduction or application) Introduces an applicant to a prospective employer. These should accompany all resumes sent by mail (including electronic transfer and fax). (Chapter 18)

Covered charges Allowable services that are outlined in dental benefits plan contracts, fee schedules, or tables of allowance, as determined by the dental provider and paid for, in whole or in part, by the third-party dental benefits plan. (Chapter 15)

CPU Central processing unit; the main operating component of a computer. (Chapter 1)

Cranium The eight bones that form a protective structure for the brain and the face. (Chapter 2)

Credibility The weight that is put on a message in accordance with the status or qualifications of the person sending the message. (Chapter 3)

Credit report A tool used to gather credit information. (Chapter 14)

Cross-referencing Method that identifies another name (or number) under which a record may be filed. (Chapter 9)

Crown The portion of the tooth covered in enamel. These come in different shapes and sizes depending on the function of the tooth. (Chapter 2)

Current Dental Terminology (CDT) Terms and codes standardized by the American Dental Association (ADA) for the purpose of consistency in reporting dental services and procedures to dental benefits plans. (Chapters 1, 15)

Current Procedural Terminology (CPT) Codes and procedures standardized by the American Medical Association (AMA) for the purpose of reporting medical treatment and services. (Chapter 15)

Cusp Pointed or rounded eminence on the surface of a tooth. (Chapter 2)

Cuspids Canines. Anterior teeth. (Chapter 2)

Customary fee Fee, as determined by the third-party administrator, from actual submitted fees, for specific dental services. (Chapter 15)

D

Daily journal Form used to record business transactions. (Chapter 7)

Daily schedule sheets Posted schedules used in treatment rooms, dentists' private offices, laboratories, and other work areas. (Chapter 10)

Darkroom Place where dental x-ray film is processed. (Chapter 10)

Data Information. (Chapter 13)

Data processor Person responsible for entering data into the computer system. (Chapter 1)

Dateline (letter writing) The date on which the letter is written. (Chapter 4)

DDS Doctor of Dental Surgery. (Chapter 4)

Deductible Service fee that the patient is responsible for paying before the third party will consider payment of additional services. It may be payable annually, over a lifetime, or as a family. (Chapter 15)

Dental arches Sections into which the anatomical structure of the mouth is divided. Each contains the same number of teeth. See Maxillary arch and *Mandibular arch.* (Chapter 2)

Dental assistant Personnel who perform vital duties in the efficient operation of successful dental practices and who provide a link between the patient and the dentist. Several different types may be available to assist patients and dentists in a practice. (Chapter 1)

Dental Assisting National Board, Inc. National testing agency for dental assisting. (Chapter 1)

Dental auxiliary Any person, other than the dentist, who provides a service in a dental practice. (Chapter 1)

Dental benefit plan Plan that provides dental service to an enrollee in exchange for a fixed, periodic payment made in advance of the dental service. Such plans often include the use of deductibles, coinsurance, and maximums to control the cost of the program to the purchaser. (Chapter 15)

Dental caries Also known as tooth decay. It is a progressive disease that demineralizes enamel, enters the dentin, and quickly reaches the pulp of the tooth. (Chapter 2)

Dental healthcare team All persons in the dental office. Someone who excels and becomes a vital member will have mastered multiple skills, will be flexible, and will work well in a team environment. (Chapter 1)

Dental history Information about previous treatment. It also alerts the dental healthcare team to fears and apprehensions that the patient may have concerning dental treatment. (Chapter 8)

Dental hygienist Professionally educated and licensed member of the dental healthcare team who provides educational, clinical, and therapeutic dental services to patients. (Chapter 1)

Dental insurance Method of financial assistance (provided by a dental benefits service) that helps to pay for specified procedures and services concerning dental disease and accidental injuries to the oral structure. (Chapter 15)

Dental Practice Act Legislation that outlines the duties that can be performed by dental auxiliaries, the type of education required, and what licensure, if any, is necessary for these duties. (Chapter 1)

Dental prophylaxis Removal of stains and hard deposits from teeth. (Chapter 2)

Dental public health Dentists who help to organize and run dental programs that address the dental health of the general public. (Chapter 1)

Dental radiographs X-rays of teeth. (Chapter 8)

Dental service corporation A legally formed, not-for-profit organization that contracts with dental providers for the sole purpose of providing dental care. Examples include Delta Dental Plans and Blue Cross/Blue Shield. (Chapter 15)

Dentin Bulk of a tooth that consists of living cellular substance similar in structure to bone and softer than the hard outer shell of the crown (enamel) and the covering of the root surface (cementum). (Chapter 2)

Dependents Persons who are covered under another person's dental benefits policy. (Chapter 15)

Diagnostic models (study models) Casts of a patient's mouth used as a tool in treatment planning. (Chapter 8)

Diastema Space created when the maxillary labial frenum is too thick or wide and it keeps the two front teeth from coming into contact. (Chapter 2)

Direct reimbursement Payment plan that allows an organization to be self-funded for the purpose of providing dental benefits. (Chapter 15)

Direct sales A process of ordering supplies by going directly to the manufacturer or by going to an online distributor (such as Amazon). (Chapter 12)

Disposable supplies Items used only once and then thrown away. (Chapter 12)

Distal The proximal surface that faces away from the midline. (Chapter 2)

Divided payment plan Plan in which payments are divided according to the length of treatment. (Chapter 4)

Doctor of Dental Medicine (DMD) and **Doctor of Dental Surgery** (DDS) An advanced degree received after graduating from an accredited dental education program. (Chapter 1)

Dominating style A style of conflict resolution that is appropriate when speed is important in making a decision and the results are trivial, when an unpopular course of action is needed, when the decisions of others will be costly to you, or when one is handling an overly aggressive subordinate. (Chapter 6)

Downcoding Method of changing a reported benefits code by third-party payers so as to reflect a lower-cost procedure. (Chapter 15)

Dual addressing When a post office box and a street address are used in the same destination address. The address listed directly above the city, state, and zip code is where the mail will be delivered. (Chapter 4)

Dual choice program An insurance policy (benefit plan) that provides the eligible individual the choice of an alternative dental benefits program or a traditional dental benefits program. (Chapter 15)

E

Educational institutes Organizations that provide career placement services for their students. (Chapter 18)

Electronic file A total picture of the patient and the patient's needs visualized through a series of forms. (Chapter 8)

Electronic ledger Computerized tool that stores all of the necessary financial information for a patient. (Chapter 17)

Electronic noise Noise from high-speed handpieces and other electronic equipment. (Chapter 6)

Electronic patient statements Statements generated by the practice management software and sent directly to the patient via e-mail or through a third-party billing service. (Chapter 17)

Electronic scheduler A computerized version of the manual appointment book. (Chapter 10)

Electronically protected health information (ePHI) Health information that is shared electronically; covered providers are required to protect the integrity, confidentiality, and availability of this information. (Chapter 1)

Electronically submitted forms Forms that contain the same information as paper dental claim forms except that they are "mailed" via electronic transfer. (Chapter 15)

Emotions (communication) Feelings, such as being upset, angry, or even happy, that can keep listeners from hearing the message (barriers to effective communication). (Chapter 3)

Employment agency Organization that offers placement services. (Chapter 18)

Employment agreement An outline of conditions for employment. May include job title and description, work schedule, salary, and benefits. (Chapter 18)

Enamel Hard, mineralized substance that covers the anatomical crown of a tooth. It consists of 99% inorganic matter and cannot regenerate. (Chapter 2)

Enclosure reminder (letter writing) Notation stating that additional documents are enclosed with the letter. (Chapter 4)

Encounter forms Forms used to communicate information that is on a dental insurance claim form. (Chapter 15)

Endodontics Root canal procedures performed to replace the pulp. (Chapter 1)

Ergonomics Science of fitting the job to the worker. When the job does not match the physical capacity of the worker, work-related musculoskeletal disorders may result. (Chapter 13)

Ethics Category of moral judgments. (Chapter 1)

Examination form Form used in a clinical record to record examination information. (Chapter 8)

Exclusion The option in a dental benefits program to exclude dental services and procedures. These services and procedures are outlined in the patient's contract (benefits book). (Chapter 15)

Exclusive provider organization (EPO) A dental benefits plan or program that will cover dental services only if they are provided by an institutional or professional provider with whom the dental benefits plan has a contract. (Chapter 15)

Expanded (extended) function assistants Assistants who have additional training and education in functions that enable more independent patient care. Functions are identified in each state's Dental Practice Act. (Chapter 1)

Expendable products Supplies and products that can be reused for a specific length of time before they have to be replaced. Instruments, handpieces, and small equipment fall into this category. (Chapter 12)

Expiration date Date that identifies when a product should no longer be used. (Chapter 15)

Express mail The fastest service offered by the U.S. Postal Service. It is guaranteed for overnight delivery, 365 days a year. (Chapter 15)

Extended payment plan One of several methods that can be used when it is necessary to extend the schedule for payment of treatment. (Chapter 14)

F

Face The front of the head, consisting of 14 bones. (Chapter 2)

Facial An interchangeable term used to describe the buccal and labial surfaces. (Chapter 2)

Family deductible A deductible that can be satisfied when combined deductibles of the family have been met. This deductible will be less than the total of the individual family members' deductibles. (Chapter 15)

Fédération Dentaire Internationale Numbering System Tooth numbering system that is widely used in countries other than the United States. In this system, the quadrants and sextants are assigned numbers. Each configuration is a two-digit number that consists of a 0 and a number from 1 through 8. (Chapter 2)

Fee for service Method of payment that compensates the dentist according to individual services and procedures. Reimbursement is determined by established fee schedules. (Chapter 15)

Fee schedule List of charges for dental services and procedures. These are established by the dentist or a dental benefits provider and are mutually agreed on. (Chapter 15)

Feedback Method for determining whether a message has been received and understood. (Chapter 3)

File folders Items used to store documents, patient record forms, and business reports. (Chapter 9)

File labels Items used to identify contents of files and indexing (filing procedure). (Chapter 9)

Filing segment One or more filing units, such as the total name, subject, or number, that is being used for filing purposes. (Chapter 9)

Filing unit A number, a letter, a word, or any combination of these used for filing. (Chapter 9)

Filtering by level (organizational communications) Process by which information sent is not received because it has been changed or stopped at one level. If, as an administrative dental assistant, you send a message or idea to the dentist and it is stopped or changed by the office manager, there is a breakdown in the upward flow of the message. (Chapter 6)

Final decision stage The stage where the patient decides on the overall impression of the dental office. The first visit, the communication skills, and the attitude and professionalism of the staff are all taken into account. (Chapter 5)

Financial reports Reports used to determine the financial health of a dental practice. Accountants use them to prepare business, income, and payroll tax reports. (Chapter 17)

Financial reports (filing procedure) Financial records filed according to subject and then subdivided chronologically. (Chapter 9)

Financially responsible Term describing the person or party who must pay any balances on the account. (Chapter 17)

First-class mail Type of mail service used for sending letters, postcards, and greeting cards that weigh less than 11 ounces. It is delivered overnight to local areas, in 2 days to locally designated states, and in 3 days to all other areas. (Chapter 17)

Fixed fee schedule Fee schedules that include established fees that are charged by all dentists, regardless of geographic area. (Chapter 15)

Fluoride treatments Treatments provided to strengthen enamel and protect teeth from developing carious lesions. (Chapter 2)

Forensic odontology Method of tooth identification based on dental conditions. (Chapter 8)

Formal downward channels (organizational communications) Communication that originates at the top of the organizational structure and filters down to the lower levels of the organization. (Chapter 6)

Franchise dentistry Method of providing dental care under a common name. Its purpose is to provide a common name, regional or national advertising, contract agreements with dental benefits providers, and financial and managerial support. (Chapter 15)

Frenum Strip of tissue that connects two structures. (Chapter 2)

Full-blocked (letter writing) Format in which all letter sections begin at the left margin and proper spacing is applied between sections. (Chapter 4)

Full denture Prosthesis used to replace all teeth in an arch. (Chapter 2)

Full gold and metal crowns Replacements for tooth structures cast from gold alloy and other metals and categorized according to the amount of gold used: high noble, noble, low noble, and nongold (analogous to the carat classification for gold jewelry: 18k, 14k, and 10k). (Chapter 2)

Functional resumes Resumes in which skills and abilities are placed first, according to importance, regardless of the time of occurrence. After the objective statement, skills and abilities are highlighted, followed by work experience, education, and miscellaneous information. (Chapter 18)

G

Gag reflex Contraction of the constrictor muscles of the pharynx in response to taste or touch on the posterior pharyngeal wall or nearby areas. (Chapter 2)

Gender rule Rule that determines the primary and secondary coverage of the child by assigning primary coverage to the father and secondary to the mother. (Chapter 15)

Geographic filing Means of categorizing records according to geographic location, such as city, zip code, area code, state, or country. Each document is coded and filed according to the selected geographic locator. (Chapter 9)

Geometric chart Method of charting by which circles are used to represent teeth; it is divided into sections that represent the surfaces of the teeth. (Chapter 2)

Gingivae Masticatory mucosa and the tissue that surrounds the teeth. Normal healthy kind is firm and attached tightly around the teeth; it is coral or salmon-pink in color (in races other than Caucasian, the color is commonly darker). (Chapter 2)

Guides Items used to divide filing systems into small sections. (Chapter 9)

H

Hard palate Hard plate or roof of the mouth, covered with masticatory mucosa. (Chapter 2)

Hardware The physical part of the computer system. In a simple computer system it includes the central processing unit (CPU), monitor, keyboard, mouse, and printer. (Chapter 13)

Hazardous communication program Method of dealing with hazardous material. Consists of five parts: written program, chemical inventory, Safety Data Sheets, container labeling, and employee training. (Chapter 12)

Health Information Technology for Economic and Clinical Health (HITECH) Act Part of the American Recovery and Reinvestment Act of 2009, it contains general incentives related to healthcare information technology and specific incentives designed to accelerate the adoption of electronic health record systems. (Chapter 1)

Health Insurance Portability and Accountability Act of 1996 Legislative Act involving health information. The *Portability* section of the Act simply guarantees that a person covered by health insurance provided by one employer can obtain health insurance through the second employer if he or she changes jobs. The *Accountability* section of the Act answers the question of who and what should be accountable for specific healthcare activities. (Chapters 1, 15)

Health maintenance organization (HMO) Healthcare delivery system composed of providers who will accept payment for services on a per capita basis or a limited fee schedule. (Chapter 15)

HIPAA Omnibus Rule Rule enacted to strengthen the privacy and security portions for health information under the Health Insurance Portability and Accountability Act (HIPAA). (Chapter 1)

Horizontal channel (organizational communications) Working across (horizontally) organizational structures, communication is transmitted between members. This type of communication occurs primarily among members at the same level. (Chapter 6)

HOSA, Future Health Professionals Student organization with a mission to promote career opportunities in healthcare and to enhance the delivery of quality healthcare to all people. (Chapter 1)

Humanistic theory Theory based on the works of Maslow and Rogers. See *Maslow, Abraham H.* and *Rogers, Carl.* (Chapter 5)

Hybrid resumes Resumes that combine the best features of chronological and functional resumes in various arrangements while focusing only on information that is relevant to the current job objective. (Chapter 18)

Hyphenated surnames (filing procedure) Two surnames joined with a hyphen, treated as one unit. (Chapter 9)

I

Inappropriate span of control (organizational communications) One person has control for too long a period. This leads to lack of trust and fuels resentment. It may be the result of poor communication, lack of direction, or poor or nonexistent policies and procedures. (Chapter 6)

Incentive program Payment schedule by which the copayment percentage changes when patients follow a preset standard of treatment. (Chapter 15)

Incisal Sharp cutting edge of anterior teeth (incisors and cuspids). (Chapter 2)

Incisive papilla The papilla located straight behind the central incisors. (Chapter 2)

Incoming mail Mail received by the dental office that requires sorting according to category and routing to the correct person or department. (Chapter 4)

Indemnity plan Dental benefit plan that uses schedules of allowances, tables of allowances, or reasonable and customary fee schedules as the bases of payment calculations. (Chapter 15)

Indexing Method used to determine placement of files in an organized system. (Chapter 9)

Individual patient file folder Organizer used to keep documents and forms (clinical record). (Chapter 8)

Individual practice association (IPA) Legally formed organization that enters into contracts with dental benefits plans to provide services to enrollees in the dental benefits plan. (Chapter 15)

Informal channel (organizational communications) Communication that takes place in an informal setting and is not the official communication of the organization. The communication can be accurate or inaccurate and is often referred to as "the grapevine." (Chapter 6)

Information system Combination of equipment, software, data, personnel, and procedures that process information. (Chapter 15)

In-house payment plans (budget plans) Financial arrangements between the dental practice and the patient. (Chapter 14)

Initial contact stage The stage in selecting a dental practice that determines whether or not the patient will make an appointment. Factors considered are how the phone was answered, the attention given to the patient during the phone call, whether or not the patient's questions were answered, whether the name was used correctly, and whether the needs were met. (Chapter 5)

Initial oral examination Examination performed during the patient's first visit to the dental practice. Consists of diagnostic aids that will help the dentist to determine existing conditions and restorations as well as the dental needs of the patient. (Chapter 14)

Inlay Partial coverage of a tooth, usually on the same surfaces as amalgam restorations. Cast from gold or composite materials. (Chapter 2)

Input devices Peripherals that transfer data into a computer system. Common versions include keyboard, mouse, and scanner. (Chapter 13)

Inside address (letter writing) Address of the person or company to whom a letter is being sent. (Chapter 4)

Inspecting (filing procedure) Checking the document to make sure it is ready to file. (Chapter 9)

Insurance biller Administrative dental assistant responsible for insurance billing. (Chapter 1)

Insurance billing Process of billing a benefits provider for services rendered to a patient. (Chapter 9)

Insurance billing plans Types of payment plans that have established policies that must be followed. (Chapter 14)

Insurance information Information needed for insurance billing. (Chapter 17)

Insurance records Records that include contracts with third-party carriers (insurance companies). (Chapter 9)

Insured A person who has enrolled with an insurer (third party) to arrange for payment for dental services and procedures. (Chapter 15)

Insurer Third party who assumes responsibility for payment for dental services and procedures on behalf of enrollees in the program. (Chapter 15)

Integrating style Style of conflict resolution that works best when time is available to address the problem. Usually, problems are complex and solving them requires the expertise of more than one person. The problem must be identified and then input from all members is needed to develop a solution. (Chapter 6)

Intergroup conflict Conflict between two or more groups because members of one group disagree with members of another group. (Chapter 6)

Intermediate (practice management) system Middle or secondary level of software used in computerized practice management systems. (Chapter 7)

International Standards Organization See *Fédération Dentaire Internationale Numbering System.* (Chapter 2)

Interorganizational conflict Conflict between two or more organizations. (Chapter 6)

Interpersonal communication Communication in which the sender and the receiver exchange information in real time. This includes face-to-face, telephone, and video conferencing. (Chapter 3)

Interpersonal conflict Conflict (between two team members) that occurs when members of the team at the same level (assistant and assistant) or at different levels (hygienist and assistant) disagree about a given matter. (Chapter 6)

Interproximal The space created by two proximal surfaces. (Chapter 2)

Intragroup conflict Conflict (within the group) that occurs when members at the same level (assistant and assistant, dentist and dentist) disagree. This conflict normally occurs when differences in goals, tasks, and procedures are discussed. (Chapter 6)

Intraorganizational conflict Conflict within the organization. (Chapter 6)

Intrapersonal conflict Conflict within oneself when one is expected to perform a task that does not meet personal goals, values, beliefs, or expertise. (Chapter 6)

Introduction (letter writing) The first paragraph in the body of a letter. It should contain a brief list of the important points discussed in the main body of the letter. (Chapter 4)

Inventory management system A manual or automated system used to track and manage inventory effectively. (Chapter 12)

Investigation stage The stage of selecting a dentist in which the patient researches the dental practice. He or she will investigate the name of the dental practice, what types of insurance plans it accepts, the advertising, and what others think of the practice. (Chapter 5)

Invoice Document that indicates charges or products sent. (Chapter 16)

J

Jargon Specialized words, acronyms (groups of initials), and other terms that are unique to a given group. (Chapter 3)

Job search log Method used to organize, plan, and follow through with employment leads. Tracks submitted resumes and identifies company names and telephone numbers of contact persons. (Chapter 18)

K

Keyboard Common type of computer input device that is similar in configuration to a typewriter. It may include a variety of function keys. (Chapter 13)

L

Labial The surface of anterior teeth that faces or touches the lips. (Chapter 2)

Labial frenum Structure that connects the tissue of the lips (labia) to the gingival tissue. (Chapter 2)

Labial vestibule Junction of the lips and the gingiva. (Chapter 2)

Laboratory (dental) Area of the dental office where nonpatient procedures can be performed. (Chapter 8)

Laboratory form Prescription used to communicate instructions to a laboratory technician. (Chapter 8)

Lack of trust and openness (organizational communications) Situation when feedback is not accepted that can occur at all levels of the organization, possibly leading to conflict. (Chapter 6)

Lateral file folders Folders used for clinical records. Tabs are located on the side of each folder. (Chapter 9)

Lateral files Open file cabinets used to store file folders and help save space. (Chapter 9)

Lateral incisors Anterior teeth characterized by thin, sharp incisal edges that aid in cutting food. (Chapter 12)

Lead time The time it takes for supplies to arrive at the office once an order has been placed. (Chapter 12)

Least expensive alternative treatment (LEAT) A provision in dental benefits plans that allows payment for dental services and procedures according to the lowest price. (Chapter 15)

Legal standards Legislation regulated by boards and commissions. (Chapter 1)

Letterhead Name, address, and telephone number of the sender. (Chapter 4)

Lettering Single spaced in the body of the letter, with double spacing between paragraphs. (Chapter 4)

Licensure Identifies members of a profession who meet minimal standards and are qualified to perform set duties outlined in regulations and standards (Dental Practice Act). (Chapter 1)

Lighting Critical factor for a comfortable and productive workstation. The correct type and optimal level depend on the task at hand. (Chapter 13)

Line spacing The number of lines between the elements of a letter. (Chapter 4)

Lingual Surface of teeth that faces the tongue or inside of the mouth. (Chapter 2)

Lingual frenum Structure that connects the tongue to the floor of the mouth. (Chapter 2)

Lining mucosa Covers the cheeks, lips, vestibule, ventral (underside) surface of the tongue, and soft palate. This tissue is very thin and can be injured easily. (Chapter 2)

Lips Tissue that surrounds the opening to the oral cavity. (Chapter 2)

Locker room Place to change from street clothes into uniforms.

Logical When writing a letter, the ideas that you wish to convey should be organized in this type of order to help the reader understand the message you are sending. (Chapter 4)

Loudness (speech) Volume of a voice. (Chapter 3)

M

Mail recall system System that requires the mailing of recall cards to patients to remind them that they are due in the dental office for an appointment. (Chapter 11)

Main body (letter writing) Details of the points stated in the introduction of a letter. One or two paragraphs in length. (Chapter 4)

Major equipment Equipment that can be depreciated, such as dental chairs, radiology units, computers, office equipment, and laboratory equipment. (Chapter 12)

Malocclusion Teeth that are out of alignment or occlusion. (Chapter 2)

Managed care Method employed by some benefits plans that is designed to contain the cost of healthcare. These methods involve limiting access to care (enrollees are assigned healthcare providers), services and procedures covered, and reimbursement amounts. (Chapter 15)

Mandibular arch Lower teeth or jaw. (Chapter 2)

Mandibular left One of the dental arches that are divided into four sections or quadrants. Each quadrant has the same number and type of teeth as the opposite quadrant. Quadrants consist of maxillary right, maxillary left, mandibular left, and mandibular right. (Chapter 2)

Mandibular right See *Mandibular left*. (Chapter 2)

Manual appointment books Tools used to organize the daily office schedule. The most common style is the week-at-a-glance. (Chapter 10)

Maslow, Abraham H. (1908–1970) Psychologist who believed that individuals have to satisfy a level of physiologic need before they are motivated to seek the next level. These levels range from the basic needs of life (food, shelter, and safety) to the higher needs of love, belonging, and self-esteem to the highest need self-actualization. (Chapter 5)

Mastication Chewing and grinding of food with the teeth. (Chapter 2)

Masticatory mucosa Thick, dense mucosa attached tightly to bone (with the exception of the tongue). It is designed to resist the pressure of chewing food and is not easily injured. This tissue type forms the gingiva (gums), the hard palate, and the dorsum (top) of the tongue. (Chapter 2)

Matrixing Outlining. (Chapter 10)

Maxillary arch Upper teeth or jaw. (Chapter 2)

Maxillary left See *Mandibular left*. (Chapter 2)

Maxillary right See *Mandibular left*. (Chapter 2)

Maximum allowance The total amount of dental benefits (dollars) that will be paid toward dental services and procedures. It is determined by the provisions of individual group contracts. (Chapter 15)

Maximum benefit The total amount of dental benefits that will be paid for an individual or family for dental services and procedures. This amount is determined by the individual group contract and may involve a yearly or lifetime cap. (Chapter 15)

Maximum fee schedule The total acceptable fee for a dental service or procedure that will be charged by a dental provider under a specific dental benefits plan. (Chapter 15)

Mechanics of scheduling Selecting the appointment book (manual or electronic), outlining

or matrixing, and entering information. (Chapter 10)

Medical history (clinical record) Comprehensive information that alerts the dentist to drug allergies and medical conditions that may be affected by certain dental procedures. (Chapter 8)

Medium (communication) Method of transferring information. Can be verbal, nonverbal, or a combination of the two. (Chapter 3)

Menu bar One of the basic elements of a software package; it lists categories of user options. (Chapter 7)

Mesial Proximal surface of a tooth that is facing toward the midline. (Chapter 2)

Message Idea to be shared with another person or group. (Chapter 3)

Mixed dentition Set of teeth in which primary and permanent teeth are both present. (Chapter 2)

Modem Unit that electronically transfers information from the CPU through a transmission line (commonly a telephone line) to another location. (Chapter 13)

Modified blocked (letter writing) A blocked format with one change: paragraphs are indented five spaces. (Chapter 4)

Molars Posterior teeth that have flat surfaces with rounded projections and are used for chewing. (Chapter 2)

Month tab Tool that makes it easy to turn to a given month in an appointment book. This is especially handy when you are scheduling a few months in advance. (Chapter 10)

Mouse Computer input device. (Chapter 13)

Mucous membrane Moist membrane that covers the inside of the cheeks. (Chapter 2)

N

National Health Information Infrastructure (NHII) A communications system designed to transmit patient health information (including dental). The system is designed to improve patient safety, improve the quality of healthcare, and better inform and empower healthcare consumers. This system will be completed in 2015. (Chapters 1, 8)

National Provider Identifier (NPI) A distinctive standard identification number issued by the U.S. government that can replace the Social Security number, individual tax ID, or other identifiers on standard electronic healthcare transactions such as dental insurance claim forms. (Chapter 15)

Necessary treatment Dental services and procedures that have been established by the dental professional as necessary for the purpose of restoring or maintaining a patient's oral health. Treatment is based on established standards of the dental profession. (Chapter 15)

Networking (employment strategy) A means of contacting other dental professionals and letting them know that you are seeking employment. This is an informal job placement service and is one of the most effective means of seeking employment. (Chapter 18)

Newspaper advertisements One of the most common ways to look for a job. Employers

place an advertisement describing the position available and inviting applicants to call for an appointment or send their resumes. (Chapter 18)

Noise (communication) Something that alters the message because the sender and the receiver cannot hear the message. When conversations take place around machinery, large groups of people, and other such areas, the message that is being sent may not be completely received. (Chapter 3)

Nomenclature The brief, literal definition provided with each procedure code. (Chapter 15)

Nonconsumable products Items that can be used for only 1 or 2 years before they must be replaced because of wear. (Chapter 12)

Nonduplication of benefits Stipulation that applies if a subscriber is covered by more than one benefit plan. In the case of dual coverage, the subscriber will never receive payment for more than 100% of the covered benefit. (Chapter 15)

Nonparticipating dentist A dental professional who is not under contract with a dental benefits plan to provide dental services and procedures to enrollees. (Chapter 15)

Nonverbal messages Method of communication in which the message is sent through facial expressions and body gestures. (Chapter 3)

Notation line The line below the enclosure reminder in a standard letter. (Chapter 4)

NSF "No significant findings"; also "nonsufficient funds." (Chapters 8, 17)

Numeric filing System in which records are filed according to an assigned number. (Chapter 9)

O

Objective (resume) Important component of your resume that identifies the position for which you are applying and is supported by the information listed in the body of your resume. (Chapter 18)

Obliging style Style of conflict resolution used when the issue is unimportant and you are willing to give in to the other party to preserve a relationship. (Chapter 6)

Occlusal The broad, flat chewing surface of posterior teeth (premolars and molars). (Chapter 2)

Occlusion Relationship between the maxillary arch and the mandibular arch and the way they meet or touch. (Chapter 2)

Occupational Safety and Health Administration (OSHA) Federal government agency that was enacted to protect the worker from workplace injury. It regulates all areas of employment. In addition, most states have their own versions, which in some cases are stricter than the federal agency. (Chapter 1)

Office letter portfolio Collection of samples of letters that can be used for different occasions. It is similar to computerized templates, with the exception that a hard copy of the letter is placed in a notebook. (Chapter 1)

Office manager Person who organizes and oversees the daily operations of the office staff. (Chapter 1)

Onlay Partial coverage of a tooth; the same as an inlay, except that it includes more tooth structure and replaces a cusp. Cast in gold or composite. (Chapter 2)

Online resume Resume that is posted on websites for prospective employers to review. (Chapter 18)

Open enrollment Period of time (occurs annually) when a member of a dental benefits program has the option of selecting the type of coverage and the provider of dental services. (Chapter 15)

Open panel Dental benefits plan in which any licensed dentist can participate. The enrollee (insured) can seek treatment from any licensed dentist with payment of benefits provided to the enrollee or the dentist. (Chapter 15)

Open punctuation (letter writing) Format in which no punctuation is used in the salutation and complimentary closing. (Punctuation is, however, used in the body of the letter.) (Chapter 4)

Operating systems software Information needed to operate and run a computer. (Chapter 13)

Oral and maxillofacial pathology Area of dentistry in which diseases of the mouth or oral structures are diagnosed and treated. (Chapter 1)

Oral and maxillofacial radiology Dental specialty that produces and interprets images and data generated by all modalities of radiant energy (x-rays and other types of imaging) that are used for the diagnosis and management of diseases, disorders, and conditions of the oral and maxillofacial region. (Chapter 1)

Oral and maxillofacial surgery Branch of surgery involving procedures of the head and neck, ranging from simple tasks such as extraction of teeth to complex surgical procedures designed to reconstruct facial structures. (Chapter 1)

Oral cavity Anatomical area in which dentistry is performed. It is also the beginning of the digestive system, contains sensory receptors, and is used to form speech patterns; it is a source of human pleasure and a weapon for defense (verbal and physical). (Chapter 2)

Oral mucosa Tissue that lines the oral cavity. (Chapter 2)

Organization A process through which you identify what you want to say and the results you hope to attain with your communication. (Chapter 4)

Orthodontics and dentofacial orthopedics Area of dentistry in which conditions of malocclusion (the way teeth meet) are diagnosed and treated. This dentist is a member of a complex team of medical and dental doctors who restore facial features and oral functions of patients. (Chapter 1)

Outgoing mail Mail sent from the dental practice. (Chapter 4)

Out-guides Tabs used to replace a file that has been removed from the system. (Chapter 9)

Outlook The presentation of information in a positive form, even when the letter contains unpleasant subject material. (Chapter 4)

Output devices Devices used to transfer data from the computer, such as monitors, printers, and peripheral storage devices. (Chapter 13)

Outside payment plans Financial arrangements made by the dental office and administered by an outside agency. (Chapter 14)

Overbilling Fraudulent practice of not disclosing to benefit plan organizations the waiver of patient copayment. (Chapter 15)

Overcoding Billing of dental benefits plans for procedures that results in higher payments than are justified by the service or procedure that was actually performed. (Chapter 15)

P

Panographic x-ray unit Machine that takes extraoral (outside the mouth) radiographic films that include a wide view of the maxilla and mandible. (Chapter 2)

Paper dental claim forms Forms generated by computer and printed in the office or typewritten by the assistant and sent from the dental office to the correct insurance carrier via mail. (Chapter 15)

Paragraphing The method of letter writing used to insert natural breaks in the flow of information. (Chapter 4)

Parotid glands Salivary glands. (Chapter 2)

Participating dentist Dentist who has a contract with a dental benefits organization to provide dental care to specific enrollees. (Chapter 15)

Patient education room Area designated for activities prepared to educate and motivate patients. (Chapter 15)

Patient information (clinical record) Information within the record that strictly pertains to the treatment of the patient. Does not include financial accounting or insurance forms. (Chapter 9)

Payer Insurance companies, dental benefits plans, or dental plan sponsors (direct reimbursement, unions) that make payments on behalf of patients. (Chapter 15)

Payment in full plan Office policy that requires the patient to pay the total amount owed after each visit. Payment may be made in the form of cash, check, or credit card. (Chapter 14)

Payroll records Documents that contain payroll information pertaining to employees. (Chapter 9)

Pediatric dentistry Area of dentistry in which dentists (pedodontists) treat patients from newborn to about the age of 15 years in all phases of dentistry. They may work in a hospital setting to provide treatment to patients under general anesthesia, work with patients with special needs, and provide treatment for children who are in need of preventive and restorative dental treatment. (Chapter 1)

Pegboard system Also referred to as a "one-write system." Components of this system consist of ledger board, daysheet, patient ledger, and receipt. Forms are arranged one on top of the other to facilitate entry of data one time only. Check-writing system components include ledger board, check register, and checks. (Chapter 17)

Periodic method (filing procedure) System by which all financial reports, payroll records, and other monthly reports are transferred to an inactive file, making room for the new year's reports and records. (Chapter 9)

Periodontal ligament Connective fibers that help to hold teeth in the alveolar socket; provide protection and nourishment for the tooth. (Chapter 2)

Periodontics Area of dentistry in which dentists (periodontists) treat patients who have diseases of the soft tissue surrounding the teeth (periodontal disease). Periodontal disease occurs in several different stages, which vary in severity. The treatment performed by a periodontist focuses on correcting and preventing the progression of disease. (Chapter 1)

Permanent dentition The second set of teeth (32 in number) that are intended to remain in the mouth for a lifetime. (Chapter 2)

Perpetual method (filing procedure) Filing method that identifies files and records that have been inactive for a predetermined length of time or that are no longer required for quick reference. (Chapter 9)

Personal career portfolio A collection of samples from your professional career. These are used as a source of information and an illustration of your skills, abilities, and strengths. (Chapter 18)

Personal letters Employment tools that help you to follow up on current leads and serve as models for future letters. They include cover letters, research letters, information interview letters, and career information request letters. (Chapter 18)

Personal names (filing procedure) Indexing method by individual names or business or organizational names, in accordance with the ARMA Simplified Filing Standard Rules.

Personnel records Nonpayroll information about employees. (Chapter 9)

Phenomenological Term that describes viewing a situation from the other person's point of view. (Chapter 5)

Pitch (voice) A quality of the sound of your voice. (Chapter 3)

Pontic Artificial replacement of a missing tooth or teeth. (Chapter 2)

Porcelain fused to metal Gold-cast crown with a porcelain cover (tooth colored). (Chapter 2)

Postage Amount of money that is required to mail an item.

Postage meter A device used to weigh items for mailing. (Chapter 4)

Postage stamp Prepaid item affixed to envelop or package for mailing. (Chapter 4)

Postal cards One-sheet items used to send short messages through the mail. (Chapter 4)

Posterior teeth Teeth toward the back of the mouth. They consist of the first premolar, second premolar (bicuspid), first molar, second molar, and third molar (wisdom tooth). (Chapter 2)

Posting transactions Placing the correct patient information on the ledger, receipt, and daysheet (manual system) or keying the information into a computerized system. (Chapter 17)

Power bars One of the basic elements of a software package that provides quick access to features or reports. (Chapter 7)

Preauthorization Certification by a dental benefits plan that a pretreatment plan has been authorized for payment in accordance with the patient's group policy. (Chapter 15)

Precertification Confirmation by a dental benefits plan that a patient is eligible to receive treatment according to the provisions of the contract. (Chapter 15)

Preconceived ideas A barrier to communication. Consists of information that has already been received and is deemed to be true. This can block or change the way a message is received. (Chapter 3)

Predated appointment book pages A manual appointment book that contains the dates. This can be helpful when schedules stay consistent. (Chapter 10)

Predetermination See *Preauthorization*. (Chapter 15)

Preexisting condition A clause in most dental benefits plans that limits coverage of dental benefits to conditions that existed before the patient was enrolled in the benefit plan. (Chapter 15)

Preferred provider organization (PPO) A contract between a dental benefits plan organization and a provider of dental care that states that, in return for the referral of dental patients, the dentist will provide dental services and procedures at a reduced fee or will adhere to an established fee schedule. (Chapter 15)

Prefiling of fees A procedure in which a dental professional files a fee schedule with the dental benefits plan organization for the purpose of gaining preauthorization of the fee schedule. (Chapter 15)

Premolars (bicuspids) Posterior teeth, smaller than molars, with two cusps, used for tearing and grinding. (Chapter 2)

Prescheduled recall system Scheduling of patients in advance of their recall. (Chapter 11)

Primary dentition A set of 20 teeth, including central, lateral, cuspid, first primary molar, and second primary molar. Often referred to as "baby teeth." (Chapter 2)

Priority mail A faster delivery service than first-class mail at a reasonable rate. (Chapter 4)

Privacy officer Person who is appointed to oversee the written policy and procedure manual for handling protected health information (PHI). (Chapter 1)

Private office A personal office. (Chapter 1)

Production reports Reports that identify what types of procedures have been performed and by whom. (Chapter 17)

Productivity Fees charged for dental treatment or monies collected. (Chapter 10)

Products Materials used in direct patient care, including dental materials and dental therapeutics. (Chapter 12)

Professional correspondence Correspondence between individuals and professional organizations. (Chapter 9)

Professional networking A means of contacting other dental professionals and letting

them know that you are seeking employment. (Chapter 18)

Professional organizations Entities that may offer placement services for their members. (Chapter 18)

Profit and loss statements Statements that identify overhead (the cost of operating a business) and determine whether the dental practice is making or losing money. (Chapter 17)

Progress notes (clinical record) Notations kept in a patient's clinical record, including those related to diagnosis, treatment, amount and type of anesthetic, and brand name of materials used. (Chapter 8)

Prosthodontics Area of dentistry for which dentists (prosthodontists) receive advanced training in performing procedures that replace lost and damaged teeth and tooth structures with partial dentures (fixed and removable), full dentures, or crowns over implants. (Chapter 1)

Protected health information (PHI) Health information that is required to be secured in all formats and in all locations; this is necessary during the transfer of information in oral, written, and electronic formats and when information is stored (paper and electronic copies). (Chapter 1)

Proximal Surfaces that are adjacent or next to another surface of a tooth. (Chapter 2)

Pulp chamber Center of the crown. (Chapter 2)

Pulpal tissue Connective tissue, blood vessels, and nerves. (Chapter 2)

Q

Quadrants The four sections of the dental arches. Each quadrant has the same number and type of teeth as the opposite quadrant. (Chapter 2)

R

Radio-frequency identification (RFID) A technology that uses radio waves to identify or track objects. (Chapter 12)

Rank and status (organizational communications) Factors that may interfere with communication in several ways. Some people use position (rank) as a means of power over others, which closes channels of communication. (Chapter 6)

Rate of use Length of time between purchase and use of a product. (Chapter 12)

Reasonable fee A determination by the third-party administrator that a specific service has been modified to take into consideration unusual complications. (Chapter 15)

Recall appointment Scheduled appointment for preventive treatment or reevaluation of dental conditions. (Chapter 11)

Recall system Method used to ensure timely scheduling of patients for preventive treatment. (Chapter 11)

Receipt Document given to a patient that shows charges and payments. (Chapter 11)

Receiver The person or place that receives the message. (Chapter 3)

Reception area The first office area to be viewed by the patient; the place where patients wait. (Chapter 1)

Receptionist Administrative dental assistant responsible for answering the telephone, greeting patients, and scheduling appointments. (Chapter 1)

Record and supply storage Areas where storage shelves and large file cabinets are maintained. (Chapter 1)

Records manager Person who organizes and maintains all aspects of patients' clinical charts according to preset standards. Establishes and maintains an efficient filing system to ensure the precise location of all clinical records. (Chapter 1)

Reference initials (letter writing) Initials of the sender of the letter (in upper case) and initials of the typist (in lower case). (Chapter 4)

Reference letters Letters written by people who know you personally and are willing to speak on your behalf. (Chapter 18)

Reference line The optional line that falls two lines below the salutation in a standard letter. (Chapter 4)

Referral letters Method for sending information about patients to other professionals. The purposes are to introduce the patient and to state the purpose of the need to send information. (Chapter 4)

Registration Form of licensure that has been established by some states as a method of protecting the public. Requirements are outlined in each state's Dental Practice Act. (Chapter 1)

Registration form (clinical record) Form that introduces the patient to the dental practice and provides demographic and financial information for insurance forms and patient billing.

Removable partial Removable prosthesis. (Chapter 8)

Resin Tooth-colored restorative material. (Chapter 2)

Resin-based composite Type of restorative material that is tooth colored and used primarily on anterior teeth. (Chapter 2)

Restorative dentistry Branch of dentistry involving procedures in which the dentist removes caries from the tooth. After the caries have been removed, the tooth is prepared to receive a material that will replace the lost tooth structure. (Chapter 2)

Resumes Personal marketing tools prepared with one goal to get a job interview. A good version will give a competitive advantage, help to organize thoughts, and make a good impression. (Chapter 18)

Retention (filing procedure) Keeping records. This varies according to the extent of treatment provided, whether radiographs have been taken, and regulations established by third-party insurance carriers. It is determined by office policy and government regulations. (Chapter 9)

Return address Text that identifies the sender of a piece of mail. Placed in the upper left corner of an envelope. (Chapter 4)

RFID tag A tag that stores information and is read using radio-frequency identification (RFID) technology. (Chapter 12)

Risk management Process that identifies conditions that may lead to alleged malpractice or procedures that are not in compliance with mandated regulations. (Chapter 8)

Rogers, Carl (1902–1987) Psychologist who theorized that each healthy individual believes in an ideal self and is constantly trying to achieve the ideal self as much as possible. (Chapter 5)

Root Anatomical portion of a tooth located in the alveolar process. (Chapter 2)

Root canal Endodontic procedure that replaces diseased pulp. (Chapter 2)

Routing slips Paper used to communicate details of patient treatment between the business office and the treatment area. (Chapter 17)

Royal and religious titles (filing procedure) Convention that states that when titles are followed by one name, they are filed as written. (Chapter 9)

Rugae Ridges located within the hard palate. (Chapter 2)

S

Safety Data Sheet (SDS) A document made available to the employer by the manufacturer of products that identifies specific safety elements of the product. (Chapter 12)

Saliva Substance produced by the salivary glands to moisturize mucous membranes, lubricate food, clean the teeth, and supply an enzyme (amylase) that begins the digestive process. (Chapter 2)

Salutation (letter writing) A greeting, such as "Dear " and "To Whom It May Concern." (Chapter 4)

Scanner Computer input device that digitizes images. (Chapter 13)

Sealant Substance that covers the chewing surfaces of teeth with a thin coat of resin. The purpose of this coating treatment is to close and protect the tooth from the effects of acid attacks, which cause demineralization of enamel and lead to carious lesions. (Chapter 2)

Semantics Meanings of words and language. (Chapter 3)

Semi-blocked (letter writing) Format that is the same as blocked with one change: paragraphs are indented five spaces. (Chapter 4)

Sender (communication) Person who has the responsibility to ensure that the proper message is sent and that the receiver understands the content of the message. (Chapter 3)

Sextants The six sections into which the dental arches are sometimes divided. This method of division is most commonly used in periodontal evaluations. The sections consist of maxillary right posterior, maxillary anterior, maxillary left posterior, mandibular left posterior, mandibular anterior, and mandibular right posterior. (Chapter 2)

Signature identification (letter writing) Text that identifies the sender of the letter. (Chapter 4)

Simple extraction Removal of one or more teeth without the need to remove bone or cut tissue. (Chapter 2)

Simplified filing standard rules for personal names Standards that can be used when filing business names. (Chapter 9)

Simplified or AMS (letter writing) Format similar to full-blocked, except that open punctuation is used, no salutation or complimentary closing is included, a subject line in all capital letters must be used, the word "subject" is omitted, the signer's identification appears in all capital letters, and lists are indented five spaces. If a numbered list is used, the period is omitted and the list is not indented. (Chapter 4)

Sincerity (communications) An emotion that patients can perceive from members of the dental healthcare team when barriers are removed and the message is interpreted as authentic. (Chapter 3)

Skip tracing Process for locating a person who has moved and not left a forwarding address. (Chapter 14)

Skull Bones in the head made up of two sections. The cranium consists of 8 bones that form a protective structure for the brain and the face consists of 14 bones. (Chapter 2)

Smile (communication) Facial expression that communicates a positive thought. (Chapter 3)

Soft palate Posterior tissue region of the roof of the mouth. This region is soft and flexible. (Chapter 2)

Soft skills A set of personal qualities, habits, attitudes, and social skills that are needed for successful job performance. (Chapter 18)

Software Instructions executed by a computer. (Chapter 13)

Software suites Applications that can create a seamless workflow, such as patient treatment, digital imaging, treatment planning, and appointment scheduling connected instantly to the patient record. (Chapter 7)

Sorting (filing procedure) Phase of the filing process during which records and documents are separated into categories according to the filing method used and the locations of files. (Chapter 9)

Speed (speech) The quickness with which a message is spoken. (Chapter 3)

Square-blocked (letter writing) The same format as full-blocked with minor changes. The date line is on the same line as the first line of the inside address and is right justified. Reference initials and enclosure reminders are typed on the same line as the signature and the signer's identification and are right justified. This style allows for squaring of the letter and is used when space is needed. (Chapter 4)

Staff room Area set aside for the exclusive use of staff for activities such as eating lunch and holding meetings. (Chapter 1)

Standard punctuation (letter writing) Type of punctuation in which the salutation is followed by a colon (:) and the complimentary closing is followed by a comma (,). (Chapter 4)

Standards for Privacy of Individually Identifiable Health Information (The Privacy Rule) Rule designed to protect health information; applies to three types of covered entities: health plans, healthcare clearinghouses, and healthcare providers who use an electronic mode to transfer information. (Chapter 1)

Standards for Security of Individually Identifiable Health Information (The Security Rule) Rule stating that covered providers must run a risk analysis to protect the integrity, confidentiality, and availability of electronic health information. (Chapter 1)

Statement Summary of individual invoices and requests for payment. (Chapter 16)

Stationery Collection of paper products that are used in correspondence. Effective professional communication combines this with messages. (Chapter 4)

Status bars One of the basic elements of a software package that identifies the current state of a task or record. (Chapter 7)

Stereotyping (communication) Attitude that blocks effective communication because assumptions are made about nonfactual information or preconceived ideas about a person, an idea, or a procedure. (Chapter 3)

Sterilization area Room in which contaminated instruments are cleaned, packaged, sterilized, and prepared for reuse. The room is separated into two areas: contaminated and clean. (Chapter 1)

Subject filing Method of storing information according to subject. In this system, files are labeled according to the subject of the contents and then filed alphabetically. (Chapter 9)

Subject lines (letter writing) Words that draw attention to the nature of the correspondence. (Chapter 4)

Subjective statement A statement that does not provide information but only an interpretation of an observation. (Chapter 8)

Sublingual gland Salivary gland. (Chapter 2)

Submandibular gland Salivary gland. (Chapter 2)

Subscriber A term used to describe the holder of a dental benefit (insurance). (Chapter 15)

Subscription services Services that provide information on a large number of insurance carriers and groups. The service compiles the same information for a wide range of third-party carriers, employers, and other dental groups into one easy reference system. (Chapter 15)

Superbills Documents used to communicate information contained on a dental insurance claim form. (Chapter 15)

Supplies Consumable goods that are used in support of dental treatment. (Chapter 12)

Surfaces of the tooth Sections into which each tooth is divided. Each has a name that is used by the dental professional to describe the exact location of tooth decay, restorations, and other conditions. (Chapter 2)

Surgical extractions Procedures that include the cutting of tissue and the removal of bone to facilitate removal of a tooth. (Chapter 2)

Symbolic numbering system Method of tooth numbering in which each tooth in a quadrant is assigned a number and the quadrant is assigned a symbol. (Chapter 2)

T

Table of allowances A list of the services and procedures that a dental benefits plan will pay for, with a dollar amount assigned to each procedure. Also referred to as a "schedule of allowances" and an "indemnity schedule." (Chapter 15)

Tax records (filing procedure) Payroll, business, and corporate tax reports that are filed by subject and then subdivided into the type of report or record. These records normally cover a specified period of time and therefore are subfiled chronologically. (Chapter 9)

Telecommunications The use of equipment to transfer information or to communicate with someone over a distance. In a dental practice, these methods include the telephone system and intraoffice memoranda. (Chapter 13)

Telephone recall system Method by which an assistant personally calls all patients before the month they are due for recall and scheduling of their appointment. (Chapter 4)

Temporary agencies Businesses that place applicants in positions for a specified length of time. They charge a fee to the employer. The applicant works in a temporary position and is paid by the agency. (Chapter 18)

Third party A group or organization that has the capacity to collect premiums, accept financial risk, and pay dental claims. In addition, this entity performs other administrative services. Also known as an administrative agent, carrier, insurer, or underwriter. (First party is the patient; second party is the healthcare provider.) (Chapter 15)

Third-party finance plans Special payment plans provided by a company via credit extension to finance dental treatment. (Chapter 14)

Third-party vendor A company that performs many tasks that could be performed by the dental practice, such as insurance verification, patient billing, marketing, and practice promotion. (Chapter 7)

Timing When and how you present an idea; determines how it is accepted. (Chapter 6)

Title bar One of the basic elements of a software package that identifies the name of the program and the mode of use. (Chapter 7)

Titles and suffixes (filing procedure) Identifying items associated with a person's name that are used as a filing unit, when they are needed to distinguish between two or more identical names. If used, they are placed in the last filing unit and filed as written but without punctuation. (Chapter 9)

Tone (communication) A quality in the sound of your voice. (Chapter 3)

Tone (letter writing) The way that words and phrases are used to convey a message. (Chapter 4)

Tongue A strong muscle in the mouth that is covered with taste buds, aids in the digestive process, and contributes to speech formation. (Chapter 3)

Tool bar One of the basic elements of a software package that uses icons to identify common functions. (Chapter 7)

Touch (communication) Nonverbal communication used to convey a message of warmth, reassurance, understanding, and caring. (Chapter 1)

Transactions and code sets Set of alpha and numeric code used to report specific treatment procedures and diagnoses to insurance carriers. (Chapter 1)

Transfer methods Methods of relocating files. A filing system works best when the location is accessible and the files are not overcrowded. Therefore this space should be used only for active files. Those that are not active are transferred to a more remote area. (Chapter 9)

Treatment plan Outline of proposed dental treatment. (Chapter 8)

Treatment rooms Areas where patients are treated by the dentist, dental hygienist, and dental assistant. Also referred to as "operatories" (although this term is fading from use because patients associate it with "surgical operating room"; some dental personnel may still use it). (Chapter 8)

U

Unconditional positive regard (communication) Total love and respect, no matter what. (Chapter 5)

Undated appointment book page A manual appointment book without dates. Used when flexibility is needed. (Chapter 10)

Union trust funds Funds that administer the distribution of their members' benefits. (Chapter 15)

Units (scheduling) Time segment into which appointment books divide the day. (Chapter 10)

Universal/National Numbering System Tooth numbering system developed in the United States to ensure consistency in identifying individual teeth. Each tooth is assigned a number, with the maxillary right third molar as tooth number 1; maxillary left third molar, tooth number 16; mandibular left third molar, tooth number 17; and mandibular right third molar, tooth number 32. (Chapter 2)

Upward channel (organizational communications) Flow of information from one level to a higher level. (Chapter 6)

Usual, customary, and reasonable (UCR) plan A dental plan that uses the following criteria to establish a fee schedule: usual fee, the fee the dentist uses most often for a given dental service; customary fee, the fee determined by the third-party administrator from actual submitted fees for specific dental services; and reasonable fee, a determination by the third-party administrator that a particular service for a given procedure has been modified to take into consideration unusual complications. This fee may vary from the dentist's usual fee and the administrator's customary fee. (Chapter 15)

Usual fee Fee that the dentist uses most often for a given dental service. (Chapter 15)

Uvula A projection of tissue located on the posterior of the soft palate that hangs down into the center of the throat. (Chapter 2)

V

Veneer crown Thin coverage on the facial surface that is made with only a cast composite or resin material. (Chapter 2)

Verbal messages Messages communicated with words, which can be divided into two categories: spoken and written. Spoken messages can be delivered face to face or transferred electronically (via telephone, voice mail, or video conferencing). Written communication may consist of letters, memos, faxes, e-mails, and newsletters. (Chapter 3)

Vermilion border The junction of the tissue of the face and the mucous membrane of the lips. (Chapter 2)

Vertical file folders Those folders used with filing systems with tabs located at the top of the file. (Chapter 9)

Vertical files Filing cabinets that consist of one to five drawers that, when pulled out, present files from the side rather than the front. When these are used for storage of business records, a frame can be inserted into each drawer that provides a means of hanging files. Hanging files can be labeled and then individual files can be organized within each hanging file. (Chapter 9)

Voice mail Recorded messages accessed by telephone. (Chapter 3)

W

Week at a glance A manual appointment book that allows the assistant to view the whole week, Monday through Saturday. (Chapter 10)

White space (letter writing) Space that surrounds the text of the letter. It should be uniform and balanced. (Chapter 4)

WNL Within normal limits. (Chapter 8)

Work overload Any amount or type of work that adds to daily stress. (Chapter 1)

A

Abutment teeth, 34
Accepted fee, 214–217b
Accepting shipments, steps in, 182b
Account aging reports, 208
Accounting, definition of, 258
Accounting tasks, performing, 93
Accounts payable, 141, 235–257
    bank statement reconciliation, 241–245, 241f
    check writing, 236–239
    definition of, 235, 258
    expenditure verification, 235
    organization of, 235
    payroll, 245–256
    reports, 271
    services, payroll, 250
Accounts receivable, 141, 258–271
    billing, 260–262
    definition of, 258
    financial records organization components,
        258–260
    HIPAA and, 263b
    managing, 205–212
        patient transactions, 263–270, 263b,
            265–267b, 265f, 266f, 267f, 268f
    report monitoring, 208, 208b
    reports for, 270–271
Active scripts, 49–50, 49b
ADA. *see* American Dental Association (ADA)
ADAA. *see* American Dental Assistants Association
    (ADAA)
Adjustments, accounts, 269, 269f
Administrative area, 15
Administrative dental assistant, 126f, 131, 201,
    202f
    career opportunities for, 273–274
    education for, 5–6
    personal traits of, 5
    roles of, 2–4, 98–101
        backup system, 101–105, 105b
        creating an account, 98, 99f
        maintaining patient records, 99, 99f, 102f
        posting transactions, 99, 102f
        processing insurance claims, 99–101
        producing reports, 101
        recording patient demographics, 98, 98f
        scheduling electronically, 101
        using general database, 99
    types of, 4–5
Administrative Management Society (AMS),
    58–59, 61f
Administrative simplification, 7
Administrator, 214–217b
Advertisements, 73, 74b
Afternoon only patient, 155
Aging, of accounts receivable, 270
Aging labels, 143–144
Allowable charges, 214–217b
Allowance, maximum, 214–217b
Alphabetic filing, 137
Amalgam restorations, 33, 33f
American Dental Assistants Association (ADAA),
    12–13
    ethics and professional conduct, 13b

American Dental Association (ADA), 82b, 127
    approved, 180b
    claim form of, 232f
    Code on Dental Procedure and Nomenclature
        (the Code), 223–224
    ethics and professional conduct, 11b
American National Standards Institute (ANSI),
    137
American Records Management Association
    (ARMA), 137
AMS. *see* Administrative Management Society
    (AMS)
Amylase, 22
Anatomical chart, 29
Angry patients, 79, 79b
Answering machines and services, 193
Apical foramen, 24
Appearance style, 55–57
Application service providers, 214–217b, 220
Application software, 191
Appointment book, 104f, 149, 149b, 150b
    columns of, 151, 151f
    features of, 150–151
    matrix, 153f
    page, anatomy of, 153f
    productivity for, 154–155
    selecting, 149–150
    time blocks, 151
    units of, 151, 151b
Appointment cards, 159, 159f
Appointment information, 164f
Appointment scheduler, 5
Appointments, 157–159
    calls for, 157–158
    codes for, 154
    missed, 132
ARMA. *see* American Records Management
    Association (ARMA)
Assignment of benefits, 214–217b
Assurance Testing System (ATS), 250
ATS. *see* Assurance Testing System (ATS)
Attending dentist's statement, 214–217b
Attitude, 77
Audit, 214–217b
Audit report, in accounts receivable, 269–270,
    270b
Audit trail, maintaining, 93
Auto accidents coverage, 218
Automated Clearing House (ACH) account, 66
Automated recall systems, 169
Availability, 275
Avoiding style, 87, 87b

B

Background noise, in office environment, 198
Backup system, 101–105, 105b
Balance, 242, 242t, 243f, 244f
Balance billing, 214–217b
Bank account reports, 271
Bank statement, 141, 141f, 241–245, 241f
    information on, 241–242
    items needed for, 242
    steps in, 242–245, 243f, 244f, 245f
Barcode, 174, 174f
Barriers, skill development, 45–46

Basic business functions, of computerized dental
    practice, 93
Basic systems, of computerized dental practice,
    92–105
    additional software suites, 93–105
        business tool applications, 94–105
        integrated clinical workstation applications,
          93–94
        patient communications applications, 93
        workflow applications, 93
    basic business functions, 93
        maintain an audit trail, 93
        perform accounting tasks, 93
        perform electronic scheduling, 93
        perform recall and reactivation
          procedures, 93
        process insurance information, 93
        provide software security, 93
        provide training and support, 93
    patient dental records management, 92
        basic patient information, 92
Benefits
    assignment of, 214–217b
    determining, 219
    payment, 214–217b
    service, 214–217b
Billing, 260–262
    balance, 214–217b
    cycles, 207
    fraudulent, 233
    statements, 207, 207f
    in cycles, 96
Birthday greetings, 62
Birthday rule, 214–217b, 218
Blocked letters, 58
Board of Dental Examiners, 10–11
Bookkeeper, 5
Bookkeeping, definition of, 258
Bookkeeping procedures
    accounts payable, 235–257
        bank statement reconciliation, 241–245, 241f
        check writing, 236–239
        definition of, 235
        expenditure verification, 235
        organization of, 235
        payroll, 245–256
        services, payroll, 250
    accounts receivable, 258–271
        billing, 260–262
        definition of, 258
        financial records organization components,
          258–260
        HIPAA and, 263b
        managing patient transactions, 263–270,
          263b, 265–267b, 265f, 266f, 267f, 268f
        reports for, 270–271
Brand name, 180b
Bridge, 35f
Buccal frena, 20
Buccal tooth, 26
Buccal vestibule, 20
Budget plans, 202
    reports, 208
Business Acceptance Testing (BAT) requirements,
    250

Business letter, anatomy of, 63f
Business manager, 4
Business office, 15, 17f
  environment, 196–198
  questions to consider, 196–198
Business principles, 201
Business records, 141
  accounts payable, 141
  accounts receivable, 141
  bank statements, 141, 141f
  business reports, 141
  confidential personnel records, 141
  financial reports, 141, 141f
  insurance records, 141
  payroll records, 141
  personnel records, 141, 141f
  professional correspondence, 141, 142f
  tax records, 141
Business telephone system, 191, 191f
Business tool applications, 94–105

C

Cafeteria plan, 214–217b
Calculators, 196, 196f
Call forwarding, 194
Call lists, 159, 159f
Call management, 194
Calls
  conference, 51
  incoming, 50
  outgoing, 50–51
  personal, 51
Canceled appointment, 156, 156b
Canceled checks verification, 242
Capitation, 214–217b
  programs, 217
Card files, 142
Card index system, 175, 177f
Cast crown restorations, 33–34
Catalog ordering, 180b
CDA. *see* Certified dental assistant (CDA)
CDT. *see* Current Dental Terminology (CDT)
Cementum, 24
Central incisors, 26
Central processing unit, 188–189, 188f
Certification, for administrative dental
  assistant, 11
Certified dental assistant (CDA), 11
Cervix, 24
Chairside dental assistant, 7
Change, communication organizational barrier
  and, 86
Change fund, 270
Channels, 83–86
  formal downward, 83, 83b, 84f
  horizontal, 84, 85b, 85f
  informal, 85–86, 85b, 86f
  upward, 84–85, 84b, 85f
Chart label, 137
Charting symbols, 29, 30b
Check writing, 236–239
  anatomy of, 237f
  electronic, 236–237, 238f, 239f
  making deposit, 236–239, 240f
  payment authorization and transfer in,
    236, 236b
  steps in, 239b
Cheeks, 20

Chronically late patient, 155–156, 156b
Chronological filing, 139, 141f
Chronological resumes, 279–280
Circulating (roving) assistant, 7
Claims, 214–217b
  payment fraud, 214–217b
  reporting fraud, 214–217b
Clinical records, 107–135, 109f
  access to, 110b
  basic elements of, 107
  collecting information, 126b, 126f, 127
  components of, 108–126, 126b
  electronic, 107–108
  function of, 107
  HIPAA and, 107, 110b
  maintaining (manual and electronic), 127–131
  manual
    incorrect and correct way in changing, 133f
    incorrect spacing of entries, 134f
  National Health Information Infrastructure
    (NHII) and, 108
  patient, 107–135
  privacy rules that apply to, 110b
  risk management of, 127–134
  safeguarding, 108f
  workflow, 109f
Closed panel, 214–217b
  programs, 217
Cloud computing, 190, 190f
COB. *see* Coordination of benefits (COB)
COBRA. *see* Consolidated Omnibus Budget
  Reconciliation Act (COBRA)
CODA. *see* Commission on Dental Accreditation
  (CODA)
Code on Dental Procedure and Nomenclature, 8,
  223–224
Coded light systems, 195
Coding, 145
  insurance, 223–233, 224b
Collection procedure, 200–212
  financial policies, 201–203
    designing, 201
  managing accounts receivable, 205–212
  placing collection calls, 211b
  process, 208–212
    collection letter, 209, 210f
    friendly reminders, 208, 208b
    roadblocks to effective collections, 211–212
    telephone reminders, 208–209
    timetable for collection levels, 211b
    turning the account over to collections,
      209–211
    ultimatum, 209, 210f
Color coding, 29, 143
Columns, of appointment book, 151, 151f
Commission on Dental Accreditation (CODA),
  11
Commissures, 20
Communication principles and practices
  patient relations, 71–81, 71b
    customer service, 79–80
    humanistic theory, 71–72
    positive image, 72–78
    problem-solving skills, 78–79
  written correspondence, 53–70
    appearance styles for, 55–57
    dictation and, 69
    format styles for, 57–59, 58f

Communication principles and practices
    (continued)
    letter writing styles, 53–55
    resources, writing, 64, 64b
    types of, 62–64, 62b
Communication process, 43f
Communication skills, 77, 279
  skill development processes
    barriers, 45–46
    communication mediums, 42–44
    elements of, 42
    interpersonal communication, 44
  and telephone techniques, 41–52
    active scripts, 49–50
    conference calls, 51
    HIPAA and, 47b, 50b, 51b
    incoming calls, 50
    outgoing calls, 50–51
    personal calls, 51
    positive image development, 47–49
    privacy rules, 47b
Communications, 83–86, 85b
  for dental healthcare team, 82–90
  mediums of, 42–44
  organizational barriers to, 86
Community standards, 201
Compensation, Workers', 218
Complaints, 78–79, 79b
Completeness, 55
Composition, resumes, 275-280. *see also*
  Resumes
Compromising style, 87, 87b
Computer integration, 194
Computer networks, 189–190
Computer screen elements, anatomy
  of, 100
Computer terminology, 192–193b
Computerized bookkeeping systems, 258
Computerized dental practice, 91–106
  administrative dental assistant, roles of,
    98–101
  basic systems of, 92–105
  daily procedures, 101–105
  functions when selecting software package,
    95–98
  practice management system of, 95
  software package basic operation, 98
Computerized system, daily procedures of,
  101–105
Concise, 55
Conference calls, 51
Confidential communications, 110b
Confidential personnel records, 141
Conflict-handling styles, 87, 87b
Conflicting interpretation, 45–46
Conflicts, organizational, 86–87
Congratulatory letters, 64
Consent form, 122f, 127
Consolidated Omnibus Budget Reconciliation Act
  (COBRA), 214–217b
Constructive conflict, 86
Consultation area, 15–16, 17f
Consulting firms, 274
Consumable supplies and products, 178, 178f
Consumer, 180b
Contract benefit level, 214–217b
Contracted dentist, 214–217b
Contracted fee, 214–217b

Conversation
    patient during, 74, 75b
    patient's name used correctly during, 75, 75b, 75f
Coordination of benefits (COB), 214–217b
Copayment, 202, 214–217b, 219
Copiers, 195
Corporate dentistry, 214–217b
Correspondence, 132
    letter writing styles, 53–55
    log, 132
    professional, 141, 142f
    between staff members, 64, 64b
    written, 53–70
        appearance styles for, 55–57
        dictation and, 69
        punctuation styles for, 59–63
        resources, writing, 64, 64b
        types of, 53b, 62–64
Cover letters, 280–281, 281f
Coverage limitation, 219
Coverage types, 218
    auto accidents, 218
    government assistance, 218
    other accidents, 218
    secondary, 218
    workers' compensation, 218
Covered charges, 214–217b
CPT codes. see Current Procedural Terminology
    (CPT codes)
Credibility, 45
Credit cards, 203
    payments, 269, 269f
    terminals, 195–196, 196f
Credit reports, 207
Cross-referencing, 139, 144
Crown, 24
Current Dental Terminology (CDT), 8, 223, 223t,
    225f
Current Procedural Terminology (CPT codes),
    214–217b
Cusp, 26
Customary fee, 213–214
Customer service, 79–80

D

Daily appointment list window, 105f
Daily journal, 262
Daily routine, 160
Daily schedule sheets, 160, 160b, 160f
DANB. see Dental Assisting National Board
    (DANB)
Data, 191
Data communication technology, 174–175
Data processor, 4–5
DDS. see Doctor of Dental Surgery (DDS)
Debit verification, in bank statement
    reconciliation, 242
Deductible, 214–217b, 219
Dental arches, 25–26
Dental assistant, 7
    concepts
        communication principles and practices,
            patient relations, 71–81
        financial management, bookkeeping
            procedures, accounts payable, 235–257
        office systems management, recall systems,
            163–172
        written correspondence, 53–70

Dental Assisting National Board (DANB), 11
Dental auxiliaries, 7, 11b, 12b
Dental basics, 15–40, 15b
    anatomy, 20–27
    chairside dental-assisting duties, 37–39
        digital images and radiographs, 38
        infection control, 39
        Occupational Safety and Health
            Administration, 38–39, 38b, 39b
        seating and dismissing a patient, 37–38, 38f
    charting methods, 29–32
    numbering systems, 27–29
    office design, 15–20, 16f
        clinical areas, 17–20
        nonclinical areas, 15–17
    procedures, 30t, 33–37
        endodontic, 36, 36f
        preventive, 33
        restorative, 33–34
        surgical, 35–36
Dental benefit plan, 214–217b
Dental benefit program, 214–217b
Dental caries, 25b
Dental chair, 179f
Dental charts, types of, 29–32
Dental claim form, 223b, 226–231f, 232f, 233b
    completing, 223
    steps in processing of, 232f, 232b
Dental film, 178f
Dental healthcare team, 3f
    communication skills for, 82–90
        communication types, 83–86
        HIPAA and, 85b
        organizational conflicts, 86–87
        procedural manuals, 82–83
        staff meetings, 87–88
    description of, 2
    members of, 6–7
    responsibility of, 107, 110b
    role of, 163
Dental history, 107
    form, 115f
Dental hygienist, 6–7
Dental instruments, 179f
Dental insurance, 214–217b
    processing, 213–234
        coding for, 223–233, 224b
        dental provider taxonomy, 232
        fraudulent insurance billing, 233
        insurance payments, 221–222
        insurance types, 213–218
        terminology of, 214–217b
Dental laboratory area, 19
Dental office systems management, recall systems,
    163–172
    classification, 164
    methods, 164–169, 164b
Dental patient scheduling, 149–162
Dental practice
    computerized, 91–106
    name of, 72–73
    procedural manual, 82–83, 82b, 83b
Dental Practice Act, 5–6
Dental procedures, 30t, 33–37
Dental profession
    administrative dental assistant
        education for, 5–6
        personal traits of, 5

Dental profession (continued)
    role of, 2–4
    types of, 4–5
    certification for, 11
    code of conduct, 11b, 13b
    dental healthcare team, members of, 6–7
    ethics of, 10–11
        American Dental Assistants Association, 13b
        American Dental Association, 11b
    Health Information Technology for Economic
        and Clinical Health Act and, 10
    Health Insurance Portability and Accountability
        Act and, 7–10
        administrative simplification, 7
        background, 7
        electronic data interchange, 8
        Omnibus Final Rule, 10
        privacy rule, 8–9
        security rule, 9
        transactions and code sets, 8, 8b
    legal standards of, 10–11
    licensure for, 10–11
    Occupational Safety and Health Administration
        and, 10–11
    organization of, 12–13
    orientation to, 1–14
    registration for, 11
Dental prophylaxis, 33
Dental provider taxonomy, 232
Dental public health, 6
Dental radiographs/images, 112f
Dental registration form, anatomy of, 131
Dental salesperson, 180b
Dental service corporation, 214–217b
"Dental shorthand," 29
Dental supply house, 180b
Dentin, 24
Dentist, 6
Dentistry
    definition of, 2
    general, 6
    objective of, 2
    pediatric, 6
    restorative, 33
Dentofacial orthopedics, 6
Dentures
    full, 35, 36f
    partial, 36f
Department of Health and Human Services, 108
Dependents, 214–217b
Deposits, 236–239, 240f
    in payroll taxes, 254–256
    verification of, in bank statement reconciliation,
        242
Destructive conflict, 86
Development processes
    barriers, 45–46
    communication mediums, 42–44
    elements of, 42
    interpersonal communication, 44
Development steps
    for employment strategies, 274–284
        information gathering, 274–275
        options assessment, 274
        self assessment, 274
    job searches, 280–283
    resume composition, 275–280
Diagnostic models, 127, 131f

Diagnostic records, 127
Diastema, 20b
Dictation, 69
Digital communications, 64–65
Diplomas, 274
Direct deposits, 220, 236
Direct mail promotions, 62
Direct reimbursement, 214–217b, 217
Direct sales, 180b
Disposable supplies, 178
Distal tooth, 26
Divided payment plan, 202
DMD. *see* Doctor of Medical Dentistry (DMD)
Doctor of Dental Surgery (DDS), 6
Doctor of Medical Dentistry (DMD), 6
Doctor's private office, 16–17
Dominating style, 87, 87b
Door signage, 76
Downcoding, 214–217b
Driver's license, 274
Dual addressing, 67
Dual choice program, 214–217b

E

E-claims service providers, 220–221
   HIPAA and, 221b
EDI. *see* Electronic data interchange (EDI)
Edit continuing care window, 105f
Educational institutes, 282
Effective scheduling, 157b
EFTPS. *see* Electronic Federal Tax Payment System
   (EFTPS)
EIN. *see* Employer identification number (EIN)
Electronic appointment book, anatomy of, 152f
Electronic business equipment, 188–191
Electronic check writing, 236–237, 238f, 239f
Electronic checking account reconciliation
   worksheet, 244f
Electronic clinical records, 107–108, 110b
Electronic data interchange (EDI), 8
Electronic Federal Tax Payment System (EFTPS),
   254
Electronic file, 107
Electronic financial record, 262–260
Electronic Fund Transfer (EFT) technology, 254
Electronic health records, 108
Electronic inventory management system, 175f
Electronic ledger, 260f, 262
Electronic mail (E-mail), 65, 65b, 195
   guidelines for, 65b
Electronic patient statements, 260
Electronic records (paperless), 108
Electronic scheduler, 97, 149–150, 150f, 151b
Electronic signature pads, 196, 196f
Electronic systems, 194–195
Electronic transactions, and code sets, 94–105b
Electronically protected health information
   (ePHI), 9, 9b, 94–105b, 136b
Electronically submitted forms, 220
Eligibility, 219
Eligibility date, 214–217b
E-mail. *see* Electronic mail (E-mail)
Embarrassment, 43
Emergency appointments, scheduling options for,
   155b
Emergency information, 274
Emergency patient, 155, 155b
Emotions, 45–46

Employee's Withholding Allowance Certificate
   (W-4 form), 245, 248f
Employer identification number (EIN), 256
Employer responsibilities, 256
Employer tax table, 252, 253f
Employer's Quarterly Federal Tax Return,
   254, 255f
Employer's tax guide, 245, 246b, 246f
Employment agency, 281
Employment Eligibility Verification form,
   245, 247f
Employment records, 275
Employment strategies, 272–285
   career opportunities
      consulting firms, 274
      insurance companies, 274
      management firms, 274
      private practice, 273
      teaching, 274
   development steps, 274–284
      information gathering, 274–275
      options assessment, 274
      resume composition, 275–280
      self assessment, 274
Employment tax rates, 250–252
Enamel, 24, 25f, 37f
Encounter forms, 221, 222f
Endodontics, 6
Enrollment, open, 214–217b
Entries, 132
Envelope preparations, 67–69, 67t, 68f, 68t, 69b
ePHI. *see* Electronically protected health
   information (ePHI)
EPO. *see* Exclusive provider organization (EPO)
Equipment, major, 178, 179f
   purchasing, 180
Ergonomic work station, anatomy of, 197f
Ergonomics, in office environment, 198
Established patient, 214–217b
Ethics, 10
Examination, oral, 33
Examination form, 118f
Exclusions, 214–217b
Exclusive provider organization (EPO),
   214–217b, 217
Expanded (extended) function assistant, 7
Expectation, patients, 77–78, 77f
Expenditures verification, 235
Expiration date, 214–217b
Extended payment plans, 202

F

Face, structures of, 20–23
Facial tooth, 26
Failure to follow instructions, 132
Fair Debt Collection Guidelines, 208–209b
Family deductible, 214–217b
Family file screen, 102f
Fax machines, 194, 194f
Federal unemployment (FUTA) taxes, 250, 252
Fédération Dentaire Internationale (FDI)
   Numbering System, 27–28, 28f
Fee for service, 213–217, 214–217b
Fee schedule, 214–217b
Feedback, 42
FICA. *see* Social Security tax (FICA)
File folders, 142
   coding the, 144

Filing
   electronic files, steps in, 145b
   equipment, 142
      card files, 142
      lateral files, 142, 143f
      Rolodex files, 142
      vertical files, 140f, 142
   label, 137–139, 143
   methods, 136–141
      alphabetic, 137–139
      chronological, 139
      electronic, 139–141, 142b
      geographic, 139
      numeric, 139
      subject, 139, 140f
   preparing paper documents for, 145–147
   procedures, 145
   segment, 137
   supplies, 142–144
   unit, 137
Filtering, 86
Final decision stage, 73b, 76–77
Financial arrangement, 200–212
   form, 124f, 203–204f
   managing accounts receivable, 205–212
   policies, 201–203
Financial data, 206–207
Financial information, 206–207, 206b, 206f
Financial management, bookkeeping procedures,
   accounts payable, 235–257
   bank statement reconciliation, 241–245, 241f
   check writing, 236–239
   expenditure verification, 235
   organization of, 235
   payroll, 245–256
   services, payroll, 250
Financial policies, 201–203
   communications, 203
   credit cards, 203
   designing, 201
   elements of, 201
   extended payment plans, 202
   insurance billing, 202
   payment in full, 202
   third-party finance plans, 202–203
Financial records organization components,
   258–260
Financial reports, 141, 141f, 270
Financial transactions, managing, 270
Fixed fee schedule, 217
Fixed prosthetics, 34
Flash drive, 190f
Flexibility/adaptability, 279
Fluoride treatments, 33
Folding letters, 69, 69f
Follow-up appointment, 158
Forensic odontology, 107
Form W-5, 245
Formal downward channels, 83, 83b, 84f
Formats, written styles, 57–59, 58f
Forms
   consent, 122f
   dental claim, 223b, 226–231f, 232f, 233b
   dental history, 115f
   examination, 118f
   financial arrangements, 124f
   laboratory, 125f
   medical history, 116f

Forms (continued)
  periodontal screening, 119f
  progress notes, 121f
  recall examination, 117f
  registration, 107, 114f
Franchise dentistry, 214–217b, 217
Fraud
  claims
    payment, 214–217b
    reporting, 214–217b
  insurance billing, 233
Frenum, 20
Full-blocked letters, 58, 59f
Fully functioning human beings, 71–72
Functional resumes, 280

G

Gag reflex, 22
Gender rule, 218
General dentistry, 6
Generic name, 180b
Geographic filing, 139
Geometric chart, 29
Gingiva, 23
Gingivitis, 23b
Gold crown, 33–34, 34f
Good listener, 47
Government assistance, 218
Greeting, 76, 76f
Guides, 143

H

Handling styles, 87, 87b
Hard palates, 22, 24f
Hardware, 188–189
Hazard communication program, 183, 184f, 185f, 186f
  effective, 186f
Head-of-house information window, 99f
Headset, 193, 193f
Health and Human Services (HHS), 7
Health Information Technology for Economic and Clinical Health Act (HITECH Act), 10
Health Insurance Portability and Accountability Act of 1996 (HIPAA), 7–10, 214–217b
  Code on Dental Procedures and Nomenclature, 225, 225b
  e-claims service provider and, 221b
  electronic clinical records
    dental healthcare team, roles and responsibilities, 110b
    privacy rules that apply to, 110b
    security standards that apply to, 110b
  National Provider Identifier and, 226b
  Omnibus Final Rule of, 10
  Privacy Rule, 107, 108f, 145b, 225b
    healthcare team-related, telephone techniques, 47b, 50b, 51b
    recall systems and, 168b
  Security Rule, 136b, 146b
  standards, 94–105b
  sets of, 7b
Health Maintenance Organization (HMO), 214–217b, 217–218
Health records, electronic, 108
Healthcare teams, communication skills for, 82–90
  communication types, 83–86
  HIPAA and, 85b

Healthcare teams, communication skills for (continued)
  organizational conflicts, 86–87
  procedural manuals, 82–83
  staff meetings, 87–88
HHS. see Health and Human Services (HHS)
Hierarchy of needs theory, 71, 72f
HIPAA. see Health Insurance Portability and Accountability Act of 1996 (HIPAA)
HITECH Act. see Health Information Technology for Economic and Clinical Health Act (HITECH Act)
Holiday greetings, 62
Horizontal channel, 84, 85b, 85f
HOSA, 13
Humanistic theory, 71–72
  in dental office, 72
Hybrid resumes, 280
Hyphenated names, 137

I

ICD. see International Classification of Disease (ICD)
Identification number, of employer, 256
Image, positive, 72–78
Imaging area, 19
Imaging equipment, 146–147
Immigration and Naturalization Service (INS)
  Form I-9, 245, 247f
Improving communication, 46–47
IMS. see Inventory management system (IMS)
Incentive program, 214–217b, 219
Incisal tooth, 26
Incisive papilla, 22, 24f
Incisor, anatomical structures of, 24f
Incoming calls, 50
Incoming mail, 65–66, 66b
Indemnity plan, 214–217b
Indexed file folder, anatomy of, 144f
Indexing, 137, 145
Individual patient file, 111f
  folder, 107
Individual Practice Association (IPA), 214–217b, 218
Informal channel, 85–86, 85b, 86f
Information
  collecting, 126b, 126f, 127, 127b, 219
  gathering strategies, 274–275
  steps for collecting, 126b
Information management, 136–148
  filing equipment for, 142
  filing methods, 136–141
  filing supplies for, 142–144
  HIPAA and, 136b, 145b, 146b
  preparing business documents for filing, 144–145, 145b
  preparing paper documents for filing, 145–147
  preparing the paper clinical record, 144
  types of, 141–142
Information system, 188, 188b
Information types, 141–142
  business records, 141
    accounts payable, 141
    accounts receivable, 141
    bank statements, 141, 141f
    business reports, 141
    confidential personnel records, 141
    financial reports, 141, 141f

Information types (continued)
    insurance records, 141
    payroll records, 141
    personnel records, 141
    professional correspondence, 141, 142f
    tax records, 141
  insurance records, 142
  patient information, 142
In-house payment plans, 202
Initial contact stage, 73–75, 73b
Initial impression stage, confirmation of, 75–76
Inlay cast restoration, 34, 35f
Input devices, 189
Inspecting documents, 145
Instructions, failure to follow, 132
Insurance
  biller, 4
  billing plans, 202
  coding, 223–233, 224b
  companies, 274
  coverage, types of, 218
  dental, 214–217b
    terminology of, 214–217b
    types of, 213–218
  payments, 221–222
  processing, 213–234
    claims, 218–221
    fraudulent billing, 233
    insurance payments, 221–222
    tracking systems for, 222, 222b
  provider claims processing, 221
Insurance information, 258
  processing, 93
Insurance plans, 73
Insurance records, 141
Insurance reports, 208, 271
Insured, 214–217b
Insurer, 214–217b
Integrated clinical workstation applications, 93–94
Integrating style, 87, 87b
Intergroup conflict, 87
Internal Revenue Service (IRS), 245, 245b, 246b, 246f
  Assurance Testing System (ATS), 250
  Business Acceptance Testing (BAT)
    requirements of, 250
International Classification of Disease (ICD), 214–217b
International Organization for Standardization (ISO), 27–28, 136
International Standards Organization Designation System, 27–28, 29t
Interorganizational conflict, 86–87
Interpersonal communication, 44, 44b
Interpersonal conflict, 86–87
Interproximal tooth, 26
Interview, 283–284
  preparation for, 283–284, 283b
    before, 284, 284b
    during, 284
    after, 284
Intragroup conflict, 87
Intraoffice communications, 194–195
Intraorganizational conflict, 86–87
Intrapersonal conflict, 86
Inventory management system (IMS)
  barcoding in, 174, 174f
  data communication technology, 174–175

Inventory management system (IMS) *(continued)*
electronic, 175f
elements of, 177b
establishing an, 173–178, 173b
key functions of, 173b
manual inventory management systems, 175–177
Occupational Safety and Health Administration (OSHA) and, 183–187
protocol, 177–178, 178b
selecting and ordering supplies, products, and equipment in, 179–183
information to consider before ordering, 181–182, 181f, 182b
purchasing major equipment, 180
receiving supplies and products, 182
selecting the vendor, 180–181
storage areas, 183, 183b, 183f
steps for, 176f
types of supplies, products, and equipment in, 178
consumable supplies and products, 178, 178f
major equipment, 178, 179f
nonconsumable products, 178
Inventory manager
duties of, 177b
personal characteristics of, 177b
selecting an, 177
Investigation stage, 72–73, 73b
Invoice, 235
IPA. *see* Individual Practice Association (IPA)
IRS. *see* Internal Revenue Service (IRS)
ISO. *see* International Organization for Standardization (ISO)

J

Jargon, 45
Job offer, 284
Job searches, 280–283
log, 282
organizing, 282

K

Keyboard, 189, 189f

L

Labels
file, 143
preparing the, 144
Labia vestibule, 20, 22f
Labial frena, 20, 20b
Labial tooth, 26
Laboratory forms, 125f
Lateral file folders, 143, 143f
Lateral files, 142, 143f
Lateral incisors, 26
Least expensive alternative treatment (LEAT), 214–217b
LEAT. *see* Least expensive alternative treatment (LEAT)
Leaving a job, 284–285
Ledger
electronic, 262
and history window, 102f
Letter head formats, 55, 56f
Letter templates, 64

Letter writing
phrases to avoid, 54b
phrases to use in, 54b
styles, 53–55, 55b
Lettering, 57
Letters
to patients, 62–64, 64b
between professionals, 64, 64b
writing styles for, 53–55
Licenses, driver's, 274
Lighting, in office environment, 198
Limitation, to coverage, 219
Line spacing, 57, 57b
Lingual frenum, 20, 20b, 23f
Lingual tooth, 26
Lining mucosa, 23
Lips and cheeks, 20, 22f
Listening and listener characteristics, 46
Logical, 55
Loudness, 47

M

Mail, 65–69, 65b
voice, 51
Mail recall system, 168–171, 168b, 168f
barrier to success of, 169–171, 169t
Malocclusion, 26
Managed care, 214–217b, 218
Managed care providers, 127
Mandibular arch, 25
Mandibular left, 25
Mandibular right, 25
Manners, professionals, 50b
Manual, procedural, 82–83
Manual accounts payable systems, deposit slip for, 240f
Manual appointment books, 150
Manual bookkeeping systems, 260, 261f
Manual inventory management systems, 175–177
inventory control card for, 177f
Manual recall system, flow chart for, 170f
Manual record, 108
Manual systems, 195, 195f
Manufacturer, 180b
Maslow's hierarchy of needs, 72f
Master application information, 274–275
Mastication, 26
Masticatory mucosa, 23
Matrixing, 149
Maxillary arch, 25
Maxillary left, 25
Maxillary right, 25
Maximum allowance, 214–217b
Maximum benefit, 214–217b
Maximum coverage, 219
Maximum fee schedule, 214–217b
Medical history, 107
form, 116f
Medicare taxes, 250, 252
Mediums, communication, 42–44
Meetings, staff, 87–88
Mesial tooth, 26
Missed appointments, 132
Mixed dentition, 26, 27t
Mobile communication devices, 194, 194f
Mobile telephones, 194
Modified blocked letters, 58, 59f, 60f

Mouse, 189
Mucous membrane, 20

N

Name as written *vs.* name as filed, 137f, 138f
Names, with prefixes, 137
National Health Information Infrastructure (NHII), 108
National Provider Identifier (NPI) standard, 10, 94–105b
HIPAA and, 226b
Necessary treatment, 214–217b
Net salary, calculation of, 252–251
Network, communication, 83
New associate/other team member, introduction of, 62
Newsletters, 74f
Newspaper advertisement, 281
NHII. *see* National Health Information Infrastructure (NHII)
No significant findings (NSF), 134
Noise, 45, 45b, 46b
Noncompliance, 78, 78b
Nonconsumable products, 178, 179f
Nonduplication of benefits, 214–217b
Nonparticipating dentist, 214–217b
Nonverbal communication, 43, 43b
Notice of privacy practices, 110b, 127, 128f
acknowledgement of receipt, 130f
NPI standard. *see* National Provider Identifier (NPI) standard
NSF. *see* No significant findings (NSF)
Numeric filing, 139
Numeric indexing, 144

O

Objective statement, 132, 275-279. *see also* Resumes
Obliging style, 87, 87b
Occlusal tooth, 26
Occlusion, 26
Occupational Safety and Health Administration (OSHA), 10–11, 38–39, 38b, 39b, 183–187, 184f, 185f, 186f
Office equipment, 188–199, 190b
Office location, 75
Office machines, 195–196
Office manager, 4
Office systems management, recall systems, 163–172
classification, 164
HIPAA and, 168b. *see also* Health Insurance Portability and Accountability Act of 1996 (HIPAA)
methods, 164–169, 164b
On-the-job training, 273
Onlay cast restoration, 34, 35f
Online resumes, 280
Open enrollment, 214–217b
Open panel, 214–217b
Open punctuation, 59–62, 62b
Operating system software, 190–191
Options assessments, 274
Oral cavity, 20, 21f
quadrants of, 25, 25f
Oral mucosa, 23
Oral pathologists, 6
Organizational communications, 83
Organizational conflicts, 86–87, 87b

Orthodontics, 6
Orthodontist, 6
Orthopedics, dentofacial, 6
OSHA. see Occupational Safety and Health Administration (OSHA)
Outgoing calls, 50–51
Outgoing mail, 66–69, 66b
Out-guides, 143, 143f
Outlook, 54
Out-of-pocket expenses, 214–217b
Output devices, 189, 190f
Outside appearance, 75–76
Overbilling, 214–217b
Overcoding, 214–217b
Overload, work, 86

P

Palmer System, 28–29
Paper clinical record, preparing the, 144
Paper dental claim forms, 221
Paper record, 108
Paragraphing, 57
Parotid glands, 22, 23f
Participating dentist, 214–217b
Password protection, 94–105b
Pathologists, oral, 6
Pathology, oral and maxillofacial, 6
Patient(s)
    accounts receivable
        identifying, 263
        information, 258, 259f
    billing, 96
    checkout, 96
    clinical records, 107–135
        collecting information, 126b, 126f, 127
        components of, 108–126, 126b
        electronic, 107–108
        HIPAA and, 107, 110b
        National Health Information Infrastructure (NHII) and, 108
        risk management for, 127–134
    communications applications, 93
    dental records management, 92
    education area, 19–20
    expectations, 77–78
    file, individual, 111f
    registration form, 206f
    relations
        customer service, 79–80
        humanistic theory, 71–72
        positive image, 72–78
        problem solving skills, 78
    statements, 96
Patient identification, 132
Patient information, 95–96
    window, 99f
Patient's rights, 11–12, 12b
Payer, 214–217b
Payment(s)
    authorization, 236, 236b
    in full, 202
    insurance, 221–222
    plans, 207
    transfer, 236, 236b
Payment Voucher (form 941-V), 255f
Payroll, 245–256, 251f, 271
    anatomy of, 249f
    calculation of, 250–252

Payroll (continued)
    computerized, 248–250
    employment tax rates, 250–252
    Immigration and Naturalization Service (INS) form I-9, 245, 247f
    Internal Revenue Service (IRS)
        Employee's Withholding Allowance Certificate (Form W-4), 245, 248f
        Form W-5, 245
        publications, 245, 246b, 246f
    net salary calculations, 252–251
    records, 141, 245–249, 248b, 250f
        creation of, 245, 245b, 247f, 248f
    services, 250
    Social Security Number (SSN) and, 245
    taxes, 254–256
Peak appointment, 156, 156b
Pediatric dentistry, 6
Pedodontists, 6
Pegboard statement, 262f
Pegboard system, 260, 262
Percentage Method of Withholding, 240f, 252, 254f
Percentage of payment, 219
Periodic method, 146
Periodontal ligament, 24
Periodontal screening examination, 119f
Periodontics, 6
Periodontists, 6
Permanent dentition, 26, 26f
Perpetual method, 146
Personal calls, 51
Personal career portfolios, 282–283, 282b
    components of, 282–283
        achievements, 283
        performance documentation, 283
        personal letters, 283
        reference letters, 283
        thank-you cards and letters, 283
        work samples, 283
Personal communications, 83
Personal name, 137
Personal strategies, for providing exceptional patient care, 80
Personal title, 137–138
Personalizing letters, 54–55, 55b
Personnel, 191
    records, 141
Petty cash, 270
PHI. see Protected health information (PHI)
Phone, answer, 74
Picture identification card, 274
Pitch, 48
Placement opportunities, in private practice, 273
Plan, dental benefit, 214–217b
Point of service, 217
Policies, financial, 201–203
Pontic, 34
Poor listener, 46
Poor scheduling, results of, 157t
Porcelain fused to metal, 34, 34f
Positive attitude, 279
Positive image, 72–78
    development of, 47–49
Positive versus negative dental terms, 48b
Post transactions, 263–270, 265–267b
Postage, 66–67

Postage meters, 195, 195f
Postal cards (postcards), 69, 69b
Posting payments, in accounts receivable, 267f, 269
PPO. see Preferred provider organization (PPO)
Practice branding, 72–78
Practice management systems, 95, 220
Preauthorization, 214–217b, 219–220, 220b
Precertification, 214–217b
Preconceived ideas, 45
Predated appointment book pages, 151
Predetermination, 214–217b
Preexisting condition, 214–217b
Preferred provider organization (PPO), 214–217b, 217
Prefiling of fees, 214–217b
Prefixes, names with, 137
Preschedule routine check-up appointment, 158–159
Prescheduled recall system, 164–165, 164b, 164f
    appointment, steps in, 165b, 165f, 166f, 167f
    barrier to success of, 164–165, 164t
Prescriptions, 132
Pretreatment, 219–220, 220b
Primary dental insurance plan, 103f
Primary dentition, 26, 26f
Privacy officer, 8–9
Privacy practices
    acknowledgement of receipt, 113f
    notice, 127
Privacy Rule, 8–9, 9b
    clinical records and, 110b
    HIPAA and, 225b
Private practice, 273
    large, 273
        benefits of, 273
    small, 273
Problem solver, 279
Problem-solving skills, 78, 78b
Procedural manual, 82–83, 83b
Procedure code editor window, 104f
Procedures, 191
Processing, insurance, 213-234. see also Financial management
    claims, 218–221
        electronic, 221
    coding for, 223–233, 224b
    documentation needed for, 224–233, 225b
    fraudulent billing, 233
    tracking systems for, 222, 222b
Production reports, 270
Products
    definition of, 179
    ordering, 177b, 180b, 182b
    receiving, 182, 182f
Professional correspondence, 141, 142f
Professional manners, 50b
Professional networking, 280–281
Professional organizations, 281
Professional titles, 137–138
Professionalism, 77
Profit and loss statements, 270
Progress notes, 132
    form, 121f
Prophylaxis, dental, 33
Prosthetic procedures, 34–35
Prosthodontics, 6
Prosthodontists, 6

Protected health information (PHI), 8–9, 85b
Provider information window, 104f
Provider specialties, 94–105b
Proximal tooth, 26
Psychology theories, 71–72
Pulp chamber, 24
Pulpal tissue, 24
Punctuation styles, 59–63, 62b

Q

Quadrants, of dental arches, 25

R

Radiofrequency identification (RFID), 174
Radiologists, 6
Radiology, oral and maxillofacial, 6
Radiology area, 19, 19f
Rank and status, communication organizational
    barrier and, 86
Rationale, 134
Reasonable fee, 213–214
Recall appointments, scheduling, 159b
Recall cards, 168f
Recall examination form, 117f
Recall systems, 163-172. see also Systems
    management
    appointment, function of, 163
    automated, 169
    benefits of, for patient, 163
    classification of, 164
    definition of, 163
    general information needed for, 164
    Health Insurance Portability and Accountability
        Act of 1996 (HIPAA) Privacy Rule and,
        168b
    maintaining successful, tips for, 169b
    methods of, 164–169, 164b
    telephone, 167–168
Receiver, 42, 47b
Reception area, 15, 17f, 76, 76f
Receptionist, 4
Reconciliation, of bank statement, 241–245, 241f
Record keeping, 256
    key elements of, 107b
Recording transactions, methods of, 258–260
Records
    clinical, 107, 108
        access to, 110b
        components of, 108–126, 126b
        electronic, 107–108, 110b
        maintaining, 127–131
        manual, 108, 133f, 134f
        privacy rules, 110b
        risk management, 127–134
        workflow, 109f
    diagnostic, 127
    electronic health, 108
    key elements of, 107b
    safeguarding, 108f
Records manager, 4
References, 275
Referral letter, 64
Regard, unconditional, 71–72
Register
    check, 242
        computer-generated, 239f
        corrections to, 242, 242t, 245f
Registration form, 107, 114f, 127, 206f

Reimbursement, direct, 214–217b, 217
Relations, patient
    customer service, 79–80
    positive image, 72–78
    problem-solving skills, 78
Religious title, 139
Removable prosthetics, 34–35, 36f
Reports
    for accounts receivable, 270–271
    financial, 141, 141f
    in payroll taxes, 254–256
Resident card, 274
Resin-based composite restorations, 33, 34f
Resources, writing, 64, 64b
Resume services, 280
Resumes, 275, 279b
    action verbs, 277–278b
    components of
        education, 279
        miscellaneous activities, 279
        skills and abilities, 279, 279b
        work experience, 279
    composition of, 275–280, 276f
    construction of, 279–280
        chronological, 279–280
        functional, 280
        hybrid, 280
        online, 280
    objective, 275–279
    organizing information for, 275–279
    services, 280
Retention record, 146
Return address, 67–69
RF tag, 174
RFID. see Radiofrequency identification (RFID)
Risk management, 127–134
Rolodex files, 142
Root, 24
Root canal, 24
Routing slips, produce of, 263, 264f
Royal title, 139
Rugae, 22

S

Safety, in office environment, 198
Safety Data Sheet (SDS), 183, 184f
Salivary glands, 22, 23f
Schedule
    fee, 214–217b
    fixed fee, 217
Scheduler, electronic, 149–150, 150f
Scheduling
    art of, 149, 151–157
    for emergency appointments, 155b
    mechanics of, 149–151, 150f
    results of, poor, 157
    scenarios for, 155–157
Scripts, active, 49–50
SDS. see Safety Data Sheet (SDS)
Sealant, application of, 36–37
Searches job. see Job searches
Secondary coverage, 218
Security rule, 9, 9b
Self-confident, 279
Semantics, 44–45
Semi-blocked letters, 58, 60f
Sender, 42, 46, 46b
Servers, 190

Sextants, 25f, 26
Short message service (SMS), 159
Signature on file, 123f
Simple extractions, 35
Simplified letters, 58–59, 61f
Sincerity, 44
Skill development processes
    barriers, 45–46
    communication mediums, 42–44
    elements of, 42
    interpersonal communication, 44
Skip tracing, 209
Skull, 20, 21f
    bones of, 20t
Smiles, 43
SMS. see Short message service (SMS)
SNODENT. see Systematized Nomenclature of
    Dentistry (SNODENT)
Social media, 280
Social Security Administration (SSA), 245
Social Security card, 274
Social Security Number (SSN), 245
Social Security tax (FICA), 250
Soft palates, 22
Software, 189–191
Software package
    basic operation of, 98
    functions to consider when selecting, 95–98
        clinical integration, 97–98
        database management, 97
        electronic scheduler, 97
        general requirements, 95
        insurance processing, 96
        management reports, 97
        patient billing, 96
        patient information, 95–96
        recall and reactivation, 96–97
        treatment planning, 96
        word processing, 97
Software security, providing, 93
Software suites, additional, 93–105
Sorting documents, 145
Speaker phones, 193
Specialization, dentist, 6
Specific tasks, procedures for, 132–134, 132b
Speed, 47–48
Speed dialing, 194
Square-blocked letters, 58
SSA. see Social Security Administration (SSA)
SSN. see Social Security Number (SSN)
Staff meetings, 87–88, 88b, 88f
Staff room, 17
Standard checking account, bank statement for,
    241f
Standard punctuation, 59–62, 62b
State dental associations, 127
Statement(s), 132, 235
    bank, 141, 141f, 241–245, 241f
Stationery, 55–57, 56f, 57b
Stereotyping, 45, 46b
Sterilization area, 19, 19f
Storage areas, 183, 183b, 183f
Strong work ethic, 279
Styles
    appearance, 55–57
    format, 57–59, 58f
    letter writing, 53–55
    punctuation, 59–63

Subject filing, 139, 140f
Subjective statement, 132
Sublingual glands, 22, 23f
Submandibular glands, 22, 23f
Subscriber, 214–217b
Superbills, 221, 221f
Supplies
 definition of, 179
 filing, 142–144
 ordering, 177b, 180b
 receiving, 182, 182f
Supply house services, 181b
Suppression, 87b
Surgeons, oral, 6
Surgery, oral and maxillofacial, 6
Surgical extractions, 35–36
Symbolic Numbering System, 23, 28–29, 28t,
 29f, 29t
Systematized Nomenclature of Dentistry
 (SNODENT), 214–217b
Systems management, recall systems, 163–172
 classification, 164
 HIPAA and, 168b. see also Health Insurance
 Portability and Accountability Act of 1996
 (HIPAA)
 methods, 164–169, 164b

T

Table of allowances, 214–217b, 217
Tax records, 141
Teaching-related opportunities, 274
Team player, 279
Team strategies, 79–80
Teams, healthcare, communication skills for,
 82–90
 communication types, 83–86
 HIPAA and, 85b
 organizational conflicts, 86–87
 procedural manuals, 82–83
 staff meetings, 87–88
Teeth
 anatomical structures of, 24
 anterior, 26
 posterior, 26
 surfaces of, 26–27, 27f, 28t
 tissues of, 24, 25f
 types of, 26
Telecommunication, 191–194
Telephone(s), 192
 conversations, 132
 recall systems, 167–168, 168b
 barriers to success of, 167–168t, 167–168
 techniques, 47b
 active scripts, 49–50
 conference calls, 51
 HIPAA and, 47b, 50b
 incoming calls, 50
 outgoing calls, 50–51
 personal calls, 51
 professional manners, 50b
Telephone system, 191–194
 features and functions of, 193–194, 193f
Telephone voice, 74–75
Temperature and humidity, in office environment,
 198–197
Temporary agencies, 281
Tenseness, 43

Terminology, of dental insurance, 214–217b
Thank you cards, 62, 62b
Theories, humanistic, 71–72
Third party, 214–217b
Third-party finance plans, 202–203
Third-party insurance carriers, 127
Time
 extra, 157
 management, 279
Time-saving functions, 159–160
 call lists, develop, 159, 159f
 daily schedule sheets, 160, 160b, 160f
Timing, 46, 86
Tone, 48, 53–54
Tongue, 20
"Tongue tied," 20b
Touch, 43
Tracking systems
 for insurance, 222, 222b
 for recalls, anatomy of, 171f
 steps of, 222b
Transfer
 of information, 42
 methods, 146–147
Treatment plan, 203, 205f, 207
 for patient, 107, 120f
Treatment room, 17–18, 19f
 furniture, 179f
 seating procedure in, 37–38b, 38f
Trust funds, union, 218
Truth-in-lending statement, 203–204f

U

UCR plans. see Usual, customary, and reasonable
 (UCR) plans
Unconditional regard, 71–72
Undated appointment book pages, 151
Understanding checks, 46
Union trust funds, 218
Units/time blocks, 151, 151f
Universal/National Numbering System, 27, 28f
Unscheduled appointment, 156–157
Upward channel, 84–85, 84b, 85f
U.S. Citizenship and Immigration Services
 Employment Eligibility Verification form,
 247f
U.S. military service, 275
Usual, customary, and reasonable (UCR) plans,
 213–214, 214–217b
Usual fee, 213–214
Uvula, 21f, 22

V

Vendor, 180b
Veneer crowns, 34, 35f
Verbal communication, 42–43
Verification, of expenditures, 235
Vermilion border, 20
Vertical file folders, 141f, 142–143
Vertical files, 140f, 142
Virtual keyboard, 189f
Vocabulary, 48–49
Voice, telephone, 74–75
Voice mail, 51, 193
Voice over Internet Protocol (VoIP), 51
VoIP. see Voice over Internet Protocol (VoIP)

W

Waiting times, 76
Web-based program appointment, 158, 158f
WEDI. see Workgroup for Electronic Data
 Interchange (WEDI)
Week at a glance, 150
Welcome letters, 62
White space, 57
Withholding taxes, 250, 252
Within normal limits (WNL), 134
WNL. see Within normal limits (WNL)
Work overload, 86
Workers' compensation, 218
Workflow applications, 93
Workgroup for Electronic Data Interchange
 (WEDI), 7
Writing resources, 64
Writing styles, 53–55
Written correspondence
 dictation and, 69
 and digital communication, 53–70
 format styles for, 57–59, 58f
 letter writing styles, 53–55
 punctuation styles for, 59–63
 resources, writing, 64
 types of, 53b, 62–64

Y

Year-end summaries, 96